PHARMACOTHERAPY

Edited by **Farid Badria**

Pharmacotherapy

Edited by Farid Badria

Published by InTech

Janeza Trdine 9, 51000 Rijeka, Croatia

Publishing Process Manager Ivona Lovric

Technical Editor Teodora Smiljanic

Cover Designer InTech Design Team

Additional hard copies can be obtained from orders@intechopen.com

Pharmacotherapy, Edited by Farid Badria
p. cm.
ISBN 978-953-51-0532-9

Meet the editor

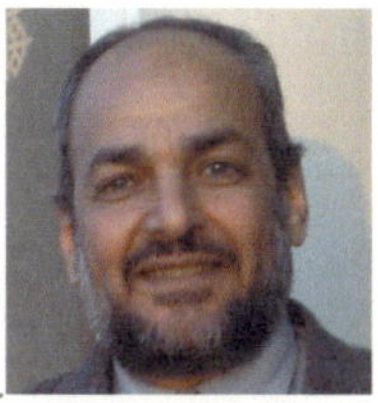

Professor Farid Badria, completed a Ph.D. in Pharmacognosy (Microbial Transformation) at the University of Mississippi, USA, with a B.Sc. in Pharmaceutical Sciences, and 2 Masters of Science in Pharmacognosy and Cell Biology from Mansoura University and the University of Minnesota. He has submitted 42 patents to the Egyptian Academy of Sciences, of which 16 had been granted with final certificates with intellectual protection for 20 years. With over 100 publications, he continues to lead research projects on: developing new therapy for liver disorders, arthritis, skin disorders, and biomarkers for cancer. Prof Badria received: World Intellectual Property Organization Gold Medal, 2011[the best Inventor in Egypt]; State Recognition Outstanding Award in Medicine (Egyptian Academy of Science) 2001; Outstanding Arab Scholar, Kuwait (2000); Khawrazmi International Award, Iran (2000).

Contents

Preface XI

Section 1 ***In Vivo* Imaging – New Diagnostic and Therapeutic Approach 1**

Chapter 1 **Small Animal Imaging in Development of New Generation Diagnostic and Therapeutic Agents 3**
Tuulia Huhtala and Ale Närvänen

Section 2 **Earthquake Medical Management 23**

Chapter 2 **Rational Drug Use in Medical Response to an Earthquake 23**
Ling-li Zhang, Yi Liang, Li-nan Zeng and Die Hu

Section 3 **Cognitive and Psychology Management 39**

Chapter 3 **Integration of Pharmacological and Psychosocial Treatment for Schizophrenia in Mexico: The Case of a Developing Country Proposal 37**
Marcelo Valencia, Alejandro Diaz and Francisco Juarez

Chapter 4 **Nicotine Addiction: Role of the Nicotinic Acetylcholine Receptors Genetic Variability in Knowledge, Prevention and Treatment 69**
Candida Nastrucci and Patrizia Russo

Chapter 5 **Psychiatric Drugs in Medical Practice 81**
María-José Martín-Vázquez

Section 4 **Up-to-Date in Anti-Inflammatory Therapy 113**

Chapter 6 **State of the Art of Anti-Inflammatory Drugs 115**
Túlio Ricardo Couto de Lima Souza, Graziella Silvestre Marques, Amanda Carla Quintas de Medeiros Vieira and Juliano Carlo Rufino de Freitas

Chapter 7 **House Dust Mite Immunotherapy in Iraqi Patients with Allergic Rhinitis and Asthma 141**
Abdulghani Mohamad Alsamarai, Amina Hamed Ahmad Alobaidi, Sami Mezher Alrefaiei and Amar Mohamed Alwan

Section 5 Up-to-Date in Antihypertensive Therapy 155

Chapter 8 **Efficacy of Aliskiren/Hydrochlorothiazide Combination for the Treatment of Hypertension: A Meta-Analytical Revision 157**
Manuel Morgado, Sandra Rolo and Miguel Castelo-Branco

Section 6 Up-to-Date in Ulcer with Venous Origin Therapy 179

Chapter 9 **LavTIME – A Brand-New Treatment Method of Lasting Wounds – A Multi-Centre Randomized Double-Blind Study on Effectiveness of Polyhexanide and Betaine in Ulcers' Healing with Venous Origin 181**
Z. Rybak, G Krasowski, R. Wajda and P. Ciesielczyk

Preface

Though Pharmacotherapy continues to be complex, it never ceases to be interesting. Pharmacotherapy is frequently combined with other treatment methods, such as physical therapy and dietotherapy. Drugs are often used in various combinations.

We have two major objectives in writing this book; firstly, to strike a balance between developments in Pharmacotherapy research and the facts that researchers must absorb, and secondly, to link scientific advances with clinical practice so that the management of diseases can be based on sound physiological concepts. Therefore, this book is a book that everybody involved in Pharmacotherapy must have. Each chapter has been reviewed and revised and new authors have brought up-to-date research to make the book better informative, illustrative, and easy to read.

The intent of this book is to provide an overview of current conceptualizations of Pharmacotherapy. The book focuses on three major areas; diagnosis, treatment, and prevention for a wide array of diseases; Cognitive and Psychological disorders (Schizophrenia and Nicotine addiction), Inflammatory disorders (New Chemical anti-inflammatory and Immunotherapy), updated antihypertensive therapy and healing of ulcers with venous origin. A separate chapter is dedicated to the rationality of drug use in earthquake injuries. The last chapter deals with Imaging of potential therapeutic or diagnostic agents in animal models in the early stage of research. This is an important step towards pre-clinical and clinical trials in human.

We hope this book is useful to a wide range of people, from students first learning about Pharmacotherapy, to advanced clinicians and researchers who are looking for a review of current treatments and conceptualizations of the condition. It is our hope that this book may motivate readers to approach the evidence on Pharmacotherapy with an open mind, and thereby spark an interest in making further contributions to the current scientific debate and treatment development efforts.

Farid A. Badria
Prof. and Head of Pharmacognosy Department
Faculty of Pharmacy, Mansoura University,
Mansoura,
Egypt

Section 1

In Vivo Imaging – New Diagnostic and Therapeutic Approach

1

Small Animal Imaging in Development of New Generation Diagnostic and Therapeutic Agents

Tuulia Huhtala and Ale Närvänen*
Biomedical Imaging Unit, A. I. Virtanen Institute for Molecular Sciences and Department of Biosciences, University of Eastern, Finland

1. Introduction

Imaging technologies form an inseparable part of molecular medicine and is a major research focus globally. Imaging of potential therapeutic or diagnostic agents in animal models in the early stage of research is an important step towards pre-clinical and clinical trials in humans. The resent achievements in molecular biology, virology and nanotechnology provide a totally new approaches to deliver therapeutic agents to the patient starting from conventional small molecules to virus based gene therapy. This creates a need for better tools for the pharmaceutical research. Small animal imaging provides excellent method for development of new generation diagnostic and therapeutic agents.

Modern transient medicine provides completely new approaches to the diagnosis and therapy of diseases. Aim of the research is to develop more specific and efficient agents with minimum side effects. Furthermore, early diagnosis of diseases and accurate follow-up is an important part of the therapy. These requirements have lead to the more complicated bioactive molecules and their carriers. Development and refinement of new bioactive agents like peptides, proteins, nanoparticles, cells or viruses to human drugs is challenged by the perplexities and instability of the complexes *in vivo*.

Due to the complexity of new diagnostic and therapeutic agents, their biodistribution and pharmacokinetic profiles *in vivo* is difficult to predict. Besides toxicity which is one of the main concerns to conventional small pharmaceutical compounds, new agents have to face defense mechanisms like reticuloendothelial system (RES), immunological response and liver as well. Larger size may also affect to the bioavailability of the agent. To overcome these problems comparative biodistribution studies *in vivo* with potential candidates should be started in early phase of the development.

Non-invasive imaging has become important part of the basic and applied research. It allows biodistribution studies within same animal in different time points and phases of the disease. This is important for accurate monitoring since variations between individuals should be minimized. In other words, using imaging applications more equal results may be achieved than with using traditional methods based on *post mortem* or dosing studies.

*Corresponding Author

Imaging is done with fewer animals which is cost-effective and also in accordance to 3R principle (Russell & Burch 1959). Appropriate dose is also easier to evaluate since behavior of the studied compound is immediately seen and changes can be done in relative short time interval compared to dosing studies which may last several months before any effects or results are obtained.

In pharmacological aspect several *in vivo* modalities for small animal imaging exist today. Magnetic resonance imaging (MRI) and resonance (MRS), single photon emission computed tomography (SPECT), positron emission tomography (PET) and optical imaging (OI) are widely used and several reviews (King et al. 2002, Gröhn & Pitkänen, 2007, Kagadis et al. 2010, Snoeks et al. 2011) have been published about these techniques, their strengths and faults. Choosing the most suitable imaging application for a certain study depends of the prioritization of features.

Our laboratory has experience to use wide range of targeting and carrier moieties in experimental animal imaging. In this review we discuss applications in different imaging moieties in development of novel diagnostic and therapeutic agents.

2. Small animal imaging

Small animal imaging provides a non-invasive method to study biodistribution and pharmacokinetics of novel bioactive agents in physiologically relevant environment. Dedicated imaging equipments for laboratory animals, mostly for rodents and rabbits, are available. Different imaging modalities produce information about anatomical structures and physiological processes. Using different modalities together and combining the information, the most accurate information of the function of studied agents with good anatomical reference is achieved.

2.1 SPECT

Single photon emission computed tomography (SPECT) is based on detection of gamma radiation from the studied object. Scanning of different projections from several angles enable three dimensional (3D) reconstruction and further analysis of the patient or animal from various planes and directions. Furthermore, using 2D planar imaging pharmacokinetics of the radiolabelled agents can be followed over the time in the same animal.

There are several radiotracers which can be used in SPECT imaging. The most used are Technetium, Indium and Iodine. Since different tracers have different physicochemical properties, labeling of the molecules or living particles for imaging purposes requires knowledge in biochemistry, traditional chemistry and radiochemistry.

Historically iodine radiolabels are the most used in biochemistry and cell biology. Over 30 isotopes of iodine have been reported of which around ten has been evaluated for biomedical applications (Welch & Redvanly 2002). Choose of the isotope depends on the purpose of the study. ^{123}Iodine decays with practical energy for imaging studies (159 and 127 keV), but its relative short half-life (13 hours) limits its usage to the transient biodistribution studies. The half life of ^{125}I is 60 days but emission energy is only 36 keV, which makes it impractical for human studies but adequate for animal experiments, especially in mice. Its long half-life enables imaging studies for several weeks with single administration of the studied agent.

For the labeling Iodine is oxidated. The target molecule typically contains benzene ring with ortho-substitution which in the most cases is OH-group, like tyrosine in the peptides or proteins. Oxidated iodine reacts to the positions 3 or 5 or both of the benzene ring. Iodine is oxidated by chloramine-T, Iodogen or lactoperoxidase in direct chemical methods (Hunter & Greenwood 1962, Fraker & Speck 1978, Marchalonis 1969). The most convenient method for iodination of biologically active molecules is commercially available Iodo-Gen tubes, which are coated with an oxidative agent 1,3,4,6-tetrachloro-3-6-diphenylglycouril. Due to the high hydrophobicity, this toxic oxidative compound is insoluble to water based buffers and remains in the walls of test tubes enabling solid phase oxidation of Sodium Iodine (NaI). Biomolecules are Iodinated in aquatic environment. The method is optimal for sensitive molecules and the toxic compound remains on the solid phase.

If the target molecule lacks a benzene ring, an additional radioiodinating reagent may be used. The most common and commercially available reagent is Bolton-Hunter reagent. This reagent is succinimidyl derivatized ortho-substituted benzene ring (*N*-succinimidyl-3-[4-hydroxyphenyl]propionate) (Bolton & Hunter 1973, Zalutsky & Narula 1987, Vaidyanathan et al. 1997, Gabel & Shapiro 1978). It reacts with primary amines, which are common in bioactive peptides, proteins, viruses and cells enabling iodination position to the target molecule.

Alternative methods for iodine tracers are ^{99m}Technetium (^{99m}Tc)and ^{111}Indium (^{111}In), which are the most used isotopes in nuclear medicine. However, these metals have to form complexes with donor ligands or chelates prior administration. If the molecule itself lacks chemical structures, which react with the metal as a ligand like sulphur fingers (Maret, 2004), the molecule has to be chelated. Diethylenetriaminepentaacetic acid (DTPA) and 1,4,7,10-tetraazacyclododecane-N,N',N,*N*'-tetraacetic acid (DOTA) are the most commonly used chelates in imaging. As with Bolton-Hunter reagent, these chelates are also available as bifunctional chelating agents (BCA) (Figure 1.) (Chakraborty & Liu 2010, Liu & Edwards 2001).

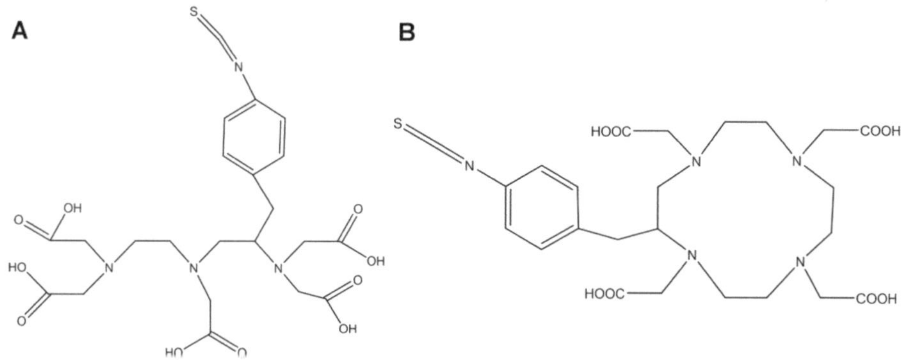

Fig. 1. Commonly used bifunctional chelating agents (BCA) in imaging. Isothiocyanate (S=CH=N-) reacts with primary amines in physiogical conditions allowing labeling of unstable peptides and proteins. A) Isothiocyanate DTPA and B) isothiocyanate DOTA.

Chelates increase the molecular weight of the target molecule and may also change the overall charge. Due to the molecular weight they may cause steric hindrances and change in total charge within small molecules. For larger molecules like peptides and proteins the use of chelates is more common. In some cases the use of the linker between chelating part and reactive part may have effect to the pharmacokinetic properties (Garrison et al. 2008, Qu et al. 2001).

2.2 PET

In positron emission tomography (PET) imaging positron emitters and the following annihilation, is used to measure radioactive accumulation or consumption in the object. Annihilation produces two gamma quanta of 511 electron volts, which are emitted to the opposite directions (180°). The gamma quanta are easily located by using a serie of stable gamma cameras around the animal. The advantage of the PET radiotracers is that radionuclides are incorporated in the molecule with minimal inference to the function of the pharmaceuticals. Also sensitivity in PET is superior to SPECT. One important limitation for PET resolution is that the localisation of positron emission is not the same that the place of annihilation. The distance between emission and annihilation depends of the energy of the particle and also the density of tissue, for example average range for ^{18}F in water is 0.064 cm (Cherry 2003).

Labeling of PET radiopharmaceuticals is complicated and requires on-site cyclotron and highly educated personnel. Due to the short half-lives of tracers the cyclotron facilities should be near the research laboratory. Only ^{18}F has adequate long half-life that the delivery time can be hours not minutes. It's also notable that even the half-lives of PET nuclides are shorter than SPECT nuclides the dose effect may be larger with PET nuclides since their emission energy of 511 electron volts is much higher than those of conventional SPECT nuclides.

In clinical PET studies ^{18}F in deoxyglucose (FDG) is the most commonly used diagnostic molecule for the functional studies in tissues. Others, such as sodium ^{18}fluoride, ^{18}fluorothymidine, ^{18}fluoromisonidazole, and ^{64}Cu-labeled diacetyl-bis N4-methylthiosemicarbazone are under evaluation for clinical use (Vallabhajosula et al. 2011).

2.3 CT

The oldest imaging modality is based on X-rays describe first by Wilhelm Röntgen already on 1895 (Röntgen, 1896). Ever since x-rays has been used to produce two dimensional images. Today X-rays are used in 3D topographic imaging. In principle, CT unit consist of high-voltage x-ray tube and oppositely located detector. Both x-ray source and detector rotate around the animal and a 3D reconstruction of the target can be made. Contrast is based on the ratio of the radiation which is passed through and absorbed in the patient. In contrast to SPECT and PET where radiation comes from the patient, in CT radiation is produced in the imaging equipment and the fraction of radiation passing through the target is measured. Since differences in linear attenuation coefficients for soft tissues are small (water = 0.21 cm^{-1}; lean tissue = 0.20 cm^{-1}; fat = 0.18 cm^{-1}; bone 0.38 cm^{-1}), contrast in the soft tissues is limited with x-ray based CT technique. Also increased resolution in CT raise significantly the radiation dose.

Although x-ray based CT is not optimal for small animal imaging this method facilitates the localization of labeleld molecules in biodistribution studies. Today there are few manufacturers, which provide combined SPECT/CT and PET/CT equipments for clinical use but also dedicated animal devices are on the market (Picler et al. 2008, Golestani et al. 2010). The advantage of these multimodality systems is the ease of imaging with different modalities without moving the object and hence the co-localization of images can be performed easily (Figure 2).

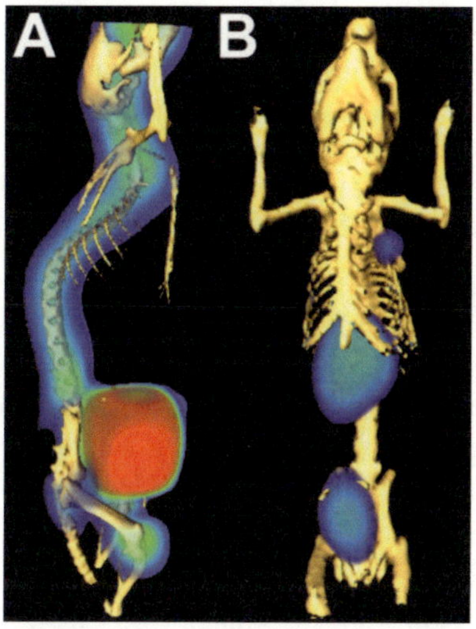

Fig. 2. Combined SPECT/CT images of mouse. A) 99mTc labeled commercially available bisphosphonate, Etidronate. Biodistribution profile studied in healthy mouse 30 min after i.v. injection. Etidronate accumulates mainly to the spine and joints of the hind limb. The image also visualizes the elimination of Etindronate through the kidneys and further excretion to the bladder (red accumulation). B) ^{111}In labeled monoclonal antibody mF4-31C1 against vascular endothelial growth factor receptor 3 (VEGFR-3) in ovarian carcinoma mouse model. Biodistribution profile studied 48 h after the single intra venous (i.v.) injection. Most of the antibodies are excreted through the liver. Signal in the lower part of the body indicates antibody's accumulation in the tumor area and the upper signal represents remote activation of VEGFR-3 in metastatic lymph nodes (Huhtala et al. 2010).

2.4 MRI/MRS

The best modality for high contrast soft tissue anatomical imaging is magnetic resonance imaging (MRI). It is based on nuclear magnetic resonance (NMR) and the nature of proton nucleus. Isotopes that contain an odd number of protons and/or neutrons and have an intrinsic magnetic moment and angular momentum, like ^{13}C, ^{2}D, ^{15}N and ^{31}P can be used for MRI. When an isotope with magnetic properties (usually a proton) is in a strong magnetic field, the nucleus of the isotope is aligned with the magnetic field. When using a short radiofrequency (RF) pulse, the nucleus will align itself with the magnetic field. After the pulse, the nucleus will return on its natural state at certain rate called relaxation time, emitting an RF signal which is recorded. The RF signal is analyzed and used to produce MR image. Since the environment of the proton affects strongly to the relaxation time, contrast is achieved between tissues. Furthermore, using Magnetic Resonance Spectroscopy (MRS) analyses the relative concentrations of molecules in the target tissue can be estimated (Liimatainen et al. 2006b, Liimatainen et al. 2006a).

In MRI fine structure investigation and spectroscopy of the tissues is performed without any tracers but biodistribution studies of active compounds are followed using contrast agents. It's notable that in small animal imaging, MRI is typically suitable to image certain part of the body and only local biodistribution e.g. the brain areas are imaged. Ferric, gadolinium or manganese are common contrast agents Ultra small superparamagnetic iron oxide (USPIO) particles, size range of 10 - 50 nm, are widely used for various applications like vascularity and macrophage content in atherosclerotic carotid plaques (Metz et al. 2011), lymph node metastasis (Lei et al. 2010), tumor vascular morphology and blood hemodynamics (Gambarota et al. 2010), diffusion in the brain disorders (Chin et al. 2009, Vellinga et al. 2009), cell number quantification (Cheung et al. 2006) and oncological studies (Gambarota et al. 2006, Baghi et al. 2005, Keller et al. 2004).

For the labeling several surface activated USPIO particles are available. The surface may contain chemically active groups like carboxylic acid, primary amines, aldehydes or isothiocyanates. Also biotinylated or avidin/streptavidin coated particles are available. Since biotin-avidin complex is one of the strongest found in nature, this phenomena can be used widely for various targeted applications or as a conjugation techniques. It should be noted that USPIO nanoparticles are several magnitudes larger than bioactive molecules and may cause sterical hindrances.

For MRI studies gadolinium and mangansese based contrast agents have also been used. They require, like Technetium and Indium, chelates for labelling. Gadolinium ion as a water soluble salt is also quite toxic to animals and chelating reduces significantly its toxicity. However, the sensitivity of these contrast agents in MRI or MRS is significantly lower than corresponding radioactive metals in SPECT or PET techniques. In MRI millimolar concentrations are needed whereas nano and even picomolar concentration of radionuclides gives reliable SPECT or PET imaging results.

Combination of PET/MRI is relatively new and rare hybrid scanning technique but very fascinating (Pichler et al. 2008, Bisdas et al. 2010, Antoch & Bockisch 2009). Especially in brain imaging combination of PET and MRI seems advantageous and promising (Heiss 2009). With combined PET and MRI imaging gives valuable information about function of the heart (PET) and also information about ventricular structure of the heart (MRI) (Nekolla et al. 2009). Combination of SPECT and MRI is available only for animal studies (Goetz et al. 2008).

2.5 Optical imaging

Compared to previously described methods advantaged of optical imaging (OI) include relatively ease usability, inexpensiveness and no need of radioactive tracers. In OI the detection is based on produced light from the tissues and monitored by common CCD camera. This method has been used for pharmacokinetic studies, angiogenesis, cancer, evaluating biodistribution or biological activity of potential therapeutic agents but also visualization of living embryos (Baker 2010, Dufort et al. 2010b, Penet et al. 2010, Eisenblatter et al. 2010, Canaria & Lansford 2010).

The OI modality uses either fluorescence of bioluminence as a tracer. The molecules are typically labelled with fluorescent molecules and their biodistribution is followed like in SPECT or PET modalities (Weissleder & Ntziachristos 2003, Napp et al. 2011). The labelling chemistry is similar as with chelates. Several fluorescence molecules like fluorescein or cyanine based molecules (Cy3, Cy5 etc.) may contain either amino or carboxylic acid groups or are pre-activated with succinimides, maleimimides or isothiocynanates for the conjugation. Another fluorescence method is based on green fluorescence protein (GFP). Using cells transfected with GFP gene, the function of the cells can be studied (Chudakov et al. 2005). However using fluorescence the depth of imaging target, surface reflectance, absorption, scattering and autofluorescence limit the sensitivity in true 3D imaging (Dufort et al. 2010a, Welsh & Kay 2005, Bremer et al. 2003).

The light emission in bioluminescence is more sensitive, mainly because it is not interfered by autofluorescence since it is based on or oxygenation of Luciferin by Luciferase enzyme. During the oxygenation Luciferin substrate produces a photon, which is measured. As with GFP the function i.e. proliferation or cell death can be studied by using transfection with Luciferase gene. Transfected cells are inoculated to the experimental animal and followed over the time with Luficerin injections. After systemic injection, luciferin circulates and internalizes in to the cells. In Luciferase expressing cells the light is lit and can be imaged. This method has successfully use i.e. in imaging of the therapeutic effect of the viruses in cancer (Heikkilä et al. 2010).

Another fascinated optical imaging application is splice correction method developed by Kole and his colleagues in 1998 (Kang et al. 1998). This method is based on transfection of a plasmid containing mutated Luciferase gene. This mutation causes an aberrant splicing of the pre-mRNA resulting non-functional mRNA. Upon the treatment with slice correcting oligonucleotide , which has complementary structure to the mutation site, the aberrant splicing is corrected and active Luciferase enzyme is expressed. This method has successfully used in cell cultures to study oligonucleotide internalisation in to the nucleus using cell penetrating peptides (CPP) (Mäe et al. 2009), but in the future it may have several applications in *in vivo* optical imaging.

3. Therapeutic and diagnostic agents in imaging

Although most of the pharmaceutical compounds are small and relatively simple structures, there are a growing number of other types of molecules for therapy and diagnostics. Exactly speaking it's inaccurate to speak novel therapeutic molecules, since there are also other solutions to deliver the therapeutic agents and affect the target tissue or cells. In recent years nanoparticles (NP), viruses and stem cells has been in focus.

What is common aim in developing novel therapeutic or diagnostic agents? The first aim is to develop specific targeting to the pathological alterations in tissues or cells. Secondly, they should be multifunctional containing several biological or chemical structures like targeting, drug, carrier and tracer moieties. Thirdly, the side effects should be minimized. Gene technology provides totally new approach to therapeutic field by delivering genes to the host cell, which transcription and translation machinery is used as "drug factory".

Small animal imaging methods are ideal to study biodistribution of various types of molecules or even viruses and cells. Since nano- and picomolar concentration of radiolabel gives adequate signal, small amounts of label is needed to preliminary results of the biodistribution, accumulation, pharmacokinetics and metabolic routes of the studied compound. Other advantages in imaging include smaller animal groups than traditional pharmacological studies since whole body results can be achieved over the time *in vivo* without sacrificing the animals.

3.1 Conventional pharmaceutical and imaging compounds

Most of the commercially available pharmaceutical compounds are small molecules below 500 Da and they typically lack homing properties but the effect is based on specific binding as an agonist or antagonist in the target tissue or cell. If small pharmaceutical compounds are used in imaging studies, in the most cases the tracer should be directly incorporated to the molecule structure like chemical labelling of Iodine for SPECT, with cyclotrone for PET or the molecule should have chelating properties, like bisphosphonates, if a radioactive metal is used.

There are several small molecules used in diagnostic imaging. One widely used imaging agent is (-)-2β-carbomethoxy-3β-(4-iodophenyl)tropane (β-CIT or RTI-55). In SPECT and PET imaging it has been used as ^{123}I labeled or ^{18}F (FP-CIT) labeled to map distribution of dopamine transporters and serotonin transporters in the brain e.g. in Parkinson's disease and supranuclear palsy (Zubal et al. 2007, Shaya et al. 1992, Shang et al. 2007, Staffen et al. 2000, Seppi et al. 2006).

For PET the small organic imaging agent ^{18}FGD, a glucose derivate, which accumulation through the body is related to tissue glucose consumption. This phenomenon is utilized in several applications of brain, tumor and myocardial metabolism (Berti et al. 2010, Miletich 2009, Chen & Chen 2011, Kopka et al. 2008). ^{18}FGD is widely used especially in neurosciences including drug research and development. With ^{18}FDG it's possible to determine activation of certain brain areas and hence applications are numerous, e.g. the sensitivity of brain areas to drugs as well as behavioral and therapeutic effects of the drug (Welch & Redvanly 2002).

^{99m}Tc is the most commonly used isotope in nuclear medicine. When it is conjugated with DTPA, it is used to measure functionality of the kidneys (Eckelman & Richards 1970), as a pyrophosphate or bisphosphonate for skeletal imaging (Thrall 1976) and with hexamethylpropyleneamine oxine (HMPAO, Ceretec™) for brain perfusion (Leonard et al. 1986a). ^{111}Indium, chelated to oxine is used in clinics to label white blood cells or platelets to study sites of acute inflammation and infection but also thrombocytopenia *in vivo* (Leonard et al. 1986b, Thakur et al. 1977, Thakur 1977, Rodrigues et al. 1999, Louwes et al. 1999).

3.2 Peptides

Although peptides and polypeptides have been used for therapeutic purposes already for over 80 years when insulin was taken in clinical use, only few novel peptide based drugs have been approved by FDA or EMEA. Most of the drugs are direct copies from nature like follitropin beta, which is a synthetic copy of follicle stimulating hormone (FSH) (Fares et al. 1992, Shome et al. 1988). Second generation peptide drugs are modified from the original molecule or are part of the larger proteins. Octreotide is a long-acting octapeptide with pharmacologic properties mimicking those of the natural hormone somatostatin (Bornschein et al. 2009, Anthony & Freda 2009, Stajich & Ashworth 2006). Fuzeon (Enfuvirtide) is a 36 residue synthetic peptide that inhibits HIV-1 fusion with CD4 cells. Enfuvirtide binds to the first heptad-repeat (HR1) in the gp41 subunit of viral envelope glycoprotein and prevents the conformational changes required for the fusion of viral and cellular membranes. It interferes the HIV-1 molecular machinery at the final stage of fusion with the target cell. Enfuvirtide is a biomimetic peptide that was rationally designed to mimic components of the HIV-1 fusion machinery and displace them, preventing normal fusion. (Joly et al. 2010, McKinnell & Saag 2009, Makinson & Reynes 2009)

The number of bioactive peptides , with potential therapeutic or diagnostic properties, will be increased due to new screening methods for novel peptides. Epitope scanning (Reece et al. 1994, Frank, 2002) and phage display libraries produce novel biologically active peptides with specific binding properties to target proteins such as receptors and proteases (Nilsson et al. 2000). Some of the identified peptides are highly specific to the receptors of the specialized tissues providing a possibility to use peptides for targeting (Laakkonen et al. 2002). These peptides serve as lead molecules for development of molecules for tumour imaging and therapy.

Both natural peptides and peptides characterized by phage display are sensitive to metabolic processes like protease activity. This limits their usefulness as diagnostic and therapeutic agents. Rationale design of chemical modifications to maximize enzymatic bioavailability while preserving the potency and specificity of the peptide is needed (Adessi & Soto 2002). Typically peptides are cyclised or the amino acid side chains or bridge structures are modulated by using unnatural structures called peptidomimetics (Pakkala et al. 2007, Pakkala et al. 2010).

Peptides and their modifications are typically produced by using solid phase peptide synthesis method (SPPS). Today synthesis is made with automated synthesiser and the time to produce a peptide is relatively short and several companies provide synthesis services for reasonable price. For labelling an additional reactive amino acid like tyrosine or cysteine are easy to add to the sequence for further labelling or conjugation purposes.

3.3 Proteins

Unlike peptides proteins are large and contain secondary, tertiary and some cases even quaternary structures on which the biological activity is based. Due to their defined tertiary structure and size, they may be sensitive to the labelling and purification methods. Furthermore, the administration route, which is mainly the systemic injection, and immunological response limits the usefulness of the proteins as drug candidates.

For the biodistribution studies the surface of the proteins contains several different chemically active amino acid side chains or polysaccharides, which can be used for labelling purposes. Typically proteins are labelled via the ortho-hydroxy benzene ring of tyrosine or via primary amino groups of either the amino terminus or the side chain of lysine. For the imaging purposes proteins are labelled with iodine or conjugated with chelates as previously described. After the conjugation proteins can be purified with conventional size-exclusion chromatography, dialysis or ultrafiltration using physiological conditions. In addition, chelate conjugated proteins can be labelled with ^{99m}Tc or ^{111}In without further purification steps (Helppolainen et al. 2007).

One of the most used group of proteins for diagnostic and therapeutic purposes are monoclonal antibodies. Already 50 products have been passed the long and very expensive way from the primary finding to the licensed drug (Biopharma, 2011). The limiting factors of antibodies are large size (150 000 Da) which may interfere penetration of the molecule to the target tissue and possible squeamishness. Large size can be bypassed with Fab1 or Fab2 fragments of the antibodies or as in human therapy using humanized monoclonal antibodies. The advantage of antibodies is high affinity compared to other protein-ligand interactions but also relatively easiness and diversity of modification chemistry without losing the binding activity.

Antibodies have been successfully used in cancer therapy. Cetuximab (Erbitux) is a humanized monoclonal antibody against epidermal growth factor receptor (EGFR) which is over-expressed in various cancers (Vincenzi et al. 2008, Rivera et al. 2008). It has been successfully used in the treatment of colon carcinoma in humans. Same antibody has been studied as versatile SPECT and PET imaging agent in several cancer models, e.g. malignant mesothelioma, prostate cancer, head-and-neck squamous cell carcinoma, ovarian carcinoma (Figure 2.), colon cancer and universally EGFR positive tumors (Nayak et al. 2011, Malmberg et al. 2011, Hoeben et al. 2011, Huhtala et al. 2010, Cho et al. 2010, Ping Li et al. 2008).

3.4 Viruses

This very exiting approach is based on natures own gene delivery method. After delivery, modified virus in target cell begins to use cell's natural amplification techniques to produce therapeutic molecules. Today there are both transient (Adenoviruses) and stable (Lentiviruses) viral delivery systems (Rissanen & Yla-Herttuala 2007, Mahonen et al. 2010, Lesch et al. 2009).

Biodistribution studies using non-invasive imaging is an important part of the development of virus based therapeutic agents. Viruses for the therapy are modified, they are unable to multiply and additional therapeutic and/or reporter genes are added to the viral genome. Expressed reporter genes can be imaged by using radiolabelled ligands. Using sodiumiodine symporter (hNIS) gene together with cancer-specific human telomerase promoter, human colocarcinoma xengraft has been imaged using radiolabelled iodine with SPECT/CT in animal model (Merron et al. 2007).

Fusion proteins composed of avidin and either macrophage scavenger or low-density lipoprotein receptors (LDLR) have been constructed in order to target biotinylated molecules to cells of desired tissues. Using adenovirus mediated gene transfer transient expression of the fusion protein on cell membrane was achieved (Lehtolainen et al. 2002, Lehtolainen et al. 2003). When biotinylated molecule binds to the fusion receptor, it is internalized into the cell. Local gene transfer to target tissues could be used as a universal tool to deliver therapeutic agents at systemic low concentrations. Using biotinylated tracers like biotin-DTPA or biotin-DOTA compelexes these cells can be imaged *in vivo* (Turhanen et al. 2011).

An alternative method to study the biodistribution of the viruses is avidin expression on the surface of the viral particle. Their homing properties to the target tissue may be enhanced using biotinylated moieties like antibodies or peptides. For imaging purposes biotinylated radiotracer is conjugated on the virus surface and biodistribution of the labelled virus is followed by SPECT (Raty et al. 2007, Raty et al. 2006, Kaikkonen et al. 2009).

Homing properties of viruses can be modified with biochemical methods using hybrid peptide with poly-lysine spacer together with cyclic peptide HWGF (His-Tyr-Gly-Phe) which binds to membrane metalloprotein receptors, MMP-2 and MMP-9 (Koivunen et al. 1999). This peptide has been conjugated with trasnglutaminase enzyme on the surface of Adenovirus. The use of enzyme for conjugation is gentle and do not decrease the infectivity of the virus. Conjugated receptor specific peptide enhanced the tropism of the virus *in vivo* in rabbits (Turunen et al. 2002).

3.5 Living cells

Nuclear medicine has been used to image leucocytes in infectious or inflammatory processes *in vivo* already over four decades. The techniques detect inflammatory processes to which leukocytes migrate, such as those associated with abscesses or other infection. During 1970's a new cell membrane tropic radioactive compound was developed. ^{111}In-oxine is a lipophilic complex and penetrates through cell membrane without interference of the membrane bound molecules like receptors. Penetration is unspecific and all cell types can be labelled (Thakur et al. 1977, Becker & Meller 2001).

Stem cells are immature cells, which have regenerative potential in various diseases. Especially neurodegradative disorders have been in the focus due to the poor regenerative properties on neuronal cells. The regenerative properties of the stems cells have been studied in Parkinson disease (PS), amyotrophic lateral sclerosis (ALS), Huntington's disease and stroke (Lindvall et al. 2004). For in vivo biodistribution studies stem cells have been labelled either with paramagnetic nanoparticles and followed with MRI (Arbab et al. 2003, Frank et al. 2003) or with ^{111}In-oxine (Figure 3.) for SPECT imaging (Lappalainen et al. 2008, Makinen et al. 2006).

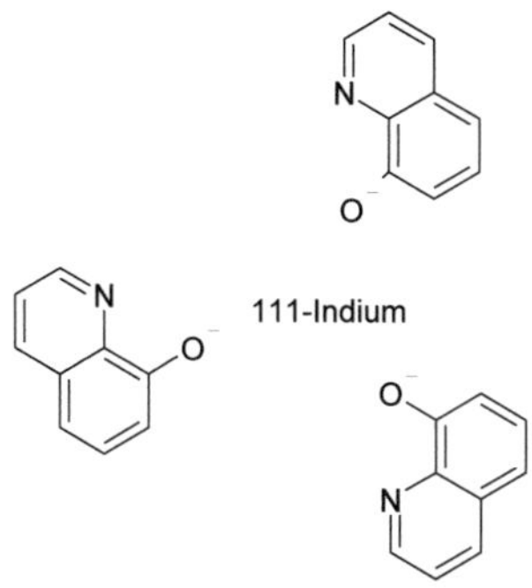

Fig. 3. ^{111}Indium oxine i.e. Indium 111 oxyquinoline. Indium is coordinating three oxyquinoline molecules. Due to the relative high hydrophobicity Indium oxine penetrates directly but unspecifically into the cytoplasm of the target cells and do not bind to the surface proteins.

Radiolabeling of living cells is probably the most challenging labeling process since several issues has to be considered. Firstly, labeling conditions have to be effective, mild, temperate, fast and without complicated purification steps. Secondly, aseptic techniques have to be followed and last, appropriate dose for the cell batch has to be evaluated avoiding too high dose for the cells. For these reasons labeling conditions must always plan carefully for each different cell type according their usual cultivation techniques. If longer (i.e. over 24 h) biodistribution studies are measured, effect of the labeling to the viability of the cells *in vitro* during timescale is worth to analyze. This is important since only the nuclide is seen in *in vivo* imaging but no information is achieved about the absolute condition of the cells viability.

3.6 Nanoparticles

There have been invasion of basic nanoparticle research in biomedicine. Many therapeutic agents like small organic compounds, nucleic acids, peptides and proteins are unstable *in vivo* and novel delivery technologies should be developed to improve their pharmacokinetic properties. Development of nanoparticle based delivery could enable sustained and hence regular release of drug. If NPs are also targeted, in the ideal case they would concentrate to the desired area and allow sustained release of the drug to the circulation or locally if needed. This would be beneficial for the patient as fewer drug intakes, steadier effect of the drug and hence milder side-effects but maybe also economically cost-effective.

The size range of nanoparticles is comparable to the viruses. Conventionally nanosized materials like polymeric nanoparticles, liposomes and micelles are prepared from organic materials although they have limited chemical and mechanical stability and inadequate control over the drug release rate (Arruebo et al. 2006). Today there are NPs made of inorganic materials like silica or silicon (Haley & Frenkel 2008, Salonen et al. 2008). Inorganic material allows the production of porous or mesoporous nanoparticles with particle size in range of 50 - 300 nm and the pore diameter in the range 5 - 50 nm. The porous structure allows high loading capacity for the therapeutic agents and/or tracers, like fluorescein, radioactive compounds or paramagnetic iron (Wiekhorst et al. 2006, Alexiou et al. 2006a, Alexiou et al. 2006b).

Furthrmore, the transportation and release of the molecules can be controlled. Mesoporous silicon nanoparticles have also shown to be non-toxic and stable (Salonen et al. 2008, Brigger et al. 2002, Limnell et al. 2007, Salonen et al. 2004). The surface of the nanoparticles can be derivatized with chemically active groups like primary amines or carboxylic acids and conjugated with several biologically and chemically active molecules (Figure 4). Large surface area allows conjugation of several different molecules on the same particle. Using targeting moieties the tropism of NPs can be modulated (Kukowska-Latallo et al. 2005, Costantino et al. 2005).

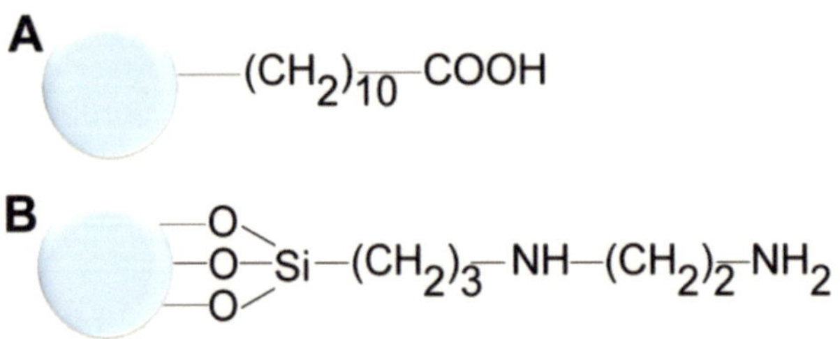

Fig. 4. Chemically modified surfcaes of the silicon based mesoporous nanoparticles for the conjugation of bioactive molecules. A) carboxylic acid derivatized nanoparticles and B) primary amino derivatized nanoparticles with alkane spacers.

4. Conclusions

Several imaging modalities for small animal pre-clinical studies have been developed. Various modalities provide different information about biodistribution, pharmacokinetics and effect of potential therapeutic agents to the target tissues and cells. Using SPECT or PET, biodistribution of the labelled agents can be easily followed over the time in animals with high sensitivity. Due to high spatial resolution, chances in fine structure and furthermore chemical chances of the target tissue can be studied using MRI and MRS. Contrast of CT is not optimal for soft tissue studies in small animals *in vivo* but using combined images with SPECT and PET it facilitates the localisation of the labelled bioactive agents. Optical imaging provides an excellent tool for the viability studies of cells and tissues. Luciferase expression based on transfected cells or whole transgenic animal gives direct information of the gene activation, growth and the death of the cells *in vivo*.

Today several new therapeutic and diagnostic agents are large and/or complexed structures especially viruses, stem cells and nanoparticles. Due to high variety of the structures in new agents, requirement of interdiscipline skills and collaboration starting from basic organic chemistry to virology and cell biology is required. Accurate information of the biodistribution and pharmacokinetics before clinical trials is needed. Using different imaging modalities and combining the information, excessive preliminary knowledge of behaviour and effect of the studied complexes *in vivo* can be achieved.

5. References

Adessi C & Soto C. Converting a peptide into a drug: strategies to improve stability and bioavailability. Current medicinal chemistry 2002;9:963-978.

Alexiou C, Jurgons R, Seliger C & Iro H. Medical applications of magnetic nanoparticles. Journal of nanoscience and nanotechnology 2006a;6:2762-2768.

Alexiou C, Schmid RJ, Jurgons R, Kremer M, Wanner G, Bergemann C, Huenges E, Nawroth T, Arnold W & Parak FG. Targeting cancer cells: magnetic nanoparticles as drug carriers. European biophysics journal : EBJ 2006b;35:446-450.

Anthony L & Freda PU. From somatostatin to octreotide LAR: evolution of a somatostatin analogue. Current medical research and opinion 2009;25:2989-2999.

Antoch G & Bockisch A. Combined PET/MRI: a new dimension in whole-body oncology imaging? European journal of nuclear medicine and molecular imaging 2009;36 Suppl 1:S113-20.

Arbab AS, Bashaw LA, Miller BR, Jordan EK, Lewis BK, Kalish H & Frank JA. Characterization of biophysical and metabolic properties of cells labeled with superparamagnetic iron oxide nanoparticles and transfection agent for cellular MR imaging. Radiology 2003;229:838-846.

Arruebo M, Fernandez-Pacheco R, Irusta S, Arbiol J, Ibarra MR & Santamaria J. Sustained release of doxorubicin from zeolite-magnetite nanocomposites prepared by mechanical activation. Nanotechnology 2006;17:4057-4064.

Baghi M, Mack MG, Hambek M, Rieger J, Vogl T, Gstoettner W & Knecht R. The efficacy of MRI with ultrasmall superparamagnetic iron oxide particles (USPIO) in head and neck cancers. Anticancer Research 2005;25:3665-3670.

Baker M. Whole-animal imaging: The whole picture. Nature 2010;463:977-980.

Becker W & Meller J. The role of nuclear medicine in infection and inflammation. The Lancet infectious diseases 2001;1:326-333.

Berti V, Osorio RS, Mosconi L, Li Y, De Santi S & de Leon MJ. Early detection of Alzheimer's disease with PET imaging. Neuro-degenerative diseases 2010;7:131-135.

Biopharma, www.biopharma.com, 6.9.2011.

Bisdas S, Nagele T, Schlemmer HP, Boss A, Claussen CD, Pichler B & Ernemann U. Switching on the lights for real-time multimodality tumor neuroimaging: The integrated positron-emission tomography/MR imaging system. AJNR.American journal of neuroradiology 2010;31:610-614.

Bolton AE & Hunter WM. The labelling of proteins to high specific radioactivities by conjugation to a 125I-containing acylating agent. The Biochemical journal 1973;133:529-539.

Bornschein J, Drozdov I & Malfertheiner P. Octreotide LAR: safety and tolerability issues. Expert opinion on drug safety 2009;8:755-768.

Bremer C, Ntziachristos V & Weissleder R. Optical-based molecular imaging: contrast agents and potential medical applications. European radiology 2003;13:231-243.

Brigger I, Dubernet C & Couvreur P. Nanoparticles in cancer therapy and diagnosis. Advanced Drug Delivery Reviews 2002;54:631-651.

Canaria CA & Lansford R. Advanced optical imaging in living embryos. Cellular and molecular life sciences : CMLS 2010;67:3489-3497.

Chakraborty S & Liu S. (99m)Tc and (111)In-labeling of small biomolecules: bifunctional chelators and related coordination chemistry. Current topics in medicinal chemistry 2010;10:1113-1134.

Chen K & Chen X. Positron emission tomography imaging of cancer biology: current status and future prospects. Seminars in oncology 2011;38:70-86.

Cherry SR. Physics in nuclear medicine. Philadelphia: Saunders 2003.

Cheung JS, Chow AM, Hui ES, Yang J, Tse HF & Wu EX. Cell number quantification of USPIO-labeled stem cells by MRI: an in vitro study. Conference proceedings: .Annual International Conference of the IEEE Engineering in Medicine and Biology Society.IEEE Engineering in Medicine and Biology Society.Conference 2006;1:476-479.

Chin CL, Pai M, Bousquet PF, Schwartz AJ, O'Connor EM, Nelson CM, Hradil VP, Cox BF, McRae BL & Fox GB. Distinct spatiotemporal pattern of CNS lesions revealed by USPIO-enhanced MRI in MOG-induced EAE rats implicates the involvement of spino-olivocerebellar pathways. Journal of neuroimmunology 2009;211:49-55.

Cho YS, Yoon TJ, Jang ES, Soo Hong K, Young Lee S, Ran Kim O, Park C, Kim YJ, Yi GC & Chang K. Cetuximab-conjugated magneto-fluorescent silica nanoparticles for in vivo colon cancer targeting and imaging. Cancer letters 2010;299:63-71.

Costantino L, Gandolfi F, Tosi G, Rivasi F, Vandelli MA & Forni F. Peptide-derivatized biodegradable nanoparticles able to cross the blood-brain barrier. Journal of controlled release : official journal of the Controlled Release Society 2005;108:84-96.

Chudakov D, Lukyanov S & Lukyanov K. Fluorescent proteins as a toolkit for in vivo imaging. Trends Biotechnol 2005; 23 (12): 605–13.

Dufort S, Sancey L, Wenk C, Josserand V & Coll JL. Optical small animal imaging in the drug discovery process. Biochimica et biophysica acta 2010a;1798:2266-2273.

Dufort S, Sancey L, Wenk C, Josserand V & Coll JL. Optical small animal imaging in the drug discovery process. Biochimica et biophysica acta 2010b;1798:2266-2273.

Eckelman W & Richards P. Instant 99mTc-DTPA. Journal of nuclear medicine : official publication, Society of Nuclear Medicine 1970;11:761.

Eisenblatter M, Holtke C, Persigehl T & Bremer C. Optical techniques for the molecular imaging of angiogenesis. European journal of nuclear medicine and molecular imaging 2010;37 Suppl 1:S127-37.

Fares FA, Suganuma N, Nishimori K, LaPolt PS, Hsueh AJ & Boime I. Design of a long-acting follitropin agonist by fusing the C-terminal sequence of the chorionic gonadotropin beta subunit to the follitropin beta subunit. Proceedings of the National Academy of Sciences of the United States of America 1992;89:4304-4308.

Fraker PJ & Speck JC,Jr. Protein and cell membrane iodinations with a sparingly soluble chloroamide, 1,3,4,6-tetrachloro-3a,6a-diphrenylglycoluril. Biochemical and biophysical research communications 1978;80:849-857.

Frank R. The SPOT-synthesis techniqueSynthetic peptide arrays on membrane supports—principles and applications J Immunol Methods 2002; 267:13-26.

Frank JA, Miller BR, Arbab AS, Zywicke HA, Jordan EK, Lewis BK, Bryant LH,Jr & Bulte JW. Clinically applicable labeling of mammalian and stem cells by combining superparamagnetic iron oxides and transfection agents. Radiology 2003;228:480-487.

Gabel CA & Shapiro BM. 125I]diiodofluorescein isothiocyanate: its synthesis and use as a reagent for labeling proteins and cells to high specific radioactivity. Analytical Biochemistry 1978;86:396-406.

Gambarota G, van Laarhoven HW, Philippens M, Lok J, van der Kogel A, Punt CJ & Heerschap A. Assessment of absolute blood volume in carcinoma by USPIO contrast-enhanced MRI. Magnetic resonance imaging 2006;24:279-286.

Gambarota G, van Laarhoven HW, Philippens M, Peeters WJ, Rijken P, van der Kogel A, Punt CJ & Heerschap A. Assessment of Blood Hemodynamics by USPIO-Induced R(1) Changes in MRI of Murine Colon Carcinoma. Applied magnetic resonance 2010;38:349-360.

Garrison JC, Rold TL, Sieckman GL, Naz F, Sublett SV, Figueroa SD, Volkert WA & Hoffman TJ. Evaluation of the pharmacokinetic effects of various linking group using the 111In-DOTA-X-BBN(7-14)NH2 structural paradigm in a prostate cancer model. Bioconjugate chemistry 2008;19:1803-1812.

Goetz C, Breton E, Choquet P, Israel-Jost V & Constantinesco A. SPECT low-field MRI system for small-animal imaging. Journal of nuclear medicine : official publication, Society of Nuclear Medicine 2008;49:88-93.

Golestani R, Wu C, Tio RA, Zeebregts CJ, Petrov AD, Beekman FJ, Dierckx RA, Boersma HH & Slart RH. Small-animal SPECT and SPECT/CT: application in cardiovascular research. Eur J Nucl Med Mol Imaging. 2010; 37(9):1766-77.

Gröhn O & Pitkänen A. Magnetic resonance imaging in animal models of epilepsy-noninvasive detection of structural alterations. Epilepsia. 2007;48 Suppl 4:3-10.

Haley B & Frenkel E. Nanoparticles for drug delivery in cancer treatment. Urologic oncology 2008;26:57-64.

Heikkilä JE, Vähä-Koskela MJ, Ruotsalainen JJ, Martikainen MW, Stanford MM, McCart JA, Bell JC & Hinkkanen AE. Intravenously administered alphavirus vector VA7 eradicates orthotopic human glioma xenografts in nude mice. PLoS One. 2010;5(1):e8603.

Heiss WD. The potential of PET/MR for brain imaging. European journal of nuclear medicine and molecular imaging 2009;36 Suppl 1:S105-12.

Helppolainen SH, Nurminen KP, Maatta JA, Halling KK, Slotte JP, Huhtala T, Liimatainen T, Yla-Herttuala S, Airenne KJ, Narvanen A, Janis J, Vainiotalo P, Valjakka J,

Kulomaa MS & Nordlund HR. Rhizavidin from Rhizobium etli: the first natural dimer in the avidin protein family. The Biochemical journal 2007;405:397-405.

Hoeben BA, Molkenboer-Kuenen JD, Oyen WJ, Peeters WJ, Kaanders JH, Bussink J & Boerman OC. Radiolabeled cetuximab: dose optimization for epidermal growth factor receptor imaging in a head-and-neck squamous cell carcinoma model. International journal of cancer.Journal international du cancer 2011;129:870-878.

Huhtala T, Laakkonen P, Sallinen H, Yla-Herttuala S & Narvanen A. In vivo SPECT/CT imaging of human orthotopic ovarian carcinoma xenografts with 111In-labeled monoclonal antibodies. Nuclear medicine and biology 2010;37:957-964.

Hunter WM & Greenwood FC. Preparation of iodine-131 labelled human growth hormone of high specific activity. Nature 1962;194:495-496.

Joly V, Jidar K, Tatay M & Yeni P. Enfuvirtide: from basic investigations to current clinical use. Expert opinion on pharmacotherapy 2010;11:2701-2713.

Kagadis GC, Loudos G, Katsanos K, Langer SG, Nikiforidis GC. In vivo small animal imaging: current status and future prospects. Med Phys. 2010 Dec;37(12):6421-42.

Kaikkonen MU, Lesch HP, Pikkarainen J, Raty JK, Vuorio T, Huhtala T, Taavitsainen M, Laitinen T, Tuunanen P, Grohn O, Narvanen A, Airenne KJ & Yla-Herttuala S. (Strept)avidin-displaying lentiviruses as versatile tools for targeting and dual imaging of gene delivery. Gene therapy 2009;16:894-904.

Kang SH, Cho MJ & Kole R. Up-regulation of luciferase gene expression with antisense oligonucleotides: implications and applications in functional assay development. Biochemistry 1998;37:6235-6239.

Keller TM, Michel SC, Frohlich J, Fink D, Caduff R, Marincek B & Kubik-Huch RA. USPIO-enhanced MRI for preoperative staging of gynecological pelvic tumors: preliminary results. European radiology 2004;14:937-944.

King MA, Pretorius PH, Farncombe T, Beekman FJ. Introduction to the physics of molecular imaging with radioactive tracers in small animals. J Cell Biochem Suppl. 2002;39:221-30.

Koivunen E, Arap W, Valtanen H, Rainisalo A, Medina OP, Heikkila P, Kantor C, Gahmberg CG, Salo T, Konttinen YT, Sorsa T, Ruoslahti E & Pasqualini R. Tumor targeting with a selective gelatinase inhibitor. Nature biotechnology 1999;17:768-774.

Kopka K, Schober O & Wagner S. (18)F-labelled cardiac PET tracers: selected probes for the molecular imaging of transporters, receptors and proteases. Basic research in cardiology 2008;103:131-143.

Kukowska-Latallo JF, Candido KA, Cao Z, Nigavekar SS, Majoros IJ, Thomas TP, Balogh LP, Khan MK & Baker JR,Jr. Nanoparticle targeting of anticancer drug improves therapeutic response in animal model of human epithelial cancer. Cancer research 2005;65:5317-5324.

Laakkonen P, Porkka K, Hoffman JA & Ruoslahti E. A tumor-homing peptide with a targeting specificity related to lymphatic vessels. Nature medicine 2002;8:751-755.

Lappalainen RS, Narkilahti S, Huhtala T, Liimatainen T, Suuronen T, Narvanen A, Suuronen R, Hovatta O & Jolkkonen J. The SPECT imaging shows the accumulation of neural progenitor cells into internal organs after systemic administration in middle cerebral artery occlusion rats. Neuroscience letters 2008;440:246-250.

Lehtolainen P, Taskinen A, Laukkanen J, Airenne KJ, Heino S, Lappalainen M, Ojala K, Marjomaki V, Martin JF, Kulomaa MS & Yla-Herttuala S. Cloning and characterization of Scavidin, a fusion protein for the targeted delivery of biotinylated molecules. The Journal of biological chemistry 2002;277:8545-8550.

Lehtolainen P, Wirth T, Taskinen AK, Lehenkari P, Leppanen O, Lappalainen M, Pulkkanen K, Marttila A, Marjomaki V, Airenne KJ, Horton M, Kulomaa MS & Yla-Herttuala S. Targeting of biotinylated compounds to its target tissue using a low-density lipoprotein receptor-avidin fusion protein. Gene therapy 2003;10:2090-2097.

Lei J, Xue HD, Li Z, Li S & Jin ZY. Possible pathological basis for false diagnoses of lymph nodes by USPIO-enhanced MRI in rabbits. Journal of magnetic resonance imaging : JMRI 2010;31:1428-1434.

Leonard JP, Nowotnik DP & Neirinckx RD. Technetium-99m-d, 1-HM-PAO: a new radiopharmaceutical for imaging regional brain perfusion using SPECT--a comparison with iodine-123 HIPDM. Journal of nuclear medicine : official publication, Society of Nuclear Medicine 1986a;27:1819-1823.

Leonard JP, Nowotnik DP & Neirinckx RD. Technetium-99m-d, 1-HM-PAO: a new radiopharmaceutical for imaging regional brain perfusion using SPECT--a comparison with iodine-123 HIPDM. Journal of nuclear medicine : official publication, Society of Nuclear Medicine 1986b;27:1819-1823.

Lesch HP, Pikkarainen JT, Kaikkonen MU, Taavitsainen M, Samaranayake H, Lehtolainen-Dalkilic P, Vuorio T, Maatta AM, Wirth T, Airenne KJ & Yla-Herttuala S. Avidin fusion protein-expressing lentiviral vector for targeted drug delivery. Human Gene Therapy 2009;20:871-882.

Liimatainen T, Hakumaki J, Tkac I & Grohn O. Ultra-short echo time spectroscopic imaging in rats: implications for monitoring lipids in glioma gene therapy. NMR in biomedicine 2006a;19:554-559.

Liimatainen T, Lehtimaki K, Ala-Korpela M & Hakumaki J. Identification of mobile cholesterol compounds in experimental gliomas by (1)H MRS in vivo: effects of ganciclovir-induced apoptosis on lipids. FEBS letters 2006b;580:4746-4750.

Limnell T, Riikonen J, Salonen J, Kaukonen AM, Laitinen L, Hirvonen J & Lehto VP. Surface chemistry and pore size affect carrier properties of mesoporous silicon microparticles. International journal of pharmaceutics 2007;343:141-147.

Lindvall O, Kokaia Z & Martinez-Serrano A. Stem cell therapy for human neurodegenerative disorders-how to make it work. Nature medicine 2004;10 Suppl:S42-50.

Liu S & Edwards DS. Bifunctional chelators for therapeutic lanthanide radiopharmaceuticals. Bioconjugate chemistry 2001;12:7-34.

Louwes H, Zeinali Lathori OA, Vellenga E & de Wolf JT. Platelet kinetic studies in patients with idiopathic thrombocytopenic purpura. The American Journal of Medicine 1999;106:430-434.

Mahonen AJ, Makkonen KE, Laakkonen JP, Ihalainen TO, Kukkonen SP, Kaikkonen MU, Vihinen-Ranta M, Yla-Herttuala S & Airenne KJ. Culture medium induced vimentin reorganization associates with enhanced baculovirus-mediated gene delivery. Journal of Biotechnology 2010;145:111-119.

Makinen S, Kekarainen T, Nystedt J, Liimatainen T, Huhtala T, Narvanen A, Laine J & Jolkkonen J. Human umbilical cord blood cells do not improve sensorimotor or cognitive outcome following transient middle cerebral artery occlusion in rats. Brain research 2006;1123:207-215.

Makinson A & Reynes J. The fusion inhibitor enfuvirtide in recent antiretroviral strategies. Current opinion in HIV and AIDS 2009;4:150-158.

Malmberg J, Tolmachev V & Orlova A. Imaging agents for in vivo molecular profiling of disseminated prostate cancer--targeting EGFR receptors in prostate cancer:

comparison of cellular processing of [111In]-labeled affibody molecule Z(EGFR:2377) and cetuximab. International journal of oncology 2011;38:1137-1143.
Marchalonis JJ. An enzymic method for the trace iodination of immunoglobulins and other proteins. The Biochemical journal 1969;113:299-305.
Maret W. Zinc and sulfur: a critical biological partnership. Biochemistry. 2004; 30;43(12):3301-3309.
McKinnell JA & Saag MS. Novel drug classes: entry inhibitors [enfuvirtide, chemokine (C-C motif) receptor 5 antagonists. Current opinion in HIV and AIDS 2009;4:513-517.
Merron A, Peerlinck I, Martin-Duque P, Burnet J, Quintanilla M, Mather S, Hingorani M, Harrington K, Iggo R & Vassaux G. SPECT/CT imaging of oncolytic adenovirus propagation in tumours in vivo using the Na/I symporter as a reporter gene. Gene therapy 2007;14:1731-1738.
Metz S, Beer AJ, Settles M, Pelisek J, Botnar RM, Rummeny EJ & Heider P. Characterization of carotid artery plaques with USPIO-enhanced MRI: assessment of inflammation and vascularity as in vivo imaging biomarkers for plaque vulnerability. The international journal of cardiovascular imaging 2011;27:901-912.
Miletich RS. Positron emission tomography for neurologists. Neurologic clinics 2009;27:61-88, viii.
Mäe M, El Andaloussi S, Lundin P, Oskolkov N, Johansson HJ, Guterstam P, Langel U. A stearylated CPP for delivery of splice correcting oligonucleotides using a non-covalent co-incubation strategy. J Control Release. 2009; 134(3):221-227.
Napp J, Mathejczyk JE & Alves F. Optical imaging in vivo with a focus on paediatric disease: technical progress, current preclinical and clinical applications and future perspectives. Pediatric radiology 2011;41:161-175.
Nayak TK, Garmestani K, Milenic DE, Baidoo KE & Brechbiel MW. HER1-targeted 86Y-panitumumab possesses superior targeting characteristics than 86Y-cetuximab for PET imaging of human malignant mesothelioma tumors xenografts. PloS one 2011;6:e18198.
Nekolla SG, Martinez-Moeller A & Saraste A. PET and MRI in cardiac imaging: from validation studies to integrated applications. European journal of nuclear medicine and molecular imaging 2009;36 Suppl 1:S121-30.
Nilsson F, Tarli L, Viti F & Neri D. The use of phage display for the development of tumour targeting agents. Advanced Drug Delivery Reviews 2000;43:165-196.
Pakkala M, Hekim C, Soininen P, Leinonen J, Koistinen H, Weisell J, Stenman UH, Vepsalainen J & Narvanen A. Activity and stability of human kallikrein-2-specific linear and cyclic peptide inhibitors. Journal of peptide science : an official publication of the European Peptide Society 2007;13:348-353.
Pakkala M, Weisell J, Hekim C, Vepsalainen J, Wallen EA, Stenman UH, Koistinen H & Narvanen A. Mimetics of the disulfide bridge between the N- and C-terminal cysteines of the KLK3-stimulating peptide B-2. Amino acids 2010;39:233-242.
Penet MF, Mikhaylova M, Li C, Krishnamachary B, Glunde K, Pathak AP & Bhujwalla ZM. Applications of molecular MRI and optical imaging in cancer. Future medicinal chemistry 2010;2:975-988.
Pichler BJ, Judenhofer MS & Wehrl HF. PET/MRI hybrid imaging: devices and initial results. European radiology 2008;18:1077-1086.
Ping Li W, Meyer LA, Capretto DA, Sherman CD & Anderson CJ. Receptor-binding, biodistribution, and metabolism studies of 64Cu-DOTA-cetuximab, a PET-imaging

agent for epidermal growth-factor receptor-positive tumors. Cancer biotherapy & radiopharmaceuticals 2008;23:158-171.

Qu T, Wang Y, Zhu Z, Rusckowski M & Hnatowich DJ. Different chelators and different peptides together influence the in vitro and mouse in vivo properties of 99Tcm. Nuclear medicine communications 2001;22:203-215.

Raty JK, Liimatainen T, Huhtala T, Kaikkonen MU, Airenne KJ, Hakumaki JM, Narvanen A & Yla-Herttuala S. SPECT/CT imaging of baculovirus biodistribution in rat. Gene therapy 2007;14:930-938.

Raty JK, Liimatainen T, Wirth T, Airenne KJ, Ihalainen TO, Huhtala T, Hamerlynck E, Vihinen-Ranta M, Narvanen A, Yla-Herttuala S & Hakumaki JM. Magnetic resonance imaging of viral particle biodistribution in vivo. Gene therapy 2006;13:1440-1446.

Reece JC, McGregor DL, Geysen HM & Rodda SJ. Scanning for T helper epitopes with human PBMC using pools of short synthetic peptides. J Immunol Methods. 1994 Jun 24;172(2):241-54.

Rissanen TT & Yla-Herttuala S. Current status of cardiovascular gene therapy. Molecular therapy : the journal of the American Society of Gene Therapy 2007;15:1233-1247.

Rivera F, Vega-Villegas ME & Lopez-Brea MF. Cetuximab, its clinical use and future perspectives. Anti-Cancer Drugs 2008;19:99-113.

Rodrigues M, Sinzinger H, Thakur M, Becker W, Dewanjee M, Ezekowitz M, Isaka Y, Martin-Comin J, Peters M, Roca M & Stratton J. Labelling of platelets with indium-111 oxine and technetium-99m hexamethylpropylene amine oxime: suggested methods. International Society of Radiolabelled Blood Elements (ISORBE). European journal of nuclear medicine 1999;26:1614-1616.

Röntgen WC. On a new kind of rays. Science. 1896;3(59):227-31.

Russell WMS & Burch RL,. The Principles of Humane Experimental Technique. England: 1959.

Salonen J, Björkqvist M, Laine E & Niinistö L. Stabilization of porous silicon surface by thermal decomposition of acetylene. Applied Surface Science 2004;225:389-394.

Salonen J, Kaukonen AM, Hirvonen J & Lehto VP. Mesoporous silicon in drug delivery applications. Journal of pharmaceutical sciences 2008;97:632-653.

Seppi K, Scherfler C, Donnemiller E, Virgolini I, Schocke MF, Goebel G, Mair KJ, Boesch S, Brenneis C, Wenning GK & Poewe W. Topography of dopamine transporter availability in progressive supranuclear palsy: a voxelwise [123I]beta-CIT SPECT analysis. Archives of Neurology 2006;63:1154-1160.

Shang Y, Gibbs MA, Marek GJ, Stiger T, Burstein AH, Marek K, Seibyl JP & Rogers JF. Displacement of serotonin and dopamine transporters by venlafaxine extended release capsule at steady state: a [123I]2beta-carbomethoxy-3beta-(4-iodophenyl)-tropane single photon emission computed tomography imaging study. Journal of clinical psychopharmacology 2007;27:71-75.

Shaya EK, Scheffel U, Dannals RF, Ricaurte GA, Carroll FI, Wagner HN,Jr, Kuhar MJ & Wong DF. In vivo imaging of dopamine reuptake sites in the primate brain using single photon emission computed tomography (SPECT) and iodine-123 labeled RTI-55. Synapse (New York, N.Y.) 1992;10:169-172.

Shome B, Parlow AF, Liu WK, Nahm HS, Wen T & Ward DN. A reevaluation of the amino acid sequence of human follitropin beta-subunit. Journal of protein chemistry 1988;7:325-339.

Snoeks TJ, Khmelinskii A, Lelieveldt BP, Kaijzel EL, Löwik CW. Optical advances in skeletal imaging applied to bone metastases. Bone. 2011 Jan;48(1):106-14.

Staffen W, Mair A, Unterrainer J, Trinka E, Bsteh C & Ladurner G. 123I] beta-CIT binding and SPET compared with clinical diagnosis in parkinsonism. Nuclear medicine communications 2000;21:417-424.

Stajich GV & Ashworth L. Octreotide. Neonatal network : NN 2006;25:365-369.

Thakur ML. Gallium-67 and indium-111 radiopharmaceuticals. The International journal of applied radiation and isotopes 1977;28:183-201.

Thakur ML, Coleman RE & Welch MJ. Indium-111-labeled leukocytes for the localization of abscesses: preparation, analysis, tissue distribution, and comparison with gallium-67 citrate in dogs. The Journal of laboratory and clinical medicine 1977;89:217-228.

Thrall JH. Technetium-99m labeled agents for skeletal imaging. CRC critical reviews in clinical radiology and nuclear medicine 1976;8:1-31.

Turhanen P, Weisell J, Lehtolainen-Dalkilic P, Määttä A-M, Vepsäläinen J, Närvänen A. A novel strategy for the synthesis of enzymatically stable biotin-DOTA conjugates for *in vivo* use. Med Chem Commun 2011; 2, 886-888.

Turunen MP, Puhakka HL, Koponen JK, Hiltunen MO, Rutanen J, Leppanen O, Turunen AM, Narvanen A, Newby AC, Baker AH & Yla-Herttuala S. Peptide-retargeted adenovirus encoding a tissue inhibitor of metalloproteinase-1 decreases restenosis after intravascular gene transfer. Molecular therapy : the journal of the American Society of Gene Therapy 2002;6:306-312.

Vaidyanathan G, Affleck DJ & Zalutsky MR. Method for radioiodination of proteins using N-succinimidyl 3-hydroxy-4-iodobenzoate. Bioconjugate chemistry 1997;8:724-729.

Vallabhajosula S, Solnes L & Vallabhajosula B. A Broad Overview of Positron Emission Tomography Radiopharmaceuticals and Clinical Applications: What Is New? Seminars in nuclear medicine 2011;41:246-264.

Vellinga MM, Vrenken H, Hulst HE, Polman CH, Uitdehaag BM, Pouwels PJ, Barkhof F & Geurts JJ. Use of ultrasmall superparamagnetic particles of iron oxide (USPIO)-enhanced MRI to demonstrate diffuse inflammation in the normal-appearing white matter (NAWM) of multiple sclerosis (MS) patients: an exploratory study. Journal of magnetic resonance imaging : JMRI 2009;29:774-779.

Vincenzi B, Schiavon G, Silletta M, Santini D & Tonini G. The biological properties of cetuximab. Critical reviews in oncology/hematology 2008;68:93-106.

Weissleder R & Ntziachristos V. Shedding light onto live molecular targets. Nature medicine 2003;9:123-128.

Welch M, J. & Redvanly C, S. Handbook of Radiopharmaceuticals: Radiochemistry and Applications England: Wiley 2002.

Welsh DK & Kay SA. Bioluminescence imaging in living organisms. Current opinion in biotechnology 2005;16:73-78.

Wiekhorst F, Seliger C, Jurgons R, Steinhoff U, Eberbeck D, Trahms L & Alexiou C. Quantification of magnetic nanoparticles by magnetorelaxometry and comparison to histology after magnetic drug targeting. Journal of nanoscience and nanotechnology 2006;6:3222-3225.

Zalutsky MR & Narula AS. A method for the radiohalogenation of proteins resulting in decreased thyroid uptake of radioiodine. International journal of radiation applications and instrumentation.Part A, Applied radiation and isotopes 1987;38:1051-1055.

Zubal IG, Early M, Yuan O, Jennings D, Marek K & Seibyl JP. Optimized, automated striatal uptake analysis applied to SPECT brain scans of Parkinson's disease patients. Journal of nuclear medicine : official publication, Society of Nuclear Medicine 2007;48:857-864.

Section 2

Earthquake Medical Management

2

Rational Drug Use in Medical Response to an Earthquake

Ling-li Zhang[1], Yi Liang[1,2], Li-nan Zeng[1] and Die Hu[1,2]
[1]*Department of Pharmacy, West China Second University Hospital, Sichuan University*
[2]*West China School of Pharmacy, Sichuan University, China*

1. Introduction

Earthquake can be defined as the shaking of earth caused by waves moving on and below the earth's surface and causing: surface faulting, tremors vibration, liquefaction, landslides, aftershocks and/or tsunamis (World Health Organization [WHO], 2011). 118 earthquakes of magnitude 7 or over occurred since 21st century all over the world, and caused millions of casualties (National Geophysical Data Centre [NGDC], 2011). In 2004, the Indian Ocean earthquake with a magnitude of 9.1 triggered a series of devastating tsunamis along the coasts, killing 230,000 people in 14 countries, which was one of the deadliest natural disasters in recorded history. In 2011, the 9.0 magnitude East Japan earthquake, which caused tsunami and nuclear crisis, killed 15,365 people.

Earthquakes cause high mortality resulting from trauma, asphyxia, dust inhalation (acute respiratory distress), or exposure to the environment (i.e. hypothermia) (WHO, 2011). Recent studies suggest that primary prevention is the most effective means of reducing earthquake casualties (Durkin & Thiel, 1992). Therefore, priority should be given to considering seismic safety in land-use planning and in building design (Coburn & Spence 1992). After an earthquake occurs, however a well-planned medical response is a key strategy for reducing mortality and disability (Schultz et al, 1996). During a medical response, drug use is an important issue in the management of the injured, especially for ones have known or suspected infections, internal injuries and crush syndrome requiring intensive drug treatment besides surgery. Therefore, the rationality of drug use in earthquake injured needs to be discussed to find whether irrationality exists and how to get improved in future medical response. In addition, there is no doubt that the pharmacists as medical professionals play an important role in promoting rational drug use in our medical service, however, what can pharmacists do to promote rational drug use in earthquake medical response? Based on these facts and questions, in this chapter we reviewed drug use and practice experience of pharmacists in management of injured in previous earthquakes, to provide evidence for better pharmacy practice in earthquake medical response in the future.

2. Death and diseases caused by earthquakes

In most earthquakes, people are injured and killed by mechanical energy as direct result of being crushed by falling building materials. Deaths caused by earthquakes can be instantaneous, rapid or delayed (Naghii, 2005). Instantaneous death can result from sever crushing injuries to the head or chest, severe external or internal bleeding, or get drowned in the tsunamis caused by the earthquake. Rapid death occurs within minutes or hours and can result from asphyxia caused by inhalation or chest compression, hypovolemic shock, or environmental exposure. Delayed death occurs within days and can result from dehydration, electrolyte disturbance, crush syndrome, or infections (Pretto et al, 1994).

Within 1 week after an earthquake occurs, the dominated disease is traumas. In the first day after Sichuan earthquake in 2008, trauma accounted for 96.8% of all the patients (Liu et al, 2011). 1 week later, number of traumas patients decreases and more patients are admitted to internal medicine, pediatrics and dermatology department for infectious diseases, in which respiratory infection, diarrhea and skin rash are more common (Ma et al, 2011). Trauma is mostly caused by the collapse of building and leads the majority of deaths and injuries in most earthquakes (Coburn & Spence 1992). Major injury requiring hospitalization includes skull fractures with intracranial hemorrhage, spine injuries, and damage to intrathorcic, intra-abdominal, and intrapelvic organs, including pneumothorax, liver lacerations, and ruptured spleen. Most seriously injured people have combination injuries, such as pneumothorax in addition to an extremity fracture (Naghii, 2005). A study based on the Spitak-88 earthquake in 1988 found that combination injuries accounted for 39.7% of the cases. Superficial trauma such as lacerations and contusions were the injuries most frequently observed (24.9%), followed by head injuries (22%), lower extremity injuries (19%), crush syndrome (11%), and upper extremity trauma (10%) (Noji, 1992). Appropriate medical and surgical treatment of these injuries is vital to improving survival, minimizing future functional impairment and disability.

3. Drug use in earthquake injured patients

There was scarcely any study investigating drug use in the earthquake injured until several studies based on data from Sichuan Earthquake in 2008 had addressed this topic. To our knowledge, there is no data on this subject from other earthquakes, we discussed drug use in earthquake injured patients based on available data from Sichuan earthquake.

3.1 Characteristics of drug use

3.1.1 Types of drugs

The study conducted by Yuan analyzed types of drugs used in injured patients in a hospital which is the nearest large general hospital to epicenter in Sichuan earthquake. This study was based on medical record of 325 patients who were admitted within 1 week after the disaster. Most patients had trauma, including bone fractures, soft tissue trauma, brain injury and other kinds of contusion/laceration. The results showed that 21 types and 433 drugs were used. The top 10 types in number of individual drugs used were listed in table 1. Among all drugs used, anti-infective drugs had the most individual drugs, in which 84 drugs were used, accounting for 19.39% of all the 433 individual drugs. 65 drugs acting on central nervous system were used, including analgetics sedatives and antianxietics. 59 cardiovascular drugs were used, most of which were calcium channel blockers, drugs for chronic cardiac insufficiency, drugs for angina, hypotensive agents, and anti-shock drugs. 36 gastrointestinal drugs were used, and most of them were drugs for peptic ulcer, prokinetic agents, antiemetic agents, catarrhectics, anti-diarrheal agent and drugs for liver and gall diseases. 34 drugs were used in respiratory disease, including expectorants, antitussives and antasthmatics. Drugs affecting blood included blood coagulants, anticoagulant drugs, blood plasma and its substitutes. Externally applied drugs included disinfectants, antiseptics and dermatological drugs. Hormones included adrenal cortex hormone and trypsin. Antiallergic agents are mainly anti-histamine drugs. These drugs are mainly administered by injection or external application (Yuan & Zhang, 2009).

Types of drugs	Number of individual drugs	Percentage (%)
Anti-infective drugs	84	19.39
Drugs acting on central nervous system	65	15.01
Cardiovascular drugs	59	13.63
Gastrointestinal drugs	36	8.31
Drugs acting on respiratory system	34	7.85
Drugs affecting the blood	26	6.00
Externally applied and ophthalmological preparations	18	4.16
Hormones	17	3.93
Antiallergic drugs	9	2.08
Drugs correcting water, electrolyte and acid-base disturbances	9	2.08

Table 1. The top 10 types in number of individual drugs used in Sichuan earthquake injured patients

Another study analyzed drug use in 329 women and children injured after Sichuan earthquake, and found that 26 types involving 398 individual drugs were used (Han et al, 2008). Anti-infective, involving 77drugs, had the most number of individual drugs, which was consistent with results found by Yuan in the general hospital (Yuan & Zhang, 2009).

These results suggest that many types involving hundreds of individual drugs might be used during the treatment of earthquake injured patients, and thus actions should be taken to ensure those essential drugs accessible in medical response. Decision makers in hospitals and local governments especially in areas where earthquakes occur frequently should make related polices, such as an essential drug list to ensure those essential drugs are well prepared when an earthquake breaks out.

3.1.2 Frequently used drugs

2 studies conducted in different hospitals analyzed the consumption of drugs in injured patients after Sichuan earthquake. The top 20 frequently used drugs in injured patients admitted in 2 hospitals were listed in table 2. Both results suggested that water and electrolyte supplements were most frequently used drugs, including glucose, sodium chloride, potassium chloride, sodium lactate Ringer's and sodium bicarbonate. Antibiotics were second frequently used, but different antibiotics were used in the 2 hospitals. Ciprofloxacin was the most frequently used antibiotic in Mian Yang Central Hospital. Metronidazole, cefazolin and ofloxacin were other frequently used antibiotics (Yuan & Zhang, 2009). Benzylpenicillin was most frequently used in West China Hospital, cefuroxime, ciprofloxacin, and clindamycin were other frequently used antibiotics (Li et al,

2009). Other frequently used drugs included hemostatic drugs (etamsylate and aminomethylbenzoic acid), dexamethasone, vitamin C, atropine, dopamine, tetanus antitoxin, ambroxol, inosine injection, lidocaine hydrochloride, and disinfectants (hydrogen peroxide solution and betagen solution) .

Rank	Drug name (specification)	
	Mian Yang Central Hospital	West China Hospital
1	Glucose injection (5% 500ml)	Benzylpenicillin (80 U)
2	Etamsylate injection (2ml 0.5g)	Sodium chloride injection (0.9% 500ml)
3	Glucose and sodium chloride injection (5% 500ml)	Sodium chloride injection (0.9% 100ml)
4	Dexamethasone sodium phosphate injection (1ml 5mg)	Vitamin C injection*
5	Potassium chloride injection (10ml 1 g)	Tetanus antitoxin (250 U)
6	Ciprofloxacin lactate injection (100ml 0.2g)	Sodium chloride injection (0.9% 250ml)
7	Vitamin C injection (2ml 0.5g)	Potassium chloride Injection (10ml)
8	Sodium chloride injection (0.9% 500ml)	Etamsylate injection*
9	Sodium lactate Ringer's injection (500ml)	Glucose injection (5% 500ml)
10	Atropine sulfate injection 2ml 1mg	Cefuroxime*
11	Metronidazole injection (100ml 0.5g)	Dexamethasone (5 ml)
12	Cefazolin injection (0.5g)	Ciprofloxacin injection*
13	Ofloxacin and glucose injection (100ml 0.2g)	Sodium lactate Ringer's injection (500ml)
14	Dopamine hydrochloride injection (2ml 20mg)	Aminomethylbenzoic acid injection*
15	Glucose injection (10% 500ml)	Glucose and sodium chloride injection (5% 500ml)
16	Hydrogen peroxide solution (3% 100ml)	Glucose injection (5% 250ml)
17	Sodium bicarbonate injection (10ml 0.5g)	Clindamycin injection*
18	Tetanus antitoxin (1500U)	Ambroxol injection*
19	Lidocaine hydrochloride injection (5ml 0.1g)	Inosine injection*
20	Betagen solution (5% 200ml)	Dopamine injection*

* Drug specifications were not given in primary studies

Table 2. Top 20 frequently used drugs in Sichuan earthquake injured patients admitted in 2 hospitals

These results provided information on drugs that frequently used and thus urgently needed by injured people, which can be important evidence for drug donation and pharmaceutical management in the earthquake disaster. Priority should be given to those drugs when purchasing and donating drugs after an earthquake, and actions should be taken in hospitals to ensure that those drugs were or can be supplied in sufficient quantity immediately.

3.1.3 Antibiotic use

Open injuries are common in trauma caused by an earthquake, and have a potential for bacterial wound infections. These in turn may lead to long term disabilities, chronic wound or bone infection, and death. As the delay between injury and treatment after an earthquake, most injury presented with infected wounds, and necessitated empirical antimicrobial treatment urgently （Miskin et al, 2010）. Appropriate management with antibiotics to prevent and control infections is criticality important to the injured.

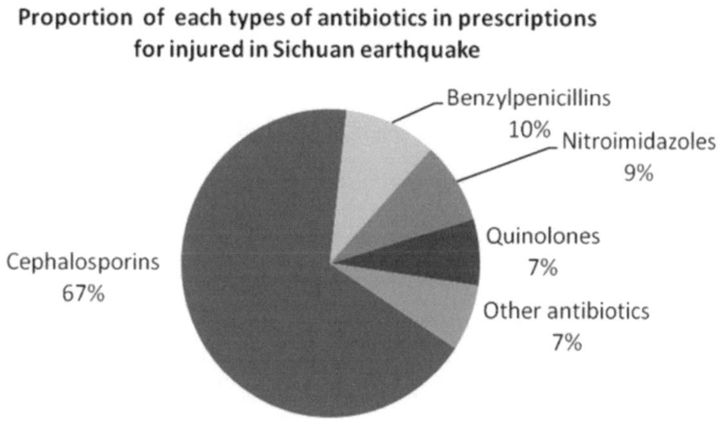

Fig. 1. Proportion of each type of antibiotics in prescriptions for injured patients in Sichuan earthquake

World Health Organization and The Centers for Disease Control and Prevention have proposed guidelines for management of wound infectious. Considering that most wound infections are due to staphylococci streptococci and anaerobe, WHO recommends penicillin G and metronidazole for empirical prophylaxis and treatment of infection (WHO, 2010). CDC recommended beta-lactam antibiotics and clindamycin for management of wound infections (Centers for Disease Control and Prevention [CDC], 2010). However, a study on Haiti earthquake injured patients found that 77% of the wound infections were poly-microbial, with 89% involving gram-negative pathogens, and these pathogens were generally resistant to the antibiotics suggested by CDC and WHO. This result exactly demonstrated the types of pathogens around injured patients in the earthquake stricken place, as the patients had not been exposed to any other health care environment since the earthquake occurred, and could not be infected by nosocomial pathogens (Miskin et al, 2010). Results of several previous studies based on data from earthquakes happened in Turkey (Keven et al, 2003), Pakistan (Kiani et al, 2009), China (Wang et al, 2008; Ran et al, 2010) and Haiti (Miskin et al, 2010) in 1999~2010 also found that most bacterial isolates that caused infection in the injured were gram-negative. The emergency-relief medical teams and hospitals should be equipped with antimicrobial drugs for treatment of gram-negative infections as well as drugs for gram-positive currently recommended.

A study analyzed the antibiotic use based on 2953 prescriptions of injured patients in Sichuan earthquake in 2008. The results showed that 2830 prescriptions included antibiotics, accounting for 98.5% of all studied prescriptions. The frequency of each type of antibiotics presented in the 2830 prescriptions is listed in Fig 1. Cephalosporin was the most frequently used antibiotic, about 2/3 prescriptions included this types of drugs, followed by Benzylpenicillins, nitroimidazoles and quinolones (Li et al, 2008). This result may suggest that the use of antibiotics for injured patients in Sichuan earthquake was consistent with the recommendation by WHO and CDC, and large quantities of beta-lactam antibiotics, nitroimidazoles and quinolones are needed for earthquake injured patients.

3.2 Irrational drug use in earthquake injured patients

Rational use of drugs requires that patients receive medications appropriate to their clinical needs, in doses that meet their own individual requirements, for an adequate period of time, and at the lowest cost to them and their community (WHO, May 2010).

The drug utilization study in 329 injured women and children in Sichuan earthquake found that over-use and under-use of drugs were very common especially in children. In women patients, over-used drugs included vitamin C, magnesium sulfate, estradiol valerate, and dexamethasone. They were prescribed in an average daily dose 7~12 times larger than the defined daily dose (DDD) which is the assumed average maintenance daily dose for its main indication (WHO,2009). Drug over-use was more serious in earthquake injured children and mostly occurred when antibiotics and hormone were used. Benzylpenicillin and oxacillin were prescribed in an average daily dose more than 6 times larger than their DDD, and prednisolone was prescribed with over-dose 40-80 times than DDD. However, drug under-use was also found, as amoxicillin and valaciclovir were far less than recommended dose, which were 0.03-0.13 times of DDD (Han et al, 2008).

Over-use of drugs increases risk of adverse effect that can be harmful and causes trouble to the treatment of injured patients. In contrast, drug under-use caused failing to achieve the intended treatment outcome. Over-use and under-use both induce waste of drugs, which can make the lack of drug resources even worse in the earthquake-stricken area. Under these circumstances, prescription during the medical care of earthquake injured patients should be monitored and regulated to improve rational drug use.

4. The role of clinical pharmacists in medical relief

Clinical pharmacists can make a difference in drug supply and use in emergency. The job of clinical pharmacists includes ensuring adequate drug supply and promoting rational drug use.

4.1 Ensuring adequate drug supply

4.1.1 Participating in making earthquake relief drug list

According to past experience and *Hospital Formulary*, hospitals could make an *Earthquake Relief Drug List*, which would act as a guide of drug supply and use during medical relief

(Rao et al 2009). The List based on the major diseases after earthquake, includes detail information of drugs, such as indication, usage, dosage, pharmacology, the main adverse reactions and precautions and warnings. Clinical pharmacists should participate in the development of the list, because they have rich pharmaceutical knowledge, basic medical knowledge and are familiar with clinical use of drugs. Furthermore, clinical pharmacists could specify first-line agents for each type of drugs in the list, which would be helpful for doctors choosing drugs rationally (Rao et al 2009).

4.1.2 Choosing suitable drugs for medical team

Choosing suitable drugs is part of the clinical pharmacists' job. Medical team could bring only limited drugs with them. In case of that, it is necessary to choose the most suitable types and formulations of drugs for easy to use in the stricken area. Additionally, the drug packaging should be considered as well. It should be convenient to transport and not be frangible. Ciprofloxacin injection was listed on the *Earthquake Relief Drug List* in a hospital, which was packaged by glass bottle (Zhang et al 2010). Levofloxacin has similar antimicrobial spectrum and anti-bacterial effect with ciprofloxacin. It needs no allergy test before use as well. What's more, Levofloxacin injection was packaged by plastic bags. Considering about the characteristics of levofloxacin, their pharmacists replaced Ciprofloxacin injection with Levofloxacin injection.

4.1.3 Choosing alternative drugs for saving the short one

After Sichuan earthquake, so many roads were blocked. It was difficult to send materials to the stricken area. In addition, there was a huge consumption of drugs. Therefore drug supply was relatively short. In this case, clinical pharmacists play a crucial role in guaranteeing drug supply by choosing alternative drugs. It is reported that in order to save injectable antibiotics during Haiti earthquake relief, pharmacists were asked to participate in rounds with doctors, and choose appropriate alternative oral antibiotics to replace injectable ones (Ferris 2010). In our hospital, albumin was once short during earthquake relief. Our pharmacists advised doctors to use Dextran and Amino acid injection for adding colloidal solution instead of albumin, and successfully saved several lives with serious crush syndrome (Chen et al 2010).

4.2 Promoting rational drug use

4.2.1 Suggesting better treatment plans

Clinical pharmacists, who are familiar with pharmacokinetics, pharmacology and pharmacy, could choose suitable drugs, adjust drug dosage and suggest better treatment plans, especially for special patients. Crush syndrome was common after earthquake, which is a serious medical condition characterized by major shock and renal failure after a crushing injury of skeletal muscle. Individualized treatment plans should be considered for those patients who had renal insufficiency. In our hospital during Sichuan earthquake relief, there was a patient who was suspected to be infected with gram-negative bacterium (Chen et al 2010). Considering about his crush syndrome, our pharmacists advised doctor to use drugs which have little effect on kidney function or failing to excrete in urine via the kidneys (e.g. cefoperazone and ceftriaxone). Apart from renal insufficiency, patients who have hepatic insufficiency or chronic disease that need long-term medications require special attention to their drug use. Additionally, clinical pharmacists should also pay attention to treatment of children, pregnant women and the elderly.

4.2.2 Prescription audit

Clinical pharmacists are responsible for drug safety monitoring. Apart from reporting adverse drug reaction (ADR), they could contribute to reducing the incidence of ADR (Chen et al 2010). Incidence of ADR is particularly higher in patients with multi diseases, because it is positively correlated with the number of administered drugs. It is difficult to make a rational treatment plan alone for multi diseases patients. In addition, in an emergency like earthquake, the efficacy of drugs is usually considered at first. And there is no time to think much about the adverse drug reaction. In order to reducing ADR, Clinical pharmacists could conduct prescription audit to prevent irrational drug use, such as over-dose drug use and negative drug interactions.

4.2.3 Providing information and guidance of drugs

Compliance of patients affects the outcome of therapy. However, there are too many factors that cause patients taking drugs not as drug therapies. In order to improve compliance of patients, clinical pharmacists could instruct patients to take drugs rationally (Chen et al 2010; Zhang et al 2010). They could provide information about the effects, proper dosage and usage, and potential adverse effect of drugs for patients. In addition, clinical pharmacists could provide information and guidance for local residents and relief workers.

Improving use of donated drugs could avoid wasting resources. But doctors are not familiar with donated drugs. Clinical pharmacists could introduce donated drugs to doctors, provide them with information on indication, efficacy, dosage, adverse effect, precautions and warnings of those drugs, and change their prescribing habits. In our hospital, the utilization rate of donated drugs was significantly improved in the effort of our clinical pharmacists (Zhang et al 2008).

4.3 Making therapeutic decisions alone

Clinical pharmacists have the ability to make and implement therapeutic decisions alone when a clear diagnosis is made by doctors (Chen et al 2010). Earthquake can cause a large number of injured. Facing too many patients after earthquake, it is crucial to distribute limited medical personnel reasonably. Optimizing the diagnosis and treatment procedures could greatly improve the efficiency of treating patients. Clinical pharmacists are familiar with clinical use of drugs and have the ability to make therapeutic decisions alone for the patients with common diseases such as diarrhea, upper respiratory tract infection and soft tissue or superficial infection, when a clear diagnosis is made. In addition, clinical pharmacists are responsible for making *the Detailed Rules of the Reasonable Application of Antimicrobial Agents* in many hospitals. They are vital in treating infective diseases which are common after earthquake. Therefore for part of medical disease, they also have the ability to make therapeutic decisions alone.

Clinical pharmacists can play an important role in medical response after an earthquake and thus should be included in the medical relief team. Hospitals especially those undertake medical relief should routinely employ clinical pharmacists. In addition, experienced clinical pharmacists can be sent to the earthquake-stricken place for the benefit of the injured to achieve a better treatment outcome.

5. Pharmaceutical administration in medical response to an earthquake

Multi-sectoral collaboration is vital in a relief operation. A survey in 2006 showed that 84% of pharmacy in the investigated hospitals had participated in emergency exercise (Hsu et al 2006). Pharmaceutical administration is a key link to keep the medical response work in an orderly way. As different influencing factors exist in earthquake stricken areas distributed all over the world and decision makers may face new problems in each disaster, there can hardly a guideline for the administration work. The past experience can be important evidence for making decisions.

5.1 Devising an emergency plan

Earthquake could occur in a sudden, and in a flash. It is difficult to take an emergency evacuation or fight against earthquake. It can cause a large number of life and material losses. Pharmacy should be prepared for disasters such as earthquake. It is necessary to devise a well-developed emergency plans for earthquake (Rao et al 2009; Tong & Xiao 2008). Once the disaster happened, pharmacy could supply drugs rapidly and timely. Firstly, an *Earthquake Relief Drug List* should be made, which is the directory for drug supply in emergency. Secondly, there should be an emergency team, which can make a response to earthquake quickly. Five parts comprise the emergency team, which is respectively responsible for clinical pharmaceutical care, controlled drug management, drug purchase, transportation and dispensing (Rao 2009). All members of emergency team must be on call at any time (Tong & Xiao 2008).

5.2 Management of drug supply

5.2.1 Core principle of drug supply

Drug supply should be based on the major diseases in different periods of earthquakes (Xing et al 2008; Xu et al 2008; Cui et al 2010). After Sichuan earthquake, drug supply respectively focused on emergency drugs for trauma, antimicrobial agents and antipsychotics in different periods. In 1995, Kobe Earthquake caused several fires. Drug supply included emergency drugs for burn (Tong & Xiao 2008). In addition, disinfectant and vaccine are necessary in earthquake relief.

5.2.2 Emergency drug purchase

Our hospital, a women and children specialized hospital, is about 100 kilometers away from the epicenter of Sichuan earthquake and closed to the affected area. A large number of the injured were accepted in our hospital. But the area of drug warehouse in our hospital is very small so that the stock of emergency drugs is serious low. In the night of the day earthquake happened, pharmacy made an emergency purchase plan based on drug use of the injured in earthquake and stock of drugs, and informed the supply companies immediately. The day after earthquake, we revised the purchase plan and decided to store 3 to 10 times of the monthly average amount for emergency drugs, and 2 times for common drugs (Xu et al 2009), considering about the major diseases after earthquake, and the characteristics of our hospital and drugs. What's more, we kept in contact with each of the supply companies during earthquake relief.

5.2.3 The way to obtaining drugs in the stricken area

There are still many situations beyond our expected, although we prepared well for medical relief. Therefore, it is an important way to obtain drugs from other organizations and help each others. It is reported that in an international relief for Haiti Earthquake, there was no pediatric formulations and some special drugs in a mobile hospital, for example, oxytocin, which is necessary for a pregnant in labor and a woman with continuous vaginal bleeding after incomplete abortion (Yang et al 2006). Fortunately, they borrowed that from local Spanish Red Cross. What's more, the hospital was seriously lack of drugs after a few days of relief operation (Yang et al 2006). But with the help of local army, non-governmental organization and international counterparts, the hospital obtained drugs for 1500 patients.

5.3 Management of donated drugs

It was estimated that about 2500 tons of drugs and medical supplies had been sent directly to Armenian by the end of 1989 after the earthquake in 1988 (Autier et al 1990). But 8% of those donations had already expired on arrival, 11% was proved to be useless, 21% was not for emergency situation, and 20% had been destroyed. Only 30% could be immediately regarded as usable drugs. These proportions were striking. In Sichuan Earthquake, there were a big difference between types of donated drugs and the actual demands in our hospital (Lin et al 2010).

Although it was recognized that the management of donated medicines is important many years ago, there are still many problems need to be pay attention. According to the reviewed papers and our own experience, we provided some suggestions for management of donated drugs in order to avoid wasting resources.

- Management of the received donated drugs, including repository, records of receiving and dispensing and the statistical data, should be separated from the common drugs in a hospital (Tong & Xiao 2008).
- Providing information of clinical drug use to the organizations or individuals who are interested in donating .
- Promoting the clinical use of the donated drugs (Zhang et al 2008).
- Selling the remainder of the donated drugs in hospitals after the permission of donors has been obtained (Lin et al 2008).

Decision makers can conduct pharmaceutical administration work based on evidence from those good experiences. In case that the disaster occurs in a sudden, an emergency plan should be made by local government and hospitals; An earthquake relief drug list can be made to ensure essential relief drugs are well prepared; The drug purchase plan can be flexible, as the types and quantity of drugs used after an earthquake may be different from routine treatment; The obtaining of drugs can vary a lot depending on different situation; The management of donated medicines should be effective to avoid waste and ensure good quality.

6. Conclusion

After an earthquake occurred, trauma is the dominated disease within the first week, during the medical response, hundreds of drugs can be involved in the treatment of injured patients, but antibiotics and drugs correcting water, electrolyte and acid-base disturbances were most frequently used. Antibiotics for gram-positive bacterium and anaerobe are recommended by WHO and CDC for prophylaxis and treatment of wound infections, but antibiotics for gram-negtive bacterium should also be equipped by medical relief teams and hospitals.

The pharmacist can play an important role in supply and rational use of drugs in an earthquake medical response, by providing drug information and participating in the decision-making. Past experience from earthquake medical relief had provided evidence for management of drug supply and donated drugs in pharmaceutical administration after an earthquake.

7. References

Autier P.; Férir MC.; Hairapetien A.; Alexanian A.; Agoudjian V.; Schmets G.; Dallemagne G.; Leva MN. & Pinel J. (1990). Drug supply in the aftermath of the 1988 Armenian earthquake. *Lancet*, Vol.9, No.335, (Jun 1990), pp. 1388-1390, ISSN 0140-6736

Centers for Disease Control and Prevention. (2010) Emergency preparedness and response: emergency wound management for healthcare professionals. Atlanta: Centers for Disease Control and Prevention. Retrieved from <http://emergency.cdc.gov/disasters/emergwoundhcp.asp#guidance or http://www.bt.cdc.gov/disasters/pdf/emergwoundhcp.pdf>

Chen L.; Guo YJ.; Lan Y. & Zhang LL. (2010). Pharmaceutical support role of clinical pharmacist in earthquake medical assistance. *China Pharmacy*, Vol.21, No.5, (2010), pp. 390-392, ISSN 1001-0408

Coburn A. & Spence R. (1992). *Earthquake protection (Second Edition)*, Wiley, ISBN 0-470-84923-1, Chichester, England

Cui J.; Zhang JH.; Wu F. & Liu AB. (2010). Drug supply during earthquake emergency rescue: experience from Haiti. *China Journal of Emergency Resuscitation and Disaster Medicine*, Vol.5, No.9, (Sep 2010), pp. 805-807, ISSN 1673-6966

Durkin ME. & Thiel CC. (1992). Improving measures to reduce earthquake casualties. *Earthquake Spectra*, Vol.8, (1992), pp. 95-113, ISSN 8755-2930

Ferris D. (2010). Pharmacist's assistance after Haiti earthquake. *American Journal of Health-System Pharmacy*, Vol.67, No.14, (Jul 2010), pp. 1138, 1141, ISSN 1079-2082

Han L, Zeng LN, Guo C, Lan Y, Wang L, Luo C, Zhang LL (2009). Utilization Analysis of Drug Efficacy of the 329 Cases of Wenchuan Earthquake Women and Children Patients. *Chinese Journal of Evidence-Based Medicine*, Vol.9, No.3, (2009), pp. 265-272, ISSN 1672-2513

Hogerzeil HV.; Couper MR. & Gray R. (1997). Guidelines for drug donations. *British Medical Journal*. Vol.314, No.8, (Mar 1997), pp. 737-740, ISSN 0959-8146

Keven K, Ates K, Sever MS, et al. (2003) Infectious complications after mass disasters: the Marmara earthquake experience. *Scandinavian Journal of Infectious Diseases*. Vol.35, No.2, (2003), pp. 110-113, ISSN 0036-5548

Kiani, QH.;Amir, M,; Ghazanfar, MA. & Iqbal, M. (2009). Microbiology of wound infections among hospitalised patients following the 2005 Pakistan earthquake. *The Journal of Hospital Infection*. Vol.73, No.1, (2009), pp. 71-78, ISSN 0195-6701

Li J.; Shang L.; Zhu P. & Tang Y. (2008). Analysis of antibiotic for the injured in the 5.12 earthquake in west china hospital. *West China Medical Journal*, Vol.23, No.5, (2008), pp. 1057, ISSN 1002-0179

Li J.; Xu T.; Liu KX. & Tang Y. (2009). Analysis of drug used in the injured within 3 weeks after Wenchuan earthquake. *China Pharmaceuticals*, Vol.18, No.15, (2009), pp. 46, ISSN 1006-4931

Lin YZ.; Xu QF.; Liu SL.; Liu YT.; Luo C. & Zhang LL. (2010). Management of donated drugs viewed from perspective of the use of the donated drugs following earthquake disaster. *China Pharmacy*, Vol.21, No.1, (2010), pp. 17-20, ISSN 1001-0408

Liu XJ.; Fan HJ.; Chen W. et al. (2011). Statistical analysis of category of earthquake related diseases. *China Journal of Emergency Resuscitation and Disaster Medicine*, Vol.6, No.2, (Feb 2011), pp. 100-101, ISSN 1673-6966

Ma MX.; Guo P.; Xiao YY. et al. (2008). Chang of patterns of diseases and medical rescuing measurement after earthquake. *Journal of Sun Yat-Sen University (Medical Sciences)*, Vol.29, No.3, (Apr 2008), pp. 372-374, ISSN 1672-3554

Miskin IN.; Ran NP.; Block C. et, al. (2010). Antimicrobial Therapy for Wound Infections after Catastrophic Earthquakes. *The New England Journal of Medicine*, Vol.363, No.26, (Dec 2010), pp. 2751-2753, ISSN 0028-4793

Naghii MR. (2005). Public health impact and medical consequences of earthquakes. *Pan American Journal of Public Health* Vol.18, No.3, (Sep 2005), pp. 216-221, ISSN 1020-4989

National Geophysical Data Center. The Significant Earthquake Database. 2011-03-13 Available from: <http://www.ngdc.noaa.gov/nndc/struts/form?t=101650&s=1&d=1>

Noji EK. (1992) Medical and health care aspects of the Spitak-88 earthquake. *Proceedings of the International Seminar on the Spitak-88 Earthquake*. Yerevan, S.S.R. of Armenia. May, 1989

Pretto EA.; Angus DC.; Abrams JI. et al. (1994). An analysis of prehospital mortality in an earthquake. *Prehospital and Disaster Medicine*, Vol.9, No.2, (Apr-Jun 1994), pp. 107-117, ISSN 1049-023X

Ran YC, Ao XX, Liu L, Fu YL, Tuo H, Xu F. (2010) Microbiological study of pathogenic bacteria isolated from paediatric wound infections following the 2008 Wenchuan earthquake. *Scandinavian Journal of Infectious Diseases*. Vol.42, No.5, pp. 347-350, ISSN 0036-5548

Rao YY.; Ning H. & Yu JP. (2009). Pharmaceutical care in disaster assistance in large earthquake. *China Pharmacy*, Vol.20, No.34, (2009), pp. 2646, 2648, ISSN 1001-0408

Schultz CH.; Koenig KL. & Noji EK. (1996). A Medical Disaster Response to Reduce Immediate Mortality after an Earthquake. *New England Journal of Medicine*, Vol.334, No.7, (Feb 1996), pp. 438-444, ISSN 0028-4793

Tong RS. & Xiao BR. (2008). Experience and thoughts on hospital pharmaceutical service after disaster outbreak. *Practical Journal of Clinical Medicine*, Vol.5, No.6, (Nov 2008), pp. 35-37, ISSN 1672-6170

Wang, Y.; Hao, P.; Lu, B.; Yu, H.; Huang, W.; Hou, H. & Dai, K. (2008) Causes of infection after earthquake, China. *Emerging Infection Disease*. Vol.16, No.6, (Jun 2010), pp. 974-5, ISSN: 1080-6059

World Health Organization. (2009). Definition and general considerations. In: DDD. 2011-06-03, Available from:
< http://www.whocc.no/ddd/definition_and_general_considera/>

World health organization. (2010). Prevention and Management of Wound Infection. World health organization. Retrieved from
<http://www.who.int/entity/hac/techguidance/tools/guidelines_prevention_and_management_wound_infection.pdf>

World Health Organization. (May 2010). Medicines: rational use of medicines. 2011-5-26, Available from:< http://www.who.int/mediacentre/factsheets/fs338/en/ >

World Health Organization (2011). Earthquakes - Technical Hazard Sheet - Natural Disaster Profile. In : health action crisis. 2011-05-01, Available from:
<http://www.who.int/hac/techguidance/ems/earthquakes/en/>

Xing M.; Wang Q.; Jiang M. & Zhang EJ. (2008). Drug supply during earthquake disaster: experience from Wenchuan Earthquake. *Acta Academiae Medicinae Militaris Tertiae*, Vol.30, No.16, (Aug 2008), pp. 1578-1579, ISSN 1000-5404

Xu QF.; Lin YZ.; Liu YT. & Zhang LL. (2009). Emergency drug supply mechanism in Women and Children's Special Hospital during earthquake disaster. *China Pharmacy*, Vol.20, No.34, (2009), pp. 2679-2681, ISSN 1001-0408

Xu Y.; Wei QZ.; Meng H. & Liu S. (2008). Drug supply of field medical team in earthquake relief. *Pharmaceutical Care and Research*, Vol. 8, No.5, (Oct 2008), pp. 385-386, ISSN 1671-2838

Yang ZC.; Peng BB.; Bai XD.; Zhang YQ. & Guan XP. (2006). Drug supply during earthquake emergency rescue in Pakistan. *Medical Journal of the Chinese People's Armed Police Forces*, Vol.17, No.2, (Feb 2006), pp. 148-149, ISSN 1004-3594

Yuan CJ. & Zhang XF. (2009). Analysis of drug application in "5.12"Wenchuan major earthquake. *China Medical Herald*, Vol.6, No.1, (2009), pp. 133-134, ISSN 1673-7210

Zhang LL.; Lin YZ.; Chen L.; Liu YT.; Liu SL.; Xu QF. & Han L. (2008). Emergency pharmaceutical administration of hospital for women and children in medical rescue after Wenchuan earthquake. *Chinese Journal of Evidence-Based Medicine*, Vol.8, No.9, (2008), pp. 692-697, ISSN 1672-2513

Zhang LP.; Zhang Y.; Tang HH.; Li J. & Yang ZW. (2010). Pharmaceutical care and drug supply in hospital during emergency disaster. *Pharmaceutical Journal of Chinese People's Liberation Army*, Vol.26, No.3, (Jun 2010), pp. 282-283, ISSN 1008-9926

Section 3

Cognitive and Psychology Management

3

Integration of Pharmacological and Psychosocial Treatment for Schizophrenia in Mexico: The Case of a Developing Country Proposal

Marcelo Valencia, Alejandro Diaz and Francisco Juarez
National Institute of Psychiatry Ramon de la Fuente
Mexico

1. Introduction

For decades, schizophrenia was considered exclusively as a biological disorder. As a result, pharmacotherapy has been considered as the predominant mode of treatment. Antipsychotic medication is indicated for first episode, acute, chronic as well as for refractory patients. So much research has been conducted to evaluate the efficacy of antipsychotics through clinical studies, randomized controlled trials and meta-analyses. Scientific journals are full of research on pharmacotherapy. According to the American Psychiatric Association [APA] (2004), a treatment plan for patients with schizophrenia should include: 1.- The reduction or elimination of symptoms, 2.- Improving quality of life and adaptive functioning, and 3.- Promote and maintain recovery. In the last decades, research in the social sciences and psychiatric rehabilitation has produced a considerable body of knowledge with respect to psychosocial factors that influence the curse of this illness. As a result psychosocial treatments have also been designed and implemented. With the beginning of the new century and after more than 60 years of research, there is a consensus that biological, psychological and social factors play a very important role in understanding and treating schizophrenia. Hence, the biopsychosocial model has been considered as the most comprehensive treatment approach for this illness. The treatment of schizophrenia has been the focus of changes since the introduction of neuroleptics in the 1950´s which initiated the transition from mental hospitals to the community, with long-stay patients confined in mental institutions going through the deinstitutionalization process, to the new millennium where the majority of them are actually living in the community. A considerable effort has been carried out in recent years to articulate the scientific basis of the treatment for people with schizophrenia. As a result evidence based treatment for schizophrenia has recommended that all persons with schizophrenia should receive the combination of: 1) optimal dose of antipsychotic medication, 2) psychosocial interventions, 3) psychoeducation for patients and carers as well as family therapy, and, 4) assertive home-based management to help prevent and resolve various issues such as: crises, relapse, medication adherence, etc, (Drake et al., 2009; Falloon et al., 2004; Fenton & Schooler, 2000; Lehman & Steinwachs, 2003; Shean, 2009; Thornicroft & Susser, 2001). In summary, scientific research indicates that the management of schizophrenia should include the following: 1) pharmacotherapy, 2) psychosocial interventions, and 3) the integration of these two approaches. The aim of this chapter is to describe a research area that integrates pharmacological and psychosocial treatment for patients with schizophrenia carried out at the National Institute of Psychiatry, in Mexico City. Based upon scientific research, the second aim consists on presenting a proposal of this integration on a comprehensive treatment approach for schizophrenia patients of a developing country as Mexico.

2. Pharmacological treatment

Schizophrenia represents a chronic and debilitating mental disorder that affects about 0.7% of general population all over the world (McGrath, 2008), which means approximately 24 million people worldwide (World Health Organization [WHO], 2011). In the case of Mexico, with a population of 112 million inhabitants, the population at risk between 15-65 years of developing schizophrenia is 63.6 millions, a one percent estimate would indicate that approximately 630,000 individuals suffer schizophrenia as to 2011. Treatment is complex and should always be initiated with pharmacological interventions. Antipsychotics are the drugs of choice (Freedman, 2005; Geddes, 2000; Kane & Marder, 1993; Kane & McGlashan, 1995; Marder, 2002) as they control most of the symptom clusters that characterize this disorder. More than 60 years ago, Jean Delay and colleagues discovered chlorpromazine (López-Muñoz et al., 2002), a then novel sedative compound, and almost at the same time Paul Janssen discovered haloperidol (Granger, 1999), a potent neuroleptic compound. Both drugs were shown to be useful to relieve psychotic symptoms, and so began a new era in the treatment of psychotic disorders, with schizophrenia as the prototype. Emergence of this 2 kind of drugs, phenothiazines and butyrophenones, placed the so called conventional antipsychotics as the first line treatment for schizophrenia for many decades (Geddes, 2000; Kane & Marder, 1993; Kane & McGlashan, 1995; Marder, 2002). Beginning with clozapine some decades ago, but mostly for the last 15 to 20 years, new antipsychotic medications have been developed (Geddes, 2000; Lehman et al., 2004). The now named atypical antipsychotics (more correctly second generation antipsychotics) represent a better said heterogeneus group of drugs (Davis et al., 2003; Geddes, 2000; Haddad & Sharma, 2007). These new agents are quite different in that, at least most of them, do not generate neuroleptization quite so much as some of the conventional medications and in that, most of them are effective antipsychotics with minimal or negligible EPS and hiperprolactinemia (García-Anaya et al., 2001, Geddes, 2000; Rosenheck, 2003). One important issue that distinguishes this group of drugs from conventional antipsychotics is the separation of their clinical efficacy from their neurotoxic effects (Posligua, 1995). Beside this advantages they also appear to have greater effectiveness than conventional antipsychotics in treating the so-called negative symptoms of schizophrenia (García-Anaya et al., 2001; Leucht, 1999; Posligua, 1995), in controlling other symptom clusters like behavioral disturbances, in having an apparent positive impact on neurocognitive functioning (Keefe, 1999, 2003; Rosenheck, 2003) and on psychosocial functioning (Swartz, 2003; Swartz et al., 2007), in lowering relapse and rehospitalisation rates (Csernansky & Schuchart, 2002) and in promoting a better quality of life for patients (Chung, 2004; Jones, 2006). This relative superiority could result from the reduction in side effects, especially EPS, but also maybe from a direct pharmacologic effect, that can explain why this group of drugs are now considered first line treatment choice and, as so, could have a relevant impact in improving social and vocational outcomes of patients with psychotic disorders like schizophrenia.

Antipsychotic	Chemical Group	Usual dose	Available since
Haloperidol*	Butyrophenone	5-20 mg/day	70's
Chlorpromazine	Phenothiazine	25-500 mg/day	70's
Sulpiride	Benzamide	50-600 mg/day	70's
Perphenazine*	Phenothiazine	4-60 mg/day	70's
Trifluoperazine	Phenothiazine	5-50 mg/day	70's
Levomepromazine	Phenothiazine	25-200 mg/day	70's
Clozapine	Thienobenzo-diazepine	25-600 mg/day	80's
Flupenthixol	Thioxanthene	5-20 mg/day	90's
Zuclopenthixol	Thioxanthene	20-60 mg/day	90's
Olanzapine*	Thienobenzo-diazepine	5-20 mg/day	90's
Risperidone*	Benzisoxazole	1-6 mg/day	90's
Quetiapine	Dibenzothiazepine	300-800 mg/day	90's
Ziprasidone*	Benzisothiazol	80-160 mg/day	90's
Amisulpiride	Benzamide	50-400 mg/day	2000's
Aripiprazole	Dichlorophenyl-piperazine	10-30 mg/day	2000's
Sertindole	Phenylindole	12-20 mg/day	2000's
Paliperidone	Benzisoxazole	3-9 mg/day	2000's

(*) Available in the Mexican public health system

Table 1. Oral antipsychotic drugs available in Mexico

2.1 Introduction and use of antipsychotic drugs in Mexico

History of Latin American countries use of antipsychotics parallels some socio-cultural and economic issues; Some cases like Cuba and some central American countries are characterized by having only available some conventional antipsychotics like haloperidol and chlorpromazine (González et al., 2004), and, in most Latin American countries, even though having second generation antipsychotics available, economic issues have limited their use. In Mexico we have had available conventional antipsychotics from the 70's, initiating with the prototypes of the first two classes of this group of drugs: the butyrophenone haloperidol and the phenothiazine chlorpromazine, and then some other phenothiazine compounds and first generation atypical drugs (Table 1). Some first generation antipsychotic drugs like fluphenazine, thioridazine and penfluridol were available in Mexico in the past but now they are not available anymore. Some of this conventional antipsychotic drugs are frequently used in most public psychiatric hospitals and institutions and even some of them are still included in the "Cuadro básico" (Basic Table of Medications) of the Mexican public health system (Secretaría de Salud, 1999). Second generation antipsychotics were introduced in Mexico in the 80's with their first representative drug, clozapine and then in the 90's, drugs like olanzapine, risperidone, quetiapine and ziprasidone were available. Finally, in the 21th century, four more second generation antipsychotic drugs are now available: amysulpiride, aripiprazole, sertindole and paliperidone. Some of this second generation antipsychotic drugs, like risperidone and olanzapine, are being introduced in the Mexican public health system, so they now are at hand for more patients.

2.2 Clinical considerations for prescribing antipsychotics

Once a diagnosis of schizophrenia is established, patient should be started on antipsychotic treatment as soon as possible, meanwhile other therapeutic measures are initiated. Election of antipsychotic drug by a physician most take into account some issues like illness related characteristics, drug efficacy, side effects and cost (Kane & McGlashan, 1995; Leuch, Corves et al., 2009), patient characteristics including age, gender, health status, other drugs being taken by the patient, history of previous use of any antipsychotic drug and some other socio-cultural aspects. In a prospective naturalistic study (Edlinger, 2009), the factors influencing physicians' choice of antipsychotic drug therapy in the treatment of patients with schizophrenia were investigated; it was concluded that antipsychotic drug side effects have a larger influence on the choice of antipsychotic than other factors like demographic or illness-related variables, with the exception of the severity of positive symptoms, which did influenced decision. As it was mentioned above, in developing countries like most Latin American countries, including Mexico, aspects like antipsychotic drug availability and drug cost should always be considered when making a choice for any antipsychotic. Some general important issues concerning the adequate use of antipsychotic drugs that should always be considered every time pharmacological treatment is started on a patient with schizophrenia include:

1. **Type of antipsychotic drug**: At this time, second generation drugs are usually considered as first line treatment for individuals with newly diagnosed schizophrenia (Leucht, 1999; Leucht, 2003; Leuch, Corves et al., 2009), even though their heterogeneity has brought some concerns about their superiority over conventional drugs (Geddes, 2000; Leucht, 1999; Leuch, Corves et al., 2009; Marder, 2002), and in between them (Leuch, Kommossa et al., 2009). In Mexico and some other developing countries, is not rare that some patients could still be started on conventional antipsychotics mostly regarding availability and cost-effectiveness issues. The choice for oral, parenteral or depot formulations will be considered later.
2. **Recommended dosage of antipsychotic drug:** Any antipsychotic drug given to treat a schizophrenic patient should be started at the lowest effective level of the recommended therapeutic range (Davis & Chen, 2004). Dosage outside of this range should be justified and documented always; "rapid neuroleptisation" is not recommended, and in case of using rapid loading doses, this manoeuvre should be made with extreme caution. Subsequent titration of antipsychotic drug on follow up should be made according to clinical response and tolerability, sometimes using blood levels as a useful manoeuvre (Citrome & Volavka, 2002).
3. **Antipsychotic drug treatment duration:** Treatment should be continued for at least 12 months, then, just in the eventual situation of the disease remitting fully, drug treatment may be ceased gradually over at least 1-2 months. In most cases, however, antipsychotic drug treatment should be continued indefinitely, as this stance represents the best option for the long standing control of symptoms.
4. **Definition and management of antipsychotic treatment resistance:** If a patient with schizophrenia has been unresponsive to at least two adequate trials (that is using therapeutic doses of the drugs, for enough time to get a response) of two different antipsychotic medications, then it can be established the diagnosis of antipsychotic treatment resistance. If so, a trial of clozapine should be offered to patients, as this second generation antipsychotic has been recognized as the drug of choice for treatment

resistant schizophrenic patients (Chakos, 2001; Lehman et al., 2004; Marder, 2002; Wahlbeck, 1999).

5. **Switching of antipsychotic drug treatment:** Reasons for switching antipsychotic drug treatment include lack of clinical response and important side effects (Essock, 2002; Lehman et al., 2004; Stroup, 2011) Treatment trial with a first prescribed antipsychotic drug should be kept for at least 4-8 weeks before considering the use of another antipsychotic medication, and only after optimizing first drug dosage, which could mean dose titrating until the maximum recommended (Essock, 2002). Two antipsychotic medications at a time, whatever second generation or conventional, should not be prescribed together, although this aspect is still controverted (Barnes & Paton, 2011; Lehman et al., 2004; Miller & Craig, 2002), with the exception of short periods to cover changeover when switching to another antipsychotic. Switching strategies of antipsychotic medications include 3 options (Weiden, 2006):

- Discontinuation: This option consists in abruptly discontinuing the first drug before starting the second medication. This method of switching minimizes risk of dosing errors and allows closer monitoring for signs of relapse and can be an appropriate choice when switching from a conventional antipsychotic to a second generation one or from a depot medication to any oral formulation. This method has the inconvenience of potentially favoring symptom exacerbation and withdrawal reactions derived from discontinuation of the previous antipsychotic.
- Cross-tapering: This option consists in gradual tapering of the first medication while starting and titrating the second antipsychotic drug, with temporal simultaneous administration of both the original and the new drug. This method of switching is suitable when stable patients are experiencing significant side effects from their previous medication. The time elapsed for the cross-titration usually goes between 1 and 4 weeks (De Nayer et al., 2003) although a slower withdrawal period is convenient when switching particular antipsychotics. This option has the inconvenience of exposing patients to subtherapeutic dosages of both medications, with risk of relapse.
- Delayed withdrawal: This option consists in starting a second antipsychotic drug, which is titraded to a therapeutic dose, before tapering of the first drug. Keeping the patient on a therapeutic dose of the new medication before reducing previous medication avoids exposure to subtherapeutic dosages, and may represent the safest switching method. This method may be suitable for patients who have not accomplished a complete stabilization following a recent relapse and for patients who are not having a good adherence to treatment. Using this method should require physicians to ensure the crossover is complete, without allowing patients to continue with both medications indefinitely. This method has the inconvenience of having patients exposed to the side effects of two antipsychotic drugs (Lehman et al., 2004).

6. **Follow-up of patients receiving antipsychotic medication:** Routine laboratory and clinical monitoring should occur before starting an antipsychotic drug and during treatment follow up as well (Marder, 2002; Lehman et al., 2004). According to toxicology and potential side effects of the drug of choice, laboratory parameters to evaluate may include Complete Blood Count (CBC), Liver Function Tests (LFT), Blood Glucose (BG), Cholesterol (Total, HDL and LDL), Triglycerides, Prolactine Blood Level (PBL) and Electrocardiogram (EKG). Clinical parameters to evaluate include Blood Pressure (BP), Weight, Body Mass Index (BMI) and Waist Circumference (WC).

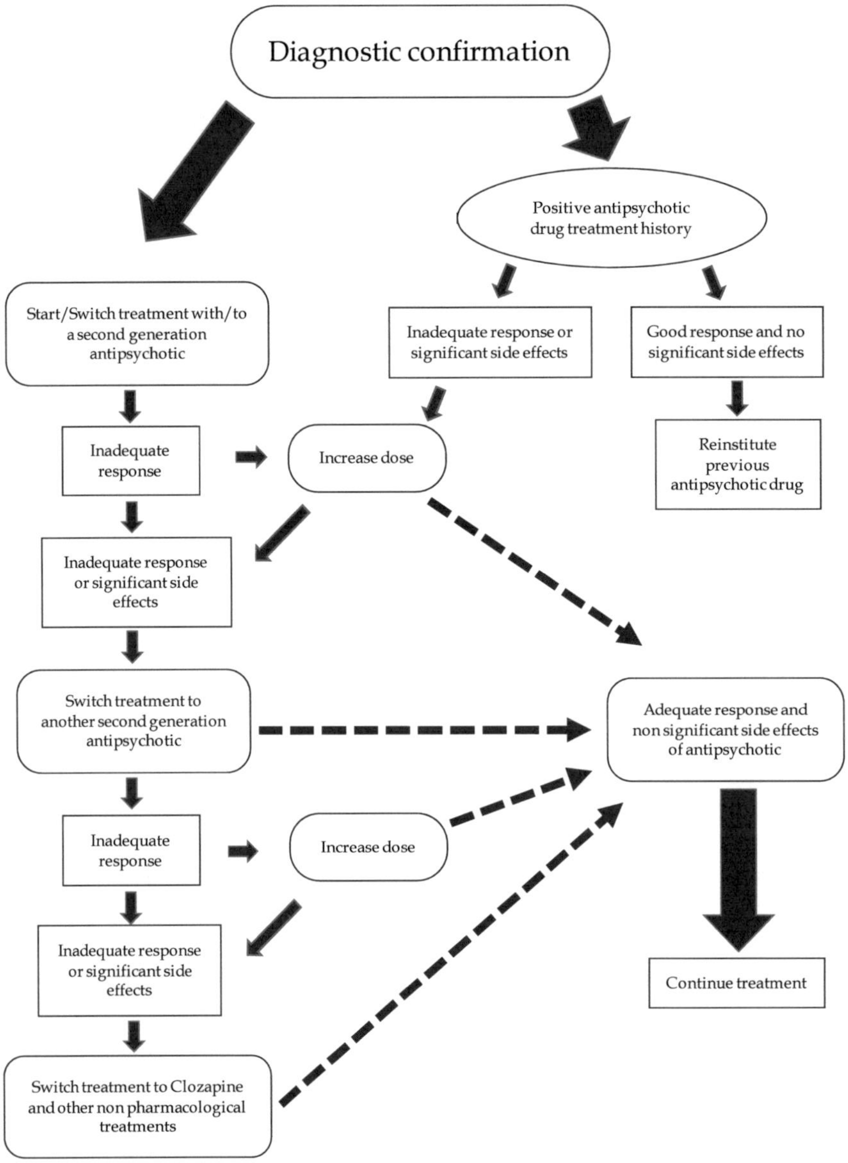

Fig. 1. Therapeutic algorithm for the use of antipsychotic drugs in the treatment of schizophrenia

7. **Tolerability and toxicologic aspects of antipsychotics:** Beyond the clear differences in side effects and toxicologic risks between antipsychotics, either conventional drugs or second generation drugs, there are common potential consequences that should be kept in mind every time an antipsychotic is prescribed to a schizophrenic patient (Haddad & Sharma, 2007; Lehman et al., 2004; Marder, 2002). Parkinsonism and other extrapyramidal side effects are common with potent conventional drugs like haloperidol and fluphenazine (Ortega-Soto et al., 1998; Ortega-Soto & Valencia, 2001), but also with some second generation antipychotics like risperidone (Haddad &

Sharma, 2007). Hyperprolactinemia is associated again with potent conventional drugs and some second generation drugs like risperidone and amysulpiride (García-Anaya et al., 2001; Haddad & Sharma, 2007). Metabolic side effects were originally described with some low potency conventional drugs but they were later evidently associated with some of the second generation drugs: Weight gain (Allison, 1999; Haddad & Sharma, 2007; Newcomer, 2005; Rosenheck, 2003); Hyperlipidemia (Haddad & Sharma, 2007; Koro, 2002; Newcomer, 2005); Glucose metabolism disturbances (Haddad & Sharma, 2007; Henderson, 2005; Newcomer, 2005), and even Diabetes Mellitus (Leslie & Rosenheck, 2004; Newcomer, 2005) have been highly associated with clozapine and olanzapine, fairly associated with quetiapine and risperidone and lightly associated with haloperidol, ziprasidone, aripiprazole, amysulpiride and paliperidone. Sedation is usually expected with Chloropromazine, Thioridazine, Clozapine, Olanzapine and Quetiapine (Haddad & Sharma, 2007; Lehman et al., 2004; Ortega-Soto & Valencia, 2001). Prolongation of QT interval (QTc) is at highest risk with thioridazine, ziprasidone and sertindole (Haddad & Sharma, 2007; Lehman et al., 2004). Other side effects reported in patients receiving antipsychotic drugs include sexual dysfunction, anticholinergic symptoms, postural hypotension, agranulocytosis, seizures and neuroleptic malignant syndrome (Haddad & Sharma, 2007; Lehman et al., 2004; Marder, 2002). Finally, cerebrovascular events have recently been associated with second generation antipsychotics (Haddad & Sharma., 2007).

Antipsychotic	Chemical Group	Usual dose	Available since
Haloperidol*	Butyrophenone	5-60 mg a day	70´s
Zuclopenthixol Acetate	Thioxanthene	50-100 mg q/2-3 d.	90´s
Olanzapine*	Thienobenzo-diazepine	10-30 mg a day	90¨s
Ziprasidone*	Benzisothiazol	10-40 mg a day	90¨s

(*) Available in Mexican Public Health System

Table 2. Parenteral antipsychotic drugs for acute states available in Mexico

Management of acute episodes: Acute states of patients with schizophrenia require initiating or adjusting antipsychotic treatment to control new and/or exacervated symptoms (Kane & McGlashan, 1995). This episodes are sometimes managed in the psychiatric hospital setting (Lehman et al., 2004) A frequent problem found in these acute descompensated patients is the lack of conciousness about the need for an acute treatment intervention and a lack of disposition for receiving pharmacological treatment as well. So patient relatives are often confronted with difficult decisions like taking the patient into a closed institution where pharmacologic and other treatment strategies could be initiated even without patient cooperation. Under these circumstances, parenteral antipsychotic drugs -usually trough intramuscular administration- are very frequently used, as they are easier to administrate to patients not accepting treatment, with lower harm risks for them. Most of these drugs should be administrated once or more times during a day, as they usually have half lives no longer than 24 hours, with the exception of Zuclopenthixol (Clopixol Aquphase), which can be administrated every 48 to 72 hrs. These drugs are useful for getting a faster control of symptoms and for facilitating treatment continuation. Table 2 shows parenteral antipsychotic drugs available in Mexico, used in acute episodes of schizophrenic patients.

Issues regarding treatment adherence: As we all know now, schizophrenic patients should keep pharmacologic treatment in the long term, as far as it has been repeatedly demonstrated that a good treatment adherence means a more complete and a more rapid control of their symptoms, a low chance for future decompensations, and, in general, a more frequent reintegration to society and a better quality of life for them. CATIE and other international studies (Lieberman et al., 2005) have shown that about 75% of schizophrenic patients stop treatment because of different reasons, including lack of clinical response and presence of side effects like sedation, EPS, weight gain, and other metabolic disturbances. This so high non-adherence rate to pharmacologic treatment means for schizophrenic patients more numerous acute decompensation states, more hospitalizations and some other negative consequences. Having said this, one important issue on pharmacologic treatment of schizophrenic patients is promoting treatment adherence. To reach the goal of keeping schizophrenic patients on treatment, depot formulations of antipsychotic drugs are becoming a very useful alternative that favors this purpose. This long acting group of antipsychotic drugs allow patients, their families and other people taking care of them, to administrate drugs at intervals of 2 to 4 weeks, instead of taking them once or even more times a day, thus facilitating and assuring adherence to treatment, First depot antipsychotic drug available in Mexico were Pipothiazine and Haloperidol Decanoate, then other depot formulations have been introduced like the two thioxanthenes Zuclopenthixol Decanoate and Flupenthixol Decanoate and more recently Risperidone and Paliperidone Palmitate.

Antipsychotic	Chemical Group	Usual dose	Available since
Pipothiazine	Phenothiazine	25-200 mg/ every 2-4 weeks	70's
Haloperidol* Decanoate	Butyrophenone	50-150 mg/ every 30 days	80's
Zuclopenthixol Decanoate	Thioxanthene	200 mg/ every 30 days	90´s
Flupenthixol Decanoate	Thioxanthene	20-100 mg/ every 2-4 weeks	90´s
Risperidone*	Benzisoxazole	25-50 mg/ every 2 weeks	2000´s
Paliperidone* palmitate	Benzisoxazole	39-234 mg/ every 30 days	2000´s

Table 3. Shows depot antipsychotics now available in Mexico

Psychothropic drugs other than antipsychotic drugs used in the pharmacologic treatment of schizophrenia in Mexico: Beside any antipsychotic drug, and mostly used as adjuvant treatment, correcting and complementary pharmacologic treatments for patients with schizophrenia, some other classes of drugs are used in the Mexican psychiatric scenarium. Litheum and some anticonvulsive drugs like carbamazepine and valproate are frequently added to antipsychotic treatment as potentiators of response, especially in patients with partial response to antipsychotic drugs alone. Anticholinergic drugs like biperiden and trihexifenidile are usually prescribed to correct EPS like parkinsonism as well as beta blockers like propranolol, mostly in the presence of acathisia. Sedative-ansiolitic drugs like clonazepam, alprazolam and bromazepam are sometimes indicated in cases of anxious states accompanying classic symptoms of schizophrenia. Finally, antidepressant drugs are used when comorbidity with depressive symptoms is detected.

3. Psychosocial treatment

3.1 Historical perspective of psychosocial treatment

The introduction of psychosocial treatment for schizophrenia is very much related to the fact that psychotic disorders produce dysfunctions, disabilities, and deficits in various domains of everyday functioning. Poor psychosocial functioning is a defining characteristic of schizophrenia. Social dysfunction is one of the most relevant factors associated with the disability of the illness (APA, 1995). Disabilities include difficulties in social and independent living skills that act as an impediment for a more normal functioning, (Kopelowicz & Liberman, 2003). From all illnesses of mankind, schizophrenia is ranked as the seventh illness that causes disability (WHO, 2001). Since schizophrenia patients are often functionally impaired, impairments in social functioning could be understood as the inability to take care for his/her self, to maintain interpersonal relationships, or the inability to work. These are important reasons for considering psychosocial functioning as an important dimension of schizophrenia, Deficits in social functioning are a core feature of schizophrenia (Burns & Patrick, 2007). Lauriello, Lenroot & Bustillo (2003), state that: "Patients with schizophrenia have limitations in their social competence and vocational functioning for a significant period. To some extent, these limitations are a consequence of the multiple symptoms and cognitive impairments of the disorder". Role functioning indicates the individual´s abilities to demonstrate role performance according to his/hers demands at work, school, social, and family situations. Even when psychotic symptoms are in remission with antipsychotic medication, approximately two-thirds of schizophrenia patients are unable to accomplish basic social roles, such as parenthood, friendship, worker, or being a spouse (Bellack et al., 2007). Schizophrenia is characterized by a deterioration, or failure to achieve adequate levels of social functioning. Because of the early illness onset many individuals with schizophrenia never learned the necessary skills required for adult functioning. The psychosocial environment that comprises family factors is another relevant component as demonstrated with a great amount of research in the area of Family Expressed Emotion (Leff et al., 1987), and family care of schizophrenia (Falloon et al., 1984; Kuipers et al., 2002). One of the most complicated challenges in schizophrenia treatment has been to restore impaired psychosocial functioning (Swartz et al., 2007), considering that current management has a strong emphasis on living in the community (Leucht & Van Os, 2009). The integration of pharmacological and psychosocial approaches has been recommended as a means of improving the outcome of patients with schizophrenia (Marder, 2000). In addition schizophrenia patients face several problems: relapse rates have been reported as high as 70% (McCann et al., 2008; Muller, 2004); even with the use of second generation antipsychotics, negatives symptoms still persist (Leucht, Corves et al., 2009; Stahl & Buckley, 2007;); approximately 50% meet criteria for substance or drug dependence (Bellack et al., 2007); cognitive deficits (Sharma & Harvey, 2000) and poor quality of life (Lehman, 1983) should also be considered. Some of these issues remain unresolved.

Psychosocial treatment aims to improve the management of schizophrenia with the use of various techniques such as coping with symptoms, medication adherence, relapse prevention, and acquisition of psychosocial skills to improve functioning in certain areas such as social relations, work, school, home, recreation, use of mental health facilities, or independent living in the community. In the last fifty years a great array of psychosocial interventions have been designed such as: social skills training (Bellack et al., 2004; Glynn et al., 2002; Liberman, 2007), supported employment (McGurk et al., 2009; Mueser et al., 2001;

Tsang, 2001), teaching illness management skills (Atkinson et al., 1996; Birchwood et al., 1989; Mueser et al., 2002), integrated psychological therapy (Briand et al., 2006; Roder et al., 2006), assertive community treatment (Bond et al., 2001; Burns et al., 1999; Thornicroft et al., 1998), cognitive rehabilitation (Bell et al., 2009; Velligan et al., 2006; Vesterager et al., 2011), integrated treatment for comorbid substance abuse (Bellack et al., 2006; Ridgely et al., 1990; Shaner et al., 2003), family psycho-education (Bauml et al, 2006; Murray & Dixon, 2004; Xia et al., 2011), and housing (McCrone & Strathdee, 1994; Harvard Medical School, 2001; Trainor et al., 1993). A large body of research supports the efficacy of psychosocial treatments, with Reviews (Bellack & Mueser,1993; Benton & Schroeder, 1990; Heinssen et al., 2000; Huxley et al., 2000; Kopelowicz et al., 2006; Penn et al., 2005); Randomized control trials (Glyn et al., 2002; Granholm et al., 2005; Guo et al 2010; Hogarty et al, 2004; Liberman, 1998); Meta-analysis (Kurtz & Mueser, 2008; Mojtabai et al., 1998; Pilling et al., 2002; Roder et al,. 2006) and Treatment recommendations (APA, 2004; Dixon et al., 2010; Kreyenbuhl et al., 2009; Lehman & Steinwaschs, 1998, 2003).

3.2 Introduction of psychosocial treatment in Mexico

The introduction, application and research in Mexico of psychosocial treatment can be divided in two stages: 1) Interventions with acute psychotic hospitalized patients, and 2) Interventions with chronic out-patients with schizophrenia.

3.2.1 Psychosocial treatment for acute psychotic hospitalized patients

In 1980, a study was conducted to assess the delivery of services of a Psychiatric Hospital for acute mentally ill patients, in Mexico City. It was found that the only treatment that patients were receiving was antipsychotic medication. As a result a proposal was made that considered the convenience to integrate pharmacological and psychosocial rehabilitation approaches, as a consequence a pilot study that was carried out between 1980 and 1984. Psychosocial treatment was included as a new component, in addition to pharmacological treatment, in a clinical trial that integrated a treatment and rehabilitation program for acute hospitalized psychotic patients. After patients were clinically stabilized with antipsychotic medication, (allowing a two week stabilization period), they participated in daily sessions during 4 weeks of the hospitalization period. Patients learned a variety of skills in various domains: 1.-Taking care of personal hygiene, appearance and clothing, 2.-Management of symptoms and medication, 3.-Occupational skills, 4.-Social skills, 5.-Communication and problem solving skills with the family, and 6.-Leisure and sports activities. Verification of the skills learned was recorded with the use of a check list. Using a quasi- experimental design, an experimental group (n=35) treated with pharmacological and psychosocial treatment was compared with a control group (n=35) that was treated with pharmacological treatment alone. Psychopathology and global functioning were assessed before and after treatment, using the Brief Psychiatric Rating Scale (BPRS) (Overall and Gorham, 1962) and the Global Assessment Scale (GAF) (Spitzer et al., 1976). Patients from the experimental group demonstrated significant improvements in symptoms such as: anxiety, tension, depression, unusual thought content and blunted affect. No improvements were found in psychopathology in the control group. These patients experienced more anxiety and tension than that reported when they started treatment. Similar results were found in global functioning since experimental patients improved their functioning: mean =52 before treatment to a mean=72 at the end of treatment. Control patients showed no improvements since they remained at the same level of functioning (51-60) with a mean=59 and a mean=58, before and after treatment. It was concluded that an integrated program that combined pharmacological and psychosocial treatment was more effective for acute hospitalized psychotic patients than pharmacological treatment alone (Valencia, 1988; Valencia, 1991). Considering the outcome of this treatment program, it was recommended that the combination of pharmacological and psychosocial treatments should be used as the best delivery approach for treating these patients. Unfortunately, the rehabilitation work could not continue due to the fact of the lack of financial funds and changes in health politics that were oriented to alcohol and drugs research at that time.

3.2.2 Psychosocial treatment for chronic outpatients

Prior to the initiation of the intervention, we consider a necessity to take into account all persons that should be involved in a treatment process. Therefore, we included patients, relatives and mental health professionals as relevant participants of this process. Patients and relatives were considered as healthy allies and collaborators of the treatment team. Relative´s participation was considered as a key element since approximately 90% of our patients live with family members (Valencia et al., 2003). Their opinions and ideas served as the background for considering the content of a psychosocial treatment program that would be offered as an add-on to pharmacotherapy. Hence, we developed a methodology for the design of integrated psychosocial and pharmacological interventions, for a developing country, as Mexico. The information came from three important sources: a) clinically stabilized chronic patients with schizophrenia, b) caregivers living with their ill relatives and aware of the patient´s, daily activities, and c) mental health professionals with experience in the treatment of schizophrenia patients and their relatives. Information was collected considering the clinical needs and psychosocial problems of our patients, as well as the caregiver´s needs and demands. The design process included seven stages: 1) Identifying clinical and psychosocial problems through two sources: a) an exploratory study including patients as participants, so, they would give their opinions about their clinical and psychosocial needs, and, b) Using focus groups with patients, relatives and mental health professionals (psychiatrists, clinical psychologists, psychiatric social workers, and psychiatric nurses), to collect information from these three sources; 2) Establishing a consensus about clinical and psychosocial problems from all sources; 3) Designing the content of the intervention, and, in addition, with the advice of clinical and social science researchers, consider the corresponding methodological issues (experimental design, study groups, instruments); 4) Implementation of the treatment program; 5) Determining its effectiveness; 6) Follow-up, and 7) Dissemination. All patients were receiving exclusively pharmacological treatment. Psychosocial and clinical problems were identified as when patients: do not have friends (60-70%); do not have a loving relationship (90-96%); unemployed (50-80%); lack of financial sources (80-90%); economically dependent upon his/her family (80-90%); do not have good family relations (70-80%); do not know the characteristics of the illness (90-95%); do not know his/her diagnosis (55-65%); consider that they do not need medication (70-80%); and, consider that they do not need psychotherapy (80-90%). In addition, the consensus indicated the presence and persistence of deficits in various skills areas that were interfering in the patient´s community functioning. It was recommended the importance of developing the following skills: the importance of effective

Treatment			
Pharmacological	Psychosocial	Psychoeducation	Family intervention
• Antipsychotic medication • First generation • Second generation • Other classes of medications: Antidepresants • Mood stabilizers • Antianxiety medications	• Symptom management • Medication management • Occupation • Social relations • Couple relations • Family relations • Money management	• Illness management • Medication management • Medication compliance • Recognition and management of warning signs of relapse	• The importance of medication • Medication compliance • Keeping appointments with treating psychiatrist • Management of warning signs of relapse • Improve communication skills • Problem solving as needed
Participants			
Patient	Patient	Relatives	Patient and relatives
Frequency			
Monthly appointments	Weekly sessions, or twice a week	Weekly sessions	After psychoeducation
Duration of sessions			
20 minutes	90 minutes	90 minutes	90 minutes
Therapeutic modality			
Individual consultation	Group sessions	Group sessions for all relatives	Family therapy for the patient and his/her relatives
Duration of treatment			
6 months or 1 year	6 months or 1 year	8 sessions or 12 sessions	4 sessions or 5 sessions

Table 4. Proposal of the integration of pharmacological and psychosocial treatment for Mexican out-patients with schizophrenia

communication with the treating psychiatrists, the need to be informed about medication benefits, learning medication side effects, learning skills to cope with persistent symptoms, planning a long term pharmacological treatment, be willing to collaborate in making decision concerning medication, learning skills for avoiding alcohol and drug abuse, learning skills to improve adherence to antipsychotic medication, identifying warning signs of relapse and developing a relapse preventive plan, developing skills to improve social relations, and learning problem-solving skills for improving family relations (Valencia et al., 2010). The consensus also recommended the inclusion of various therapeutic modalities integrated in a comprehensive biopsychosocial service delivery system including: pharmacotherapy, psychosocial therapy, psychoeducation, and family therapy. The content of these modalities are shown on table 4. After the study protocol was approved by the Scientific Research Committee, and for the Ethics Committee of the National Institute of

Psychiatry, stages 4) Implementation, and 5) Determining treatment effectiveness were tested. A research area was developed where various experimental trials were conducted comparing experimental and control groups, or four treatment groups: psychosocial treatment, musictherapy, multimodal therapies, and a control group, including 4, 5 or 7 psychosocial treatment areas, either during a one year or during six months of treatment. In all trials pharmacological treatment was delivered once a month, psychosocial treatment included one or two sessions per week, 8 or 12 sessions were conducted for psychoeducation, 4 or 5 sessions for family therapy, in the last trials, the assessment of the level of expressed emotion was also included as an important variable to determine the emotional environment in the home as expressed by relatives. (Valencia et al., 2004a, 2004b, 2006, 2007, 2010)

In this chapter we describe the results of a research program that integrated pharmacological and psychosocial treatments that was carried out at the National Institute of Psychiatry in Mexico City. Out-patients diagnosed with schizophrenia according to the DSM-IV (APA, 1995) that was corroborated with the CIDI (Robins et al., 1988) participated in the study according to the following inclusion criteria: women or men, between 16 to 50 years, with at least six years of education, living with their relatives in Mexico City or the metropolitan area. Patients had to be under pharmacological treatment and therefore demonstrate to be clinically stable as regards to their psychotic symptoms according to the PANSS within a range of 60-90 before the initiation of treatment. One hundred and fifty six out-patients attending the Schizophrenia Clinic were randomly assigned, in an alternate order, to two treatment conditions: a study group (n=78), or to a comparison group (n=78). Of the 156 patients initially included in the study, 10 from the study group (12.8%) and 17 from the comparison group (21.7%) corresponding to a total of 17 patients (17.3%) of the sample, failed to complete the study, leaving a final sample of 129 patients: n=68, in the study group and n=61, in the comparison group. Patients of the study group received psychosocial treatment, specifically, psychosocial skills training and psychoeducation for their relatives, while the comparison group received the standard pharmacological treatment alone. Both groups completed one year of treatments. Pharmacological treatment for the two groups under study was provided at the Schizophrenia Clinic of the Institute, once a month, during twenty minutes, by two psychiatrists, who prescribed antipsychotics, verified medication compliance, keep a record of the attendance to appointments, and registered relapse and rehospitalizations. The treating psychiatrists were blind to the two treatment conditions. Psychosocial treatment included seven treatment areas as specified in Table 4. The aims of the intervention were: 1) facilitate patients' acquisition of psychosocial skills; 2) improve psychosocial and global functioning, 3) prevent relapse and rehospitalizations, 4) promote compliance with medication and treatment adherence. A team of two therapists trained in psychosocial skills training held weekly group sessions during 90 minutes. To carry out the therapeutic work with the patients, therapists had to follow the therapist´s manual that describes the training strategies for all sessions (Valencia et al., 2001). For acquisition of the skills, a technique known as the "learning activities" was utilized and modified for our patients (Valencia et al., 2007). This technique was developed and empirically validated for schizophrenia patients (Liberman, 2007; Wallace et al., 1992), as well as for Latinos with schizophrenia in the United States (Kopelowicz et al., 2003). A check list was also available to verify that patients learned the corresponding skills for each treatment area. A research assistant utilized a therapist fidelity evaluation check list to assure that each learning activity included in the training manual was taught competently during treatment. Psychoeducation provided information for relatives about the management of schizophrenia, coping with the illness, antipsychotic medications and its side effects, compliance with medication, and with psychiatric consultations, and understanding and management of signs of relapse. This intervention was held during ten sessions in a group format. The two groups under study were evaluated before and after treatment. The Positive and Negative Syndrome Scale [PANSS], Spanish adaptation, (Kay et al., 1990), and the Global Assessment of Functioning Scale [GAF] (APA, 1995), were used to assess psychopathology and psychosocial functioning. Relapse, and rehospitalization rates, compliance with antipsychotic medication and adherence to treatment were also assessed.

	Study Group n = 68	Comparison Groupl n = 61
Gender, *n (%)*		
Male	50 (73.5)	47 (77.0)
Female	18 (26.5)	14 (23.0)
Marital status, *n (%)*		
Single	65 (95.6)	55 (90.2)
Married	2 (2.9)	3 (4.9)
Speratated/divorced	1 (1.5)	3 (4.9)
Occupation, *n (%)*		
Employed	9 (13.2)	16 (26.2)
Housewife	2 (2.9)	4 (6.6)
Student	2 (2.9)	8 (13.1)
Unemployed	55 (80.9)	33 (54.1)
Age, years, $\bar{X}$ (s)	29.6 (6.9)	29.5 (7.1)
Education, years, $\bar{X}$ (s)	11.2 (2.1)	11.1 (2.1)
Age at onset $\bar{X}$ (s)	21.6 (6.5)	21.2 (4.6)

Table 5. Participants demographic and clinical data at baseline

All participants expressed in a written informed consent their desire to participate in the research project. Data analysis included the following: Descriptive and Chi square analysis to compare percentages, Student *t* tests to verify that there were no significant differences between the two groups under study in their initial levels of psychopatology, and psychosocial functioning, Analysis of variance for repeated measures (ANOVA) to detect pre-post differences within and between the two study groups. For the assessment of effect size, three levels were considered: small= .25, medium= .50 and large= 1.00 irrespective of the sign (+ or -) of the number (Kazdin & Bass, 1999). Standardized estimate of effect sizes were calculated using Cohen´s (1977) *d* formula defined as: $d = \bar{x}_1 - \bar{x}_2 / s$. Where $\bar{x}_1$ and $\bar{x}_2$ are the means at baseline and at the end of treatment of the two groups under study, and *s* is the pooled within-group standard deviation (*SD*). At baseline, no statistically significant differences were found between the two groups under study in psychopathology, (PANSS) or psychosocial functioning (GAF), or in their doses of antipsychotic medication as determined by calculation of chlorpromazine equivalents. Participant´s demographic and clinical data at baseline is shown in table 5. Patients in both treatment conditions were similar with no differences on any of these variables, except for the occupational status with a minor percentage of unemployed patients in the comparison group.

	Study Group n = 68	Comparison Group n = 61	Statistics [b] Main effect for time	Main effect for group	Interaction of group and time
PANSS[a] overall score, $\bar{X}$ (s)					
Baseline	92.6 (41.6)	83.5 (33.9)	p < .001	--	p < .001
Post	43.4 (13.0)	55.7 (16.4)			
Effect size	-1.2	-.80			
PANSS positive[a], $\bar{X}$ (s)					
Baseline	21.1 (11.5)	18.3 (9.8)	p < .001	--	p < .01
Post	9.1 (2.8)	11.6 (4.5)			
Effect size	-1.0	-.70			
PANSS negative[a], $\bar{X}$ (s)					
Baseline	24.4 (11.2)	22.4 (9.4)	p < .001	--	p < .001
Post	11.6 (5.2)	15.0 (6.3)			
Effect size	-1.1	-.80			
PANSS GPS[a, c], $\bar{X}$ (s)					
Baseline	47.1 (20.5)	42.8 (16.4)	p < .001	--	p < .001
Post	22.7 (6.0)	29.1 (8.3)			
Effect size	-1.2	-.80			
Level of global functionig[d] (GAF) , $\bar{X}$ (s)					
Baseline	43.1 (6.4)	43.1 (6.8)	p < .001	p < .001	p < .001
Post	67.0 (9.2)	43.7 (9.2)			
Effect size	3.8	.10			

[a] Higher scores indicate more severe symptoms. [b] Analysis of variance for repeated measures.[c] GPS, General Psychopathology Scale. [d] Higher scores indicate better global functioning. Effect size levels: small=0.25; medium=0.50; large=1.00

Table 6. Psychopatology and Psychosocial Functioning of the Study and Comparison Group

When considering the mean change scores, over one year of treatment, the results indicated that statistically significant improvements in psychopatology, as rated by the PANSS, were observed in positive and negative symptoms, general psychopathology and in total PANSS score for both groups under study. Group-by-time analysis demonstrated significantly greater improvement in psychopatology in patients of the study group when compared with patients receiving standard pharmacological treatment. Comparison of the effect sizes were large for the study group on the total PANSS score, positive scale, negative scale, and in the general psychopathology scale. Effect sizes were medium for all score scales of the comparison group. Significant improvement in psychosocial functioning was also found for patients of the study group but not for patients under standard pharmacological care since they remained at the same level of functioning (41-50) from baseline to post treatment assessment. Patients of the study group improved two levels of functioning from 41-50 at baseline to 61-70 at the end of treatment. Effect size was large for the study group and small for the comparison group (Table 6).

	Study group n = 68	Comparison group n = 61	Statistics [b] Main effect for time	Main effect for group	Interaction of group and time
Antipsychotic medication dose, [a] $\bar{X}$ (s)					
Baseline	300.8 (286.4)	328.1 (265.4)	p < .05		
Post	367.0 (167.5)	408.8 (336.6)			
Dose Range, lower – higher					
Baseline	14 - 1600	25 – 1200			
Post	29 - 1000	50 – 2400			

[a] Chlorpromazine equivalents in mg per day. [b] Analysis of variance for repeated measures.

Table 7. Antipsychotic dosage of the Study and comparison Group [a]

Table 7, illustrates that patients in the two treatment conditions had significant increases in the dosage of antipsychotic medication from baseline to post-treatment. At the end of treatment, the variability on medication dosage was much higher in patients who received standard care. Of the total sample, 65.8% were taking first-generation and 34.2% second-generation antipsychotics. The three most prescribed medications were: First generation: Haloperidol (21.4%), Trifluoperazine (18.8%), and Sulpiride (9.4%). Second generation: Risperidone (21.4%), Clozapine (14.3%), and Olanzapine (3.6%).

	Study Group n=68		Comparison Group N=61		
Variable	*n*	%	*n*	%	X^2
Relapse	8	11.8	17	33.3	p < .01
Rehospitalizations	3	4.4	7	13.7	--
Compliance with medication	62	91.2	40	78.4	--

Table 8. Relapse, rehospitalizations and adherence

Lower relapse (11.8%) and rehospitalization rates (4.4%) were found in the study group compared to 33.3% and 13.7% respectively for the group that received medication alone. Compliance with antipsychotic medication was higher in the study group (91.2% versus 78.4%) of the comparison group, (Table 8)

3.2.3 Integrating pharmacological and psychosocial treatment

We conclude that a therapeutic approach that included the integration of pharmacological and psychosocial treatments for schizophrenia patients can be effective in a developing country as Mexico. Patients that received this integrated approach demonstrated significant improvements in psychopathology, psychosocial functioning, lower relapse and rehospitalisation rates, and higher compliance with antipsychotic medication, as compared with their counterparts that received pharmacotherapy alone. The proposal of integrating pharmacological and psychosocial approaches has been described throughout this chapter and illustrated in table 4. Of the seven stages developed for designing the interventions, five stages were accomplished that ended up with their implementation. We had certain limitations with stage 6 since we could not carry out the patient´s "follow-up" due to the lack of financial funds. We still have a long way to go since stage 7 "dissemination" is also a pendant task for all schizophrenia patients of our Institute as well for all schizophrenia patients in Mexico that would be willing to participate in integrated treatment approaches. To accomplish "dissemination", we could face some complications", if we consider that only 0.36% of the Gross Internal Product (GIP) in Mexico is allocated to scientific research, compared to 0.49 % in Argentina, 1.11% in Brazil, 2.61% in the United States, 3.22% in Japan, and 3.32% in South Korea. It seems that scientific research is not considered a priority in Mexico, as a result schizophrenia research neither. However, we have high hopes as being optimistic. We expect the necessary support to continue our efforts. When connecting clinical practice with scientific research through research protocols, we were able to carry out this type of research at the National Institute of Psychiatry whose main goals are to conduct research, provide treatment for mental disorders, and training for mental health professionals. The Institute belongs to the Coordination of National Research Institutes of Mexico that includes 13 Institutes dedicated to treatment and scientific research. Financial support for this project was possible with funds from the Institute and a grant from the National Council on Science and Technology of Mexico. It was interesting to find out that the areas where Mexican patients had psychosocial problem skills were similar to those utilized in psychosocial treatment programs in first world countries (Liberman, 2007, Roder et al., 2006; Thornicroft & Susser, 2001). It seems that schizophrenia patients share similar problems all over the world. Above all, evidence indicates that psychosocial approaches when combined with pharmacotherapy results in better outcomes, than either antipsychotic medication alone or psychosocial treatment alone. For example, when these two approaches are integrated, relapse rates can be reduces as less than 20% (Hogarty, 1993). Understanding what bio psychosocial approaches can do for persons with schizophrenia could help us to face a new reality that indicates that although there is not a "total cure" for this disease research indicates that substantial advances have been made for improving the life of people with schizophrenia in the community with the integration of pharmacological and psychosocial approaches.

4. Pharmacological and psychosocial treatment in Latin America

Research on integrated pharmacological and psychosocial treatment for schizophrenia has been carried out mostly in developed countries. We wondered what would be the situation in Latin America as to find out what treatments are actually available in this region of the world. In order to get a complete picture we searched the following electronic bibliographic databases: Medline, Psychiatry, EBM Reviews, PsychINFO-APA, Psychology & Behavioral Sciences, Base Salud en Español, CC Clinical Medicine, CC Social and Behabioral Sciences, Medic Latina, Elsevier Science Direct, LILACS, SciELO, MEDCaribe, ISI Current Contents, PAHO Catalog, The Cochrane Library, Biblioteca Cochrane Plus, Ciencias de la Salud-BIREME, Organización Mundial de la Salud, WHOLIS, and Science Electronic Library On

Line. We used the following key words: schizophrenia, pharmacological treatment, antipsychotic medication, psychosocial treatment, psychological therapy, psychosocial intervention, psychosocial rehabilitation, psychoeducation, and family therapy. We searched the literature with publications in Spanish, Portuguese and English from January 1970 to July 2011. We found that in addition to Mexico, integrated approaches have been carried out in two countries: Brazil (Zimmer et al., 2003, 2006, 2007), and Peru (Sotillo, et al., 1998). It is worth mentioning that since the early 1950´s, the first generation "conventional" antipsychotic medication, and later on, the second generation, or "atypical", have been considered as the only traditional treatment in Latin America for persons suffering from schizophrenia. For the year 2011, this approach continues as the customary treatment in most Latin American countries. Twenty five years ago, rehabilitation and psychosocial treatments were nonexistent in this region of the world; however, in the last twenty years some changes have occurred at least in three countries: Brazil (2003-2007); Mexico (1982-2011) and Peru (1998). The most reasonable explanation why psychosocial treatments have not been carried out is because of the lack of economic or financial funds. If clinical services still face serious deficits: old and huge hospitals, too many patients and a reduced staff, it is not difficult to understand why research on behavioural or psychosocial treatments is practically nonexistent. With this scenario there is no doubt that the situation in Latin America is quite different than first world countries. We have a long way to go.

5. Conclusion

Based upon international evidenced-based practices, treatment recommendations and practice guidelines for schizophrenia, an area of research that integrated pharmacotherapy and psychosocial therapies was implemented for Mexican patients with schizophrenia. Valuable contributions from patients, relatives, mental health professionals, as well as cultural considerations were taken into account for the design of the interventions. What is good to consider was to find out the effectiveness of these therapeutic modalities as described in this chapter as a comprehensive care system for people with schizophrenia in Mexico. What is new to consider is that these interventions are available for a developing Latin American country. However, reality indicates that the great majority of schizophrenia patients in Mexico and Latin America do not receive integrated approaches. We recommend the implementation of these therapeutic modalities for all schizophrenia patients in Mexico and in Latin America, because patients deserve to receive the best quality of service that goes beyond the traditional and exclusively approach of pharmacotherapy. Limitations in the implementation in clinical settings as well as problems in translating research into everyday practice should be considered (Margison, 2003). Although, antipsychotic medication can usually help to stabilize symptoms, impairments and disabilities still persist. Wouldn't it be nice if medication could help to restore the individual suffering from schizophrenia, to "normal" life, and regain his/her ability to function in society, to make up for lost time. However, patients could never learn new skills for their survival in the "real world" by taking medication. They need medication as well as psychosocial services. Living in the community independently and successfully should be a goal to pursue. The purpose is the re-integration of persons with schizophrenia in the community. Future research should focus on an independent living-beyond medication- in the community. To reach this goal, patients should go through various conditions that include new and resent proposals: 1) the achievement of "symptomatic remission" (Andreasen et al., 2005), with the use if antipsychotic medication. 2) psychosocial improvements, such as "psychosocial remission", (Barak et al., 2010), with psychosocial approaches, and, 3) the combination of these two variables that would led to "recovery" (Leucht & Lasser, 2006; Liberman, et al., 2002; Liberman & Kopelowicz, 2005; Liberman, 2008; Torgalsboen & Rund 2010). Understanding "functional recovery"as the ultimate goal for an independent living in the community. To complete the puzzle, the family must be considered as an important component. Patients and relatives can become active participants in the "recovery process" since it has been demonstrated that with the use of psychoeducation and family approaches, expressed emotion can be reduced, so patients and their carers could live in a less stressful psychosocial environment. Enhanced monitoring practices could also help for patients, relatives and the treatment team, to be in close contact, as demonstrating "good therapeutic alliance" to intervene when necessary, and also verifying that patients are not only "getting well", but also "staying well" in the community (Yeomans et al., 2010). This general picture indicates that some patients with schizophrenia are still unable to cope with tasks such as having friends, holding a job or living independently. Others have demonstrated that they could experience periods of symptomatic relief and enhanced functioning as being "in recovery", considering the notion that recovering from schizophrenia is possible. Recovery should be a goal to pursue for the future.

6. References

Allison, D. B. (1999). Antipsychotic-induced weight gain: a comprehensive research synthesis. *The American journal of psychiatry*, vol. 156, pp. 1686-1696, ISSN 0002-953X

American Psychiatric Association. (1995). Manual diagnóstico y estadístico de los trastornos mentales, DSM-IV. Editorial Masson, ISBN 84-458-0297-6, Barcelona España

American Psychiatric Association. (2004). Practice Guideline for the Treatment of Patients with Schizophrenia. *The American Journal of Psychiatry*, Vol. 161, No.2, pp. 1-56, ISSN 0002-953X

Andreasen, N. C., Carpenter, W. & Kane, J. (2005). Remission in Schizophrenia: Proposed Criteria and Rationale for Consensus. *The American Journal of Psychiatry*, Vol. 162, pp. 441-449, ISSN 0002-953X

Atkinson, J. M.; Coia, D. A.; Gilmur, W. H. & Harper, J. M. (1996). The impact of education groups for people with schizophrenia on social functioning and quality of life. *British Psychiatry*, Vol. 168, pp. 199-204, ISSN 1472-1465

Barak Y., Bleich, A. & Aizenberg D, (2010) Psychosocial remission in Schizophrenia: developing a clinician-rated scale. *Comprehensive Psychiatry*, Vol. 51, pp. 94-98, ISSN 0010-440X

Barnes, T. R. E. & Paton, C. (2011). Antipsychotic Polypharmacy in Schizophrenia Benefits and Risks. *CNS Drugs*, Vol. 25, pp. 383-399, ISSN 1172-7047

Bauml, J.; Frobose, T.; Sibylle, K. & Rentrop, M. (2006). Psychoeducation: a basic psychotherapeutic intervention for patients with schizophrenia and their families. *Schizophrenia Bulletin*, Vol.32, No. S1, pp. S1-S9, ISSN 0586-7614

Bell, M.; Tsang, H. W. H.; Tamasine, G. & Bryson, G. J. (2009). Neurocognition, social cognition, perceived social discomfort, and vocational outcomes in schizophrenia. *Schizophrenia Bulletin*, Vol. 35, No. 4, pp. 738-747, ISSN 0586-7614

Bellack, A. S. & Mueser, K. T. (1993) Psychosocial Treatment for Schizophrenia. *Schizophrenia Bulletin*, Vol. 19, pp. 317-336, ISSN 0586-7614

Bellack, A. S.; Bennett, M. E.; Gearson, J. S.; Brown, C. H. & Yang, Y. (2006). A randomized clinical trial of a new behavioural treatment for drug abuse in people with severe persistent mental illness. *Archives of General Psychiatry*, Vol. 63, pp. 426-432, ISSN 0099-5355

Bellack, A. S.; Green, M. F.; Cook, J. A.; Fenton, W.; Harvey, P. D.; Heaton, R. K. et al. (2007). Assessment of community functioning in people with schizophrenia and other severe mental illness; A white paper based on an NIMH-sponsored workshop. *Schizophrenia Bulletin*, Vol. 33, No. 3, pp. 805-822, ISSN 0586-7614

Bellack, A. S.; Mueser, K. T.; Gingerch, S. & Agresta, J. (2004). *Social skills training for schizophrenia. A step by step guide*. Guildford Press, ISBN 1-57230-846-X, New York, USA

Benton, M. K. & Schoroeder, H. E. (1990). Social skills training with schizophrenics, meta-analytic evaluation. *Journal of Consulting and Clinical Psychology*, Vol. 58, pp. 741-747, ISSN 002-006X

Birchwood, M.; Smith, J. & MacMillan, F. (1989). Predicting relapse in schizophrenia; the Development and implementation of an early signs monitoring system using patients and family as observers, a preliminary investigaction. *Psychological Medicine*, Vol 19, pp. 649-656, ISSN 0033-2917

Bond, G. R.; Decker, D. R. & Drake, R. E. (2001). Implementing supported employment as an evidence-based practice. *Psychiatric Services*, Vol.51, pp. 313-322, ISSN 1075-273

Briand, C.; Vasiliadis, H. M.; Lesage, A.; Lalonde, P.; Stip, E. & Nicole, L. (2006). Including integrated psychological treatment as part of standard medical therapy for patients with schizophrenia: Clinical outcomes. *Journal of Nervous and Mental Disease*, Vol. 194, No. 7, pp. 463-70, ISSN 0022-3018

Burns, T.; Creed, F.; Fahy, T.; Thompson, S.; Tyrer, P. &White, I. (1999) Intensive versus standard case management for severe psychotic: a randomized trial. *Lancet*, Vol. 353, pp. 2158-2189, ISSN 0099-5355

Burns, T. & Patrick, D. (2007). Social functioning as an outcome measure in schizophrenia studies. *Acta Psychiatrica Scandinavica*, Vol. 116, pp. 403-418, ISSN 0001-690X

Chakos, M. (2001). Effectiveness of second-generation antipsychotics in patients with treatment-resistant schizophrenia: a review and meta-analysis of randomized trials. *The American Journal of Psychiatry*, Vol. 158, pp. 518-526, ISSN 0002-953

Chung, I. W. (2004). Effect of antipsychotics on the quality of life of schizophrenic patients in community mental health centers: conventional versus atypical antipsychotics. *Clinical Psychopharmacology and Neuroscience*, Vol. 2, pp. 16-22, ISSN 1738108

Citrome, L. & Volavka, J. (2002). Optimal dosing of atypical antipsychotics in adults: a review of the current evidence. *Harvard Review of Psychiatry*, Vol. 10, pp. 280-291, ISSN 1067-322

Cohen, J. (1977). *Statistical power analysis for the behavioral sciences*. Academia Press, New York, NY, USA.

Csernansky, J. G. & Schuchart, E. K. (2002). Relapse and rehospitalisation rates in patients with schizophrenia effects of second generation antipsychotics. *CNS Drugs*, Vol. 16, pp. 473-484, ISSN 1172-7047

Davis, J. M.; Chen, N. & Glick, I. D. (2003). A meta-analysis of the efficacy of second-generation antipsychotics. *Archives of General Psychiatry*, Vol. 60, pp, 553-564, ISSN 0003-990X

Davis, J. M. & Chen, N. (2004). Dose response and dose equivalence of antipsychotics. *Journal of Clinical Pharmacology*. Vol. 24, pp. 192-208, ISSN 0271-0749

De Nayer, A. (2003). Efficacy and tolerability of quetiapine in patients with schizophrenia switched from other antipsychotics. *nternational Journal of Psychiatry in Clinical Practice*, Vol. 7, pp. 59–66, ISSN 1365-1501

Dixon, L. B.; Dickerson, F. & Bellack, A. S. (2010). The 2009 Schizophrenia PORT psychosocial treatment recommendations and summary statements. *Schizophrenia Bulletin*, Vol. 36, No. 1, pp. 48-70, ISSN 0586-7614

Drake, R. E.; Bond, G. R. & Essock, S. M. (2009) Implementing evidence-based practices for people with schizophrenia. *Schizophrenia Bulletin*, Vol. 35, No. 4, pp. 704-713, ISSN 0586-7614

Edlinger, M. (2009). Factors influencing the choice of new generation antipsychotic medication in the treatment of patients with schizophrenia. *Schizophrenia Research*, Vol. 113, pp. 246–251, ISSN 0920-9964

Edlinger, M., Baumgartner, S., Eltanaihi-Furtmuller, N.; Hummer, M. & Fleischhacker, W. W. (2005). Switching between second-generation antipsychotics: Why and how? *CNS Drugs*, Vol. 19, pp. 27–42, ISSN 1172-7047

Essock, S. M. (2002). Editor's Introduction: Antipsychotic Prescribing Practices. *Schizophrenia Bulletin*, Vol. 28, pp. 1-4, ISSN 0586-7614

Falloon, I. R. H.; Boyd, J. L. & McGill, C. W. (1984). *Family care of schizophrenia*. Guildford Press. ISBN 89862-923-3, New York, USA

Falloon, I. R. H.; Montero, I.; Sungur, M.; Maestroeni, A.; Malm, U., Economu, M. et al. (2004). Implementation of evidence-based treatment for schizophrenia disorders: two-year outcome of an international field trial of optimal treatment. *World Psychiatry*, Vol. 3, No. 2, pp, 104-109, ISSN: 1723-8617

Fenton, W. S. & Schooler, N. R. (2000). Editor's introduction: Evidence-based psychosocial treatment for schizophrenia. *Schizophrenia Bulletin*, Vol. 26, No. 1, pp. 1-3, ISSN 0586-7614

Freedman, R. (2005). The choice of antipsychotic drugs for schizophrenia. The New England Journal of Medicine. Vol. 353, pp. 1286-1288, ISSN 0193-953X

García-Anaya, M.; Apiquián, R. & Fresán, A. (2001). Los antipsicóticos atípicos: una revisión *Salud Mental*, Vol. 24, pp. 37-43, ISSN 1139-9287

Geddes, J. (2000). Atypical antipsychotics in the treatment of schizophrenia: systematic overview and meta-regression analysis. *BMJ*, Vol. 321, pp. 1371-1376, ISSN 0959-8138

Glynn, S. M.; Marder, S. R.; Liberman, R. P.; Blair, K.; Wirshing., D. A. & Mintz, J. (2002). Supplementing clinic based skills training for schizophrenia with manualized community support: effects on social adjustment. *American Journal of Psychiatry*, Vol. 159, pp. 829-837, ISSN 1535-7228

González, I.; Cáceres, M. C.; Llerena, A.; Berezc, R. & Kiivet, R. (2004). Estudio de utilización de antipsicóticos en la esquizofrenia en Hospitales de España, Estonia, Hungría y Cuba. *Revista del Hospital Psiquiátrico de la Habana*, Vol. 1, No. 2-3, pp. ISSN 1813-6257, 06.09.2011, Available from http://www.revistahph.sld.cu/hph0204/hph02204.htm

Granger, B. (1999). The discovery of haloperidol. *Encephale*, Vol. 25, pp. 59-66, ISSN 0013-7006

Granholm, E.; McQuaid, J. R. & McClure, F. S. (2005). A randomized controlled trial of cognitive behavioural socials skills training for middle-aged and older outpatients with chronic schizophrenia. *American Journal of Psychiatry*, Vol. 162, pp. 520-529, ISSN 1535-7228

Guo, X.; Zhai, J.; Liu, Z.; Fang, M. & Wang, B. (2010). Effects of antipsychotic medication alone vs combined with psychosocial intervention on outcomes of early-stage schizophrenia. *Archives of General Psychiatry*, Vol. 67, No. 9, pp, 895-904, ISSN 0003-990X

Haddad, P. M. & Sharma, S. G. (2007). Adverse Effects of Atypical Antipsychotics Differential Risk and Clinical Implications. *CNS Drugs*, Vol. 21, pp. 911-936, ISSN 1172-7047

Harvard Medical School. (2001). The psychosocial treatment of schizophrenia-Part II, *Harvard Mental Health Letter*, Vol. 18, No. 3, pp. 1-8, ISSN 0884-3783

Heinssen, R. K, Liberman, R. P. & Kopelowicz, A. (2000) Psychosocial skills training for schizophrenia: Lessons from the laboratory. *Schizophrenia Bulletin*, Vol. 26, No. 1, pp. 21-46, ISSN 0586-7614

Henderson, D. C. (2005). Glucose metabolism in patients with schizophrenia treated with atypical antipsychotic agents: a frequently sampled intravenous glucose tolerance test and minimal model analysis. *Archives of General Psychiatry*, Vol. 62, pp. 19-28, ISSN 0003-990X

Hogarty, G. E. (1993). Prevention of Relapse in Chronic Schizophrenia Patients. *The Journal of Clinical Psychiatry*, Vol. 54, No. Suppl. 3, pp.18-23, ISSN 0160-6689

Hogarty, G. E.; Flesher, S.; Ulrich, R.; Carter, M.; Greenwald, D.; Pogue-Geile, M. et al. (2004). Cognitive enhancement therapy for schizophrenia, effects of a 2- year randomized trial on cognition and behavior. *Archives of General Psychiatry, Vol.* 6, pp. 866-876, ISSN 0003-990X

Huxley, N., Rendall, M. & Sederer, L. L. (2000). Psychosocial treatments in schizophrenia. A review of the past 20 years. *The Journal of Nervous and Mental Disease*, Vol. 188, pp. 187-201, ISSN 0022-3018

Jones, P. B. (2006). Randomized controlled trial of the effect on quality of life of second vs. first generation antipsychotic drugs in schizophrenia: cost utility of the latest antipsychotic drugs in schizophrenia study (CUtLASS 1). *Archives of General Psychiatry*, Vol. 63, pp. 1079–1087, ISSN 0003-990X

Kane, J. M. & Marder, S. R. (1993). Psychopharmacologic treatment of schizophrenia. *Schizophrenia Bulletin*, Vol. 19, No. 2, pp. 287-302, ISSN 0586-7614

Kane, J. M. & McGlashan, T. H. (1995). Treatment of schizophrenia. *Lancet*, Vol. 346, pp. 820-825, ISSN 0099-5355

Kay, S.; Fizben, A.; Vital-Herne, M. & Silva, L. (1990). The positive and negative syndrome scale-spanish adaptation. *Journal of Nervous and Mental Diseases*. Vol. 178, pp. 510-517, ISSN 0022-3018

Kazdin, A. & Bass, D. (1999). Power to detect differences between alternative treatments in comparative psychotherapy outcome research. *Journal of Consulting and Clinical Psychology*, Vol. 57, No. 1, pp. 138-147, ISSN 0022-006X

Keefe, R. S. (1999). The effects of atypical antipsychotic drugs on neurocognitive impairment in schizophrenia: a review and meta-analysis. *Schizophrenia Bulletin*, Vol. 25, pp. 201-222, ISSN 0586-7614

Keefe, R. S. (2003). Neurocognitive assessment in the Clinical Antipsychotic Trials of Intervention Effectiveness (CATIE) project schizophrenia trial: development, methodology, and rationale. *Schizophrenia Bulletin*, Vol. 29, pp. 45-55, ISSN 0586-7614

Kopelowicz, A. & Liberman, R. P. (2003). Integrating treatment with rehabilitation for persons with major mental illnesses. *Psychiatric Services*, Vol. 54, No. 11, pp. 1491-1498, ISSN 1075-2730

Kopelowicz, A.; Liberman, R. P. & Zarate, R. (2006). Recent advances in social skills training for schizophrenia. *Schizophrenia Bulletin*, Vol. 32, No. S1, pp. S12-S23, ISSN 0586-7614

Kopelowicz, A., Zarate, R., Gonzalez, V., Mintz, J. & Liberman, R. P. (2003). Disease management in latinos with schizophrenia: a family-assisted, skills training approach. *Schizophrenia Bulletin*, Voñ. 29, No. 2, pp. 211-227, ISSN 0586-7614

Koro, C. E. (2002). An assessment of the independent effects of olanzapine and risperidone exposure on the risk of hyperlipidemia in schizophrenic patients. *Archives of General Psychiatry*, Vol. 59, pp. 1021-1026, ISSN 0003-990

Kreyenbuhl, J. K.; Buchanan, R. W.; Dickerson, F. B. & Dixon, L. B. (2009). The schizophrenia patient outcomes research team (PORT): updated treatment recommendations 2009. *Schizophrenia Bulletin*, Vol. 36, No 1, pp. 94-103, ISSN 0586-7614

Kuipers, E.; Leff, J. & Lam, D. (2004). *Esquizofrenia. Guía práctica de trabajo con las familias.* Editorial Paidos, ISBN 84-493-1629-4, Barcelona, España

Kurtz, M. M. & Mueser, K. T. (2008). A Meta-Analysis of Controlled Research on Social Skills Training. *Journal of Consulting and Clinical Psychology*, Vol. 76, No. 3, pp. 491-504, ISSN 0022-006X

Lauriello, J.; Lenroot, R. & Bustillo, J. R. (2003). Maximizing the synergy between pharmacotherapy and psychosocial therapies for schizophrenia. *Psychiatric Clinics of North America*, Vol. 26, pp. 191-211, ISSN 0193-953X

Leff, J.; Wig, N. N. & Ghosh, A. (1987). Expressed emotion in schizophrenia in North India. III. Influence of relative´s expressed emotion on the course of schizophrenia in Chandigarh. *British Journal of Psychiatry*, Vol. 151, pp. 166-173, ISSN 0007-1250

Lehman, A. F. (1983). The well-being of chronic mental patients: assessing their quality of life. *Archives of General Psychiatry*, Vol. 40, pp. 369-373, ISSN 0003-990X

Lehman, A. F.; Lieberman, J. A.; Dixon, L. B.; McGlashan, T. H.; Miller, A. L.; Perkins, D. O. et al. (2004). Practice guidelines for the treatment of patients with schizophrenia, second edition. *Supplement to The American Journal of Psychiatry*, Vol. 161, No. 2., pp. 1-56, ISSN 0002-953X

Lehman, A. F. & Steinwaschs, D. M. (1998). Translating research into practice: the schizophrenia patient outcomes research team (PORT) treatment recommendations. *Schizophrenia Bulletin*, Vol. 24, pp. 1-10, ISSN 0586-7614

Lehman, A. F. & Steinwachs, D. M. (2003). Evidence based psychosocial treatment practice in schizophrenia: lessons from the patient outcomes research team (PORT) project. *Journal of the American Academy of Psychoanalysis and Dynamic Psychiatry*, Vol. 31, No. 1, pp. 141-154, ISSN 1546-0371

Leslie D. L. & Rosenheck, R. A. (2004). Incidence of Newly Diagnosed Diabetes Attributable to Atypical Antipsychotic Medications. *The American Journal of Psychiatry*, 161, pp. 1709–1711), ISSN 0002-953X

Leucht, S. (1999). Efficacy and extrapyramidal side-effects of the new antipsychotics olanzapine, quetiapine, risperidone, and sertindole compared to conventional antipsychotics and placebo: a meta-analysis of randomized controlled trials *Schizophrenia Research*, Vol. 35, pp. 51-68, ISSN 0920-9964

Leucht, S. (2003) New generation antipsychotics versus low-potency conventional antipsychotics: a systematic review and meta-analysis. *Lancet*, Vol. 2003, No. 361, pp. 1581-1589, ISSN 0099-5355

Leucht, S.; Corves, C.; Arbter, D.; Engel, R.; Li, C. & Davis, J. M. (2009). Second-generation versus first-generation antipsychotic drugs for schizophrenia: a meta-analysis. *Lancet*, Vol. 373, No. 9657, pp. 31-41, ISSN 0099-5355

Leucht, S.; Komossa, K.; Rummel-Kluge, Ch.; Corves, C.; Hunger, H.; Schmid, F. et al. (2009) A Meta-Analysis of Head-to-Head Comparisons of Second-Generation Antipsychotics in the Treatment of Schizophrenia. *The American Journal of Psychiatry*, Vol. 166, pp. 152–163, ISSN 0002-953X

Leucht, S. & Lasser, R. (2006). The concepts of remission and recovery in schizophrenia. *Pharmacopsychiatry*, Vol. 39, pp. 161-170, ISSN 0176-379

Leucht, S & Van Os, J. (2009). Preface: Treatment optimization in schizophrenia through active patient management-proceedings from two European consensus meetings. *Acta Psychiatrica Scandinavica*, Vol. 119, No. Suppl. 438, pp. 5-6, ISSN 0001-690X

Liberman, R. P. (1998). Skills training versus psychosocial occupational therapy for persons with persistent schizophrenia. *American Journal of Psychiatry*, Vol. 155, pp. 1087-1091, ISSN 0002-953X

Liberman, R. P. (2007). Dissemination and adoption of social skills training: social validation of an evidence-based of an evidence-based treatment for the mentally disabled. *Journal of Mental Health*, Vol. 16, pp. 595-623, ISSN 0963-8237

Liberman, R. P. (2008). *Recovery from disability Manual of Psychiatric Rehabilitation*. American Psychiatric Publishing, Inc., ISBN 978-1-58562-205-4, Washington, D. C.

Liberman, R. P. & Kopelowicz, A. (2005). Recovery from schizophrenia: a concept in search of research. *Psychiatric Services*, Vol. 56, No. 6, pp. 735-742, ISSN 1075-2730

Liberman, R. P.; Kopelowicz, A.; Ventura, J. & Gutkind, D. (2002). Operational criteria and factors related to recovery from schizophrenia. *International Review of Psychiatry*, Vol. 14, No. 4, pp. 256-272, ISSN 0954-0261

Lieberman, J.; Stroup, S.; McEvoy, J. P.; Swartz, M.; Rosenheck, R. A. & Perkins, D. O. (2005). Effectiveness of antipsychotic drugs in patients with chronic schizophrenia. *The New England Journal of Medicine*, Vol. 353, Vol. 12, pp. 1209-1223. ISSN 0028-4793

López-Muñoz, F.; Alamo, C. & Cuenca, E. (2002). Aspectos históricos del descubrimiento y de la introducción clínica de la cloropromazina: medio siglo de psicofarmacología. *Frenia*, Vol. 2, pp, 77-107, ISSN 1852-4680

Marder, S. R. (2000). Integrating pharmacological and psychosocial treatments for schizophrenia. *Acta Psychiatrica Scandinavica*, Vol. 407, pp. 87-90, ISSN 0001-69X

Marder, S. R. (2002) The Mount Sinai Conference on the Pharmacotherapy of Schizophrenia. *Schizophrenia Bulletin*, Vol. 28, pp. 5-16, ISSN 0586-7614

Margison, F. (2003). Evidence-based medicine in the psychological treatment of schizophrenia. *Journal of the American Academy of Psychoanalysis and Dynamic Psychiatry*, Vol. 31, No. 1, pp. 177-190, ISSN 1546-0371

McCann, T. V.; Boardman, G.; Clark, E. & Lu, S. (2008). Risk profiles for non-adherence to anti psychotic medication. *Journal of Psychiatric and Mental Health Nursing*, Vol. 15, pp. 622-629, ISSN 1351-0126

McCrone, P. & Strathdee, G. (1994). Needs not diagnosis: towards a more rational approach to community mental health resourcing in Britain. *The International Journal of Social Psychiatry*, Vol. 40, pp. 79-86, ISSN 0020-7640

McGrath, J. (2008). Schizophrenia: A Concise Overview of Incidence. *Prevalence, and Mortality, Epidemiol* Rev, 30, pp, 67-76, ISSN 0193-936X

McGurk, R.; Mueser, K. T.; DeRosa, T. J. & Wolfe, R. (2009). Work, recover, and comorbidity in schizophrenia: a randomized controlled trial of cognitive remediation. *Schizophrenia Bulletin*, Vol. 35, No. 2, pp. 319-335, ISSN 0586-7614

Miller, A. L. & Craig, C. S. (2002). Combination antipsychotics: pros, cons, and questions. Schizophrenia Bulletin, Vol. 28, pp. 105-109, ISSN 0586-7614

Mojtabai, R., Nicholson, R. & Carpenter, B. (1998). Role of psychosocial treatments in the management of schizophrenia: a meta-analytic review of controlled outcome studies. *Schizophrenia Bulletin*, Vol. 24, pp. 569-87, ISSN 0586-7614

Mueller, N. (2004). Mechanism of relapse prevention in schizophrenia. *Pharmacopsychiatry*, Vol. 37, No. Suppl 2, S141-S147, ISSN 0176-3679

Mueser, K. T.; Corrigan, P. W.; Hilton, D.; Tanzman B., Schaub, A., Gingeric, S. et al. (2002). Illness management and recovery: a review of the research. *Psychiatric Services*, Vol. 53, No. 10, pp. 1272-1284, ISSN 1075-2730

Mueser, K. T.; Salyers, M. P. & Mueser, P. R. (2001). A prospective analysis of work in schizophrenia. *Schizophrenia Bulletin*, Vol. 27, pp. 281-296, ISSN 0586-7614

Murray-Swank, A. B. & Dixon, L. B. (2004). Family psychoeducation as an evidence-base practice. CNS Spectrums, Vol. 9, No. 12, pp. 905-912, ISSN 1092-8529

Newcomer, J. W. (2005). Second-Generation (Atypical) Antipsychotics and Metabolic Effects A Comprehensive Literature Review. *CNS Drugs*, Vol. 19, No. Suppl. 1, pp. 1-93, ISSN 1172-7047

Ortega-Soto, H. A.; Herrera, M. A. & Ortiz, C. (1998) Tratamiento farmacológico de la esquizofrenia. *Psicología Iberoamericana*, Vol. 6, pp. 4-17, ISSN: 1405-0943

Ortega-Soto, H. A. & Valencia, M. (2001). El tratamiento farmacológico de la esquizofrenia, In: *Esquizofrenia estado actual y perspectivas*, H. A. Ortega-Soto & M. Valencia (eds.), 349-398, Editorial Láser, ISBN 968-7652-31-4, Mexico City, Mexico

Overall, J. E. & Gorham, O. R. (1962). The Brief Psychiatric Rating Scale. *Psychological Reports*, Vol. 10, pp. 799-812

Penn, D., Waldheter, E. & Perkins, D. O. (2005). Psychosocial treatment for first-episode psychosis: a research update. *The American Journal of Psychiatry*, Vol. 16, pp. 2220-2232, ISSN 1535-7228

Pilling, S.; Bebbington, P.; Kuipers, E.; Garety, P.; Geddes, J.; Martindale, B. et al. (2002). Psychological treatments in schizophrenia: II. Meta-analyses of randomized controlled trials of social skills training and cognitive remediation. *Psychological Medicine*, Vol. 32, pp. 783-791, ISSN 0033-2917

Posligua, P. B. (1995). El tratamiento de la esquizofrenia: up to date. *Alcmeon*, Vol. 4, pp. 14, ISSN 0327-3954

Ridgely, M. S.; Goldman, H. H. & Willenbring, M. (1990). Barriers to the care of persons with dual diagnosis: organizational and financing issues. *Schizophrenia Bulletin*, Vol.16, pp. 123-132 , ISSN 0586-7614

Robins, L. N.; Wing, J. K. & Witchen, H. U. (1988). The composite international diagnostic interview: an epidemiological instrument suitable for use in conjunction with different diagnostic systems and in different cultures. *Archives of General Psychiatry*, Vol. 45,pp. 1069-1077, ISSN 0003-990X

Roder, V.; Mueller, D.; Mueser, K. & Brenner, H. (2006). Integrated psychological therapy (IPT) for schizophrenia. Is it effective. *Schizophrenia Bulletin*, Vol. 32, No. Suppl. 1, pp. S1-S93, ISSN 0586-7614

Rosenheck, R. A.; Perlick, D.; Bingham, S.; Liu-Mares, W.; Collins, J.; Warren, S. et al. (2003). Effectiveness and cost of olanzapine and haloperidol in the treatment of schizophrenia: a randomized controlled trial. *JAMA*, Vol. 290, pp. 2693-2702, ISSN 0098-7484

Secretaría de Salud. (1999). *Cuadro Básico y Catálogo de Medicamentos*, Consejo de Salubridad General, Secretaría de Salud, ISBN 968-811-775-7, México, D.F, México

Shaner, A.; Eckman, T.; Roberts, L. J. & Fuller, T. (2003). Feasibility of a skills training approach to reduce substance dependence among individuals with schizophrenia. *Psychiatric Services*, Vol. 54, pp. 1287-1289, ISSN 1075-2730

Sharma, D. & Harvey, P. (2000). *Cognition in schizophrenia*. Oxford University Press, ISBN 19262993X, New Yor, USA.

Shean, G. D. (2009). Evidence-based psychosocial practices and recovery from schizophrenia. *Psychiatry*, Vol. 72, No 4, pp. 307-320, ISSN 00033-2747

Sotillo, C.; Rodriguez, C. & Salazar, V. (1998). Dissemination of a social skills training program for chronic schizophrenic patients in Peru. *International Review of Psychiatry*, Vol. 10, pp. 51-53, ISSN 0954-0261

Spitzer, R. L.; Gibbon, J. & Endicott, J. (1976). The global assessment scale. *Archives of General Psychiatry*, Vol. 4, No. 33, pp. 766-771, ISSN 0003-990X

Stahl, S. & Buckley, P. (2007). Negative symptoms of Schizophrenia: a problem that will not go away. *Acta Psychiatrica Scandinavica*, Vol. 7, pp. 6-11, ISSN 0001-690X

Stroup, T. S.; McEvoy, J. P.; Ring, K. D.; Hamer, R. H., LaVange, L. M., Swartz, M. S. et al. (2011). A randomized trial examining the effectiveness of switching from olanzapine, quetiapine, or risperidone to aripiprazole to reduce metabolic risk: Comparison of Antipsychotics for Metabolic Problems (CAMP). *The American Journal of Psychiatry*, Vol. 168, pp. 947-956, ISSN 0002-953X

Swartz, M. S (2003). Assessing clinical and functional outcomes in the Clinical Antipsychotic Trials of Intervention Effectiveness (CATIE) schizophrenia trial. *Schizophrenia Bulletin*, Vol. 29, pp. 33-43, ISSN 0586-7614

Swartz, M.S.; Perkins, D. O. & Stroup, T. S. (2007). Effects of antipsychotic medications on psychosocial functioning in patients with chronic schizophrenia: findings from the NIMH CATIE study. *American Journal of Psychiatry*, Vol. 164, No. 3, pp. 428-436, ISSN 0002-953X

Thornicroft, G.; Sttathdee, G. & Phelan, M. (1998). Rationale and design: PriSM psychosis study 1. The British Journal of Psychiatry: The Journal of Mental Science, Vol. 173, pp. 363-370, ISSN 0007-1250

Thornicroft, G. & Susser, E. (2001). Evidence-based psychotherapeutic interventions in the community care of schizophrenia. *British Journal of Psychiatry*, Vol. 176, pp. 2-4, ISSN 0007-1250

Torgalsboen, A. K. & Rund, B. (2010). Maintenance of recovery from schizophrenia at 20 year follow-up: what happened?. *Psychiatry*, Vol. 73, No. 1, pp. 70-83, ISSN 00033-2747

Trainor, J. N.; Morell-Bellai, T.L.; Ballantyne, R. & Boydell, K. M. (1993). Housing for people with mental illnesses: a comparison of models and an examination of the growth of alternating housing in Canada. *Canadian Journal of Psychiatry*, Vol. 38, pp. 494-501, ISSN 0703-7437

Tsang, W. H. H. (2001). Social skills training to help mentally ill persons find and keep a job. *Psychiatric Services*, Vol. 52, pp. 891-894, ISSN 1557-9706

Valencia, M. (1988). Un programa de tratamiento psicosocial para pacientes psicóticos agudos hospitalizados. *Revista Psiquiatría*, Vol. 4, No. 4, pp. 71-96, ISSN 0187-4543

Valencia, M. (1991). El hospital mental como instrumento terapéutico: el rol del psicólogo en la práctica clínica institucional. *Revista Mexicana de Psicología, Vol.* 8, pp. 99-107, ISSN 0185-6073

Valencia, M.; Murow, E. & Rascón, M. L. (2006). Comparación de tres modalidades de intervención en esquizofrenia: la terapia psicosocial, la musicoterapia y las terapias múltiples. *Revista Latinoamericana de Psicología*, Vol. 38, No. 3, pp. 535-549, ISSN 0120-0534

Valencia, M.; Ortega-Soto, H. A.; Rodríguez, M. S. & Gómez, L. (2004a). Estudio comparativo de consideraciones clínicas y psicoterapéuticas en el tratamiento biopsicosocial de la esquizofrenia. Primera Parte. *Salud Mental*, Vol. 27, No. 3, pp. 47-53, ISSN 0185-3325

Valencia, M.; Ortega-Soto, H. A.; Rodríguez, M. S. & Gómez, L. (2004b) Estudio comparativo respecto a consideraciones clínicas y psicoterapéuticas en el tratamiento biopsicosocial de la esquizofrenia. Parte II. *Salud Mental*, Vol. 27, No. 4, pp. 35-43, ISSN 0185-3325

Valencia, M.; Rascón, M. L. & Quiroga, H. (2003). Aportaciones de la investigación respecto al tratamiento psicosocial y familiar de pacientes con esquizofrenia. *Salud Mental*, Vol. 26, No. 5, pp. 1-18, ISSN 0185-3325

Valencia, M.; Rascón, M. L.; Juárez, F.; Escamilla, R.; Saracco, R. & Liberman, R. P. (2010). Application in Mexico of psychosocial rehabilitation with schizophrenia patients. *Psychiatry*, Vol. 73, No. 3, pp. 248-263, ISSN 00033-2747

Valencia, M.; Rascón, M. L.; Juárez, F. & Murow, E. (2007). A psychosocial skills training approach in Mexican out-patients with schizophrenia. *Psychological Medicine*, Vol. 37, pp. 1393-1402, ISSN 0033-2917

Valencia, M., Rascón, M. L. & Ortega-Soto, H. A. (2001). Tratamiento psicosocial en pacientes con esquizofrenia. In In: *Esquizofrenia estado actual y perspectivas*, H. A. Ortega-Soto & M. Valencia (eds.), 399-454, Editorial Láser, ISBN 968-7652-31-4, Mexico City, Mexico

Velligan, D. I.; Kern, R. & Gold, J. M. (2006). Cognitive rehabilitation for schizophrenia and the putative role of motivation and expectancies. *Schizophrenia Bulletin*, Vol. 32, No. 3, pp. 474-485, ISSN 0586-7614

Vesterager, L.; Christensen, T.; Olsen, B. B.; Kraup, G.; Forchhammer, H. B.; Melau, M.; Gluu, C. & Nordentoft, M. (2011). Cognitive training plus a comprehensive psychosocial programme (OPUS) versus the comprehensive psychosocial programme alone for patients with first-episode schizophrenia (the NEUROCOM trial): A study protocol for a centrally randomized, observer-blinded multicentre clinical trial. *Bio Med Central*, Vol.12, No.35, pp. 1-9, ISSN 1745-6215

Wahlbeck, K. (1999). Evidence of clozapine's effectiveness in schizophrenia: a systematic review and meta-analysis of randomized trials. *The American Journal of Psychiatry*, Vol. 1 56, pp. 990-999, ISSN 0002-953X

Wallace, C. J.; Liberman, R. P.; MacKain, S. J.; Blackwell, G. & Eckman, T. E. (1992). Effectiveness and replicability of modules for teaching social and instrumental skills to the severely mentally ill. *American Journal of Psychiatry*, Vol. 149, pp. 654-658, ISSN 0002-953X

Weiden, P. J. (2006). Switching antipsychotics: an updated review with a focus on quetiapine. *Journal of Psychopharmacology*, vol.20, pp. 104-118, ISSN 0271-0749

World Health Organization. (2001). *World health report mental health: new understanding, new hope*. World health organization, ISBN 1562013, Geneve

World Health Organization. (2011). Schizophrenia, In: *Mental Health*, 06.09.2011, Available from http://www.who.int/mental_health/management/schizophrenia/en/

Xia, J.; Bertil-Merinder, L. & Belgamwar M. R. (2011). Psychoeducation for schizophrenia. *Schizophrenia Bulletin*, Vol. 37, No. 1, pp. 21-22, ISSN 0586-7614

Yeomans, D.; Taylor, M.; Currie, A.; Whale, R.; Ford, K. & Fear, C. (2010). Resolution and remission in schizophrenia: getting well and staying well. *Advances in Psychiatric Treatment*, Vol. 16, pp. 86-95, ISSN 1355-5146

Zimmer, M.; Godoy, L. A.; Godoy, J. & .Belmonte-de Abreu, P. (2003). Mudanca no funcionamiento social e occupational de portadores de esquizofrenia e trastorno de humor expostos ao programa de psicoterapia congnitivo-compotamental derivada de Roder: um estudi naturalistico de 3 años. *Revista Brasileira de Psicoterapia*, Vol. 5, No. 1, pp. 3-18, ISSN 1516-8530

Zimmer, M.; Verissimo, A. & Belmonte-de Abreu, P. (2006). Análise qualitativa de variáveis relevantes para a aplicacao do programa de terapia psicológica integrada emj pacientes com esquizofrenia de tres centros do Sul do Brasil. *Revista de Psiquiatria do Rio Grande do Sul*, Vol. 28, No. 3, pp. 256-264, ISSN 0187-4543

Zimmer, M.; Verissimo, A.; .Laitano, D.; Ferreira, E. E. & Belmonte-de Abreu, P. (2007). A twelve-week randomized controlled study of the cognitive-behavioral integrated psychosocial therapy program: posite effect on the social functioning of schizophrenic patients. *Revista Brasileira de Psiquiatria*, Vol. 29, No. 2, pp. 140-147, ISSN 1516-4466

4

Nicotine Addiction: Role of the Nicotinic Acetylcholine Receptors Genetic Variability in Knowledge, Prevention and Treatment

Candida Nastrucci and Patrizia Russo
Laboratory of Systems Approaches and Non Communicable Diseases,
IRCCS "San Raffaele Pisana"
Italy

1. Introduction

In 1988 the US Surgeon General's report stated that tobacco use, in any form, is addicting as a result of its nicotine content and defined the processes determining tobacco addiction as "*similar to those that determine addiction to drugs such as heroin and cocaine*" (U.S. Surgeon General, 1988). Tobacco smoking has been classified by the WHO International Classification of Diseases (ICD-10) under the "Mental and behavioural disorders" (F00-F99 (http://apps.who.int/classifications/apps/icd/icd10online/). Continuous use of nicotine induces adaptive changes in the CNS leading to tolerance, physical or physiological dependence, sensitization, craving, reward and relapse. Drug addiction has been defined by Koob (2008) as "*a chronically relapsing disorder characterized by compulsive drug use and loss of control over drug intake*". Indeed Koob (2008) proposed that addiction includes three different stages, which are: "*preoccupation/anticipation, binge/intoxication, and withdrawal/negative affect*". As a final result chronic use of nicotine produces 'tolerance', an occurrence that reduces the effect of a drug given dose (Fig. 1.).

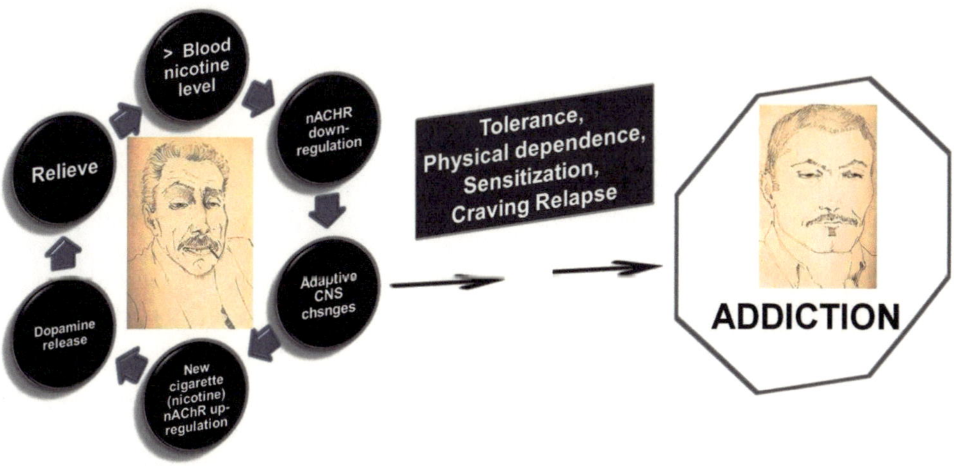

Fig. 1. Steps signals involved in the circuit of nicotine addiction (adapted from Russo, 2011).

Cessation of tobacco use determines a withdrawal syndrome, characterized by agitation, irritation, frustration or anger, concentration difficulty, depressed mood, anxiety, restlessness, decreased heart rate and increased appetite or weight gain (Benowitz, 2010; Perkins, 2002; Shiffman et al., 2004). These symptoms occur after four to twelve hours, peak after one week and decrease progressively over time (Perkins, 2002). Nicotine addiction is sustained by the individual positive effects experienced during smoking, and by the wish to hold off the negative symptoms of nicotine withdrawal. Thus, episodic and repetitive doses of nicotine are indispensable to maintain normal levels of functioning. Moreover, stress conditions, processes concerning consciousness, evaluation and response to negative, threatening or, challenging events or stimuli have been found to exacerbate nicotine withdrawal symptoms and increase vulnerability to relapse (Morissette et al., 2007).

2. Neurochemistry of Nicotinic receptor (nAChR)

The functional properties of nicotine are related to its interaction with the nicotine receptors (nAChR). nAChR are acetylcholine gated ion channels consisting of homo- or hetero-pentamers subunits arranged symmetrically around a membrane perpendicular axis, outlining the ionic hole (Russo et al., 2006; Taly et al., 2009) (Fig. 2.).

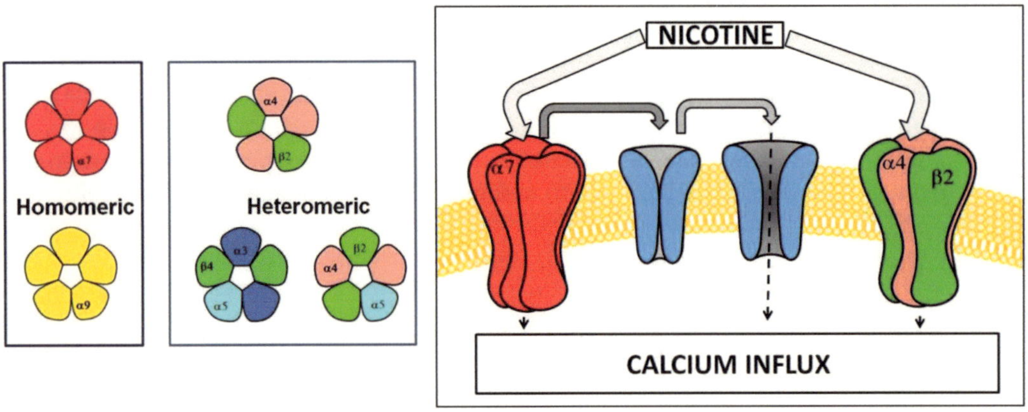

Fig. 2. Nicotinic Receptors. nAChR consist of homo- (e.g. α7 or a9, non the left) or hetero-pentamer (e.g. $(\alpha4)_3(\beta2)_2$, $\alpha5(\alpha3)_2(\beta4)_2$,, $\alpha5(\alpha4)_2(\beta4)_2$), composed of the various subunits (α1–α10; β1–β4) that are arranged symmetrically around an axis perpendicular to the membrane, thus delineating the ionic pore. The α subunits are distinguished by the presence of adjacent (vicinal) Cysteine residues in loop C, and this originally defined α subunits as agonist-binding subunits. The homomeric α7 nAChR is a special case, since having five agonist-binding sites per receptor can bind from two to five molecules of agonist. α7-nAChR utilizes multiple calcium amplification pathways to efficiently raise the intracellular calcium levels by subsequent activation of voltage-gated calcium channels as well as calcium release from the endoplasmic reticulum (Russo et al., 2006; Taly et al., 2009).

The composition and stoichiometry of the pentamer determines receptor pharmacology, cations selectivity, desensitization kinetics and spatial distribution. Receptors containing α4 and β2 subunits are the most abundant in the CNS accounting for the majority of nicotine high affinity binding sites (Flores et al., 1992; Schoepfer et al., 1988). It has been shown, by pharmacological and ligand-binding experiments, that nAChR containing the β2-subunit (β2*nAChR, the asterisk indicates the possibility of other subunits to be incorporated in the receptors) bind to nicotine with high affinity (Changeux et al., 1998). β2-containing nAChR, which have been implicated in nicotine self-administration (Picciotto et al., 1998), do not influence the onset of nicotine withdrawal symptoms (Salas et al., 2004). Evidence shows that acute nicotine self-administration is absent if the α4* receptors are deleted (Marubio et al., 2003; Pons et al., 2008). Activation of α4 nAChR is sufficient to sustain nicotine-induced reward, tolerance and sensitization (Tapper et al., 2004). Since the α3 and α5 subunits are coexpressed within α4 in the medial habenula (MHb), in the interpeduncular nucleus (IPN) and in the peripheral ganglia, it is likely that α3* and α5* nAChR may be involved in the mechanisms of nicotine withdrawal. It has been shown that α6β2* nAChR expressed in the VTA (ventral tegmental area) are necessary for the effects of systemic nicotine on DA (dopamine) neuron activity and DA-dependent behaviours, such as locomotion and reinforcement. It was proposed that both α6β2 and α4β2 receptors are necessary for (at least some of) the effects of nicotine on the DA system. In the brain, the homomeric α7 subtype is the most abundant and widespread nAChR (Breese et al., 1997; Quik et al., 2000), being involved in the modulation of glutamatergic and cholinergic neurotransmitter release, in the synaptic plasticity, in the regulation of neuronal growth, in the differentiation and survival, in the regulation of calcium-dependent gene expression and in the mediation of circuit excitability (reviewed in Gotti & Clementi, 2004). New data support a model in which the α7 nAChR, found on glutamate terminals, increases glutamate release contributing to presynaptic facilitation and synaptic plasticity and enhancing dopamine release from neighbouring boutons (Livingstone et al., 2010). The regulation of the nAChR is linked to their intrinsic property of being allosteric receptors. (Changeux & Edelstein, 2005). Thus nAChR are susceptible to desensitization and inactivation following, or in some cases independent of, channel opening (Giniatullin et al., 2005). Desensitization represents a decrease or loss of biological response after prolonged or repetitive stimulation by an agonist, such as nicotine, or a neurotransmitter. Indeed, when nicotine is continuously applied, nAChR become 'desensitized' (i.e. temporarily inactive) (Katz & Thesleff, 1957; Quick & Lester, 2002). The sensitisation-desensitization is correlated to the property of nAChR to increase their expression (upregulation) when exposed to nicotine (Vallejo et al., 2005; Gahring et al., 2010). Subtypes containing α2, α3 and α5 are not up-regulated by chronic nicotine administration (Mao et al., 2008; Marks et al., 1992), whereas α4- or β2–containing nAChR (Tapper et al., 2004; Nashmi et al., 2007), containing subunits are up-regulated following repeated nicotine administration (McCallum et al., 2006). α7 upregulation occurs at higher nicotine concentrations than are required to increase α4β2 nAChR (Pauly et al., 1991; Rasmussen & Perry, 2006; Kawai & Berg, 2001). Up-regulation of α6-containing receptors, after nicotine administration, is a process which less clear, since studies report either upregulation (Parker et al. 2004), down-regulation (Lai et al., 2005; Perry et al., 2007) or no change (Drenan et al., 2008, McCallum et al., 2006).

3. Mechanism of nicotine addiction

Although the molecular mechanisms leading to and maintaining NA are not completely understood, they involve the regulation of brain monoamines levels and in particular DA (Benowitz, 2010; Changeux, 2009). Nicotine stimulates those nAChR placed principally in the ventral tegmental area, in the nucleus accumbens and in the pedunculopontine and laterodorsal tegmental nuclei, important neuronal structures of the mesolimbic reward pathway (Brunzell et al., 2009; Dani, 2003; Exley & Cragg, 2008; Sharma & Brody, 2009; Schiltzet al., 2005). It has been proposed that the change from voluntary drug use to a more habitual and compulsive drug use, corresponds to a transition, at the neural level, from prefrontal cortical to striatal control, as well a progression from ventral to more dorsal domains of the striatum, involving its dopaminergic innervation (Everitt & Robbins, 2005). These neural transitions may themselves depend on the neuroplasticity in both cortical and striatal structures that is induced by chronic self-administration of drugs. Several nAChR subtypes such as: $\alpha4\alpha6\beta2\beta3$, $\alpha4\beta2$, $\alpha4\alpha5\beta2$, $\alpha6\beta2\beta3$ and $\alpha6\beta2$ are expressed on dopamine nerve terminals (Grady et al., 2007). Converging indication proposes that the dopaminergic system is important in mediating the pleasurable feelings of reward when activated by nicotine (Soderpalm et al., 2000; Zoli et al., 2002). It has been hypothesized that exposure to nicotine may initially increases the firing of ventral tegmental area GABAergic neurons through $\alpha7$ nAChR activation, followed by $\alpha7$ nAChR desensitization, that leads the disinhibition and firing of DA neurons. This latter event might be also enabled by a more prolonged activation of the $\alpha7$ nAChR expressed on glutamatergic terminals (Wonnacott et al., 2005). At the molecular level, several studies have suggested that ERK1/2 activation followed by phosphorylation of Cyclic AMP Response Element Binding protein (CREB) at Ser^{133} and the activity of Fos gene are highly involved in many forms of experience dependent plasticity, such as long-term potentiation (LTP; Wu et al., 2007). ΔFosB, a long-lived truncated isoform of the FosB protein, accumulates within the striatum of rats treated repeatedly with either cocaine or nicotine, for several weeks and suggesting a sustained molecular change initiated by drug experience (Nestler, 2001), although not sufficient to account for the perseverance of drug dependence. CREB may play an important role in the rewarding and reinforcing effects of many drugs of abuse (Nestler, 2001, 2002), since pCREB is required in the NAc to establish nicotine-conditioned place preference (CPP) in mice (Brunzell et al., 2009).

4. Genetic of nicotine addiction

Meta-analysis of studies on twins showed that both genes and environment are important in smoking-related behaviours, with an estimated mean heritability of 0.50 for smoking initiation and 0.59 for nicotine dependence (Li et al., 2003). In women, genetic factors have a larger role in initiation than in persistence, whereas the opposite is observed in men (Li et al., 2003; Madden et al., 1999). Recent genome-wide association studies (GWAS) have shown that the CHRNA5-A3-B4 region, on chromosome 15q24-25.1, encoding the $\alpha3$, $\alpha5$ and $\beta4$ subunits, is strongly associated with nicotine dependence, as well as alcohol and cocaine dependence and lung cancer susceptibility (Amos et al., 2008; Amos et al., 2010; Bierut, 2010; Caporaso et al., 2009; Saccone et al., 2010; Spitz et al., 2008; Thorgeirsson et al., 2008). One of the strongest association within the 15q24-25.1 region is the rs16969968, located in exon 4 of CHRNA5, which causes an aminoacid substitution from an aspartic acid (D) to asparagine (N) (missense mutation) (D398N). This change reduces the $\alpha4\beta2\alpha5$ receptor function (Saccone et al. ,2007), as found by *in vitro* functional studies, which shown that $\alpha4\alpha5\beta2$ receptors, containing the N substitution, exhibited a weaker response to nicotine compared to the D variant in $\alpha5$ (Bierut et al., 2008). Other nAChR gene variants associated to ND are reported in Table 1.

Gene	SNP	Chromosome number/ position (base pairs)	Major/Minor Allele
CHRNA3	rs1051730	15/76681394	C/T
CHRNA3	rs11637630	15/76686774	A/G
CHRNA3	rs3743078	15/76681814	C/G
CHRNA3	rs578776	15/76675455	C/T
CHRNA3	rs7177514	15/76694461	C/G
CHRNA3/B4	rs8023462	15/76701789	C/T
CHRNA4	rs1044394	20/61452529	C/T
CHRNA4	rs2236196	20/61448006	A/G
CHRNA4	rs2273504	20/61458505	A/G
CHRNA4	rs6122429	15/76701810	C/T
CHRNA5	rs16969968	15/76669680	G/A
CHRNA5	*rs17486278*	15/76654537	A/C
CHRNA5	*rs2036527*	15/7663870	C/T
CHRNA5	*rs569207*	15/76660174	GA
CHRNA5	*rs637137*	15/7661031	T/A
CHRNA5	*rs8034191*	15/45468658	G/A
CHRNA6	*rs1072003*	8/42729008	C/G
CHRNA6	rs2304297	8/42725148	C/G
CHRNA6	rs892413	8/42727356	A/C
CHRNB2	rs2072658	1/152806850	A/G
CHRNB2	rs2072660	1/152815345	C/T
CHRNB2	rs2072661	1/152815504	A/G
CHRNB3	rs13280604	8/ 42678742	A/G
CHRNB3	rs4950	8/42671789	C/T
CHRNB4	rs1948	15/76704500	C/T

Table 1. Association Results for Significant SNP–Phenotype Associations 'Current Frequent Smokers', Reviewed in Russo, 2011.

5. Drugs in smoking cessation

The drugs for smoking cessation currently approved by the FDA (Hurt et al., 2009) include nicotine-replacement therapy (NRT), Bupropion and Varenicline. A Cochrane Database of Systematic Reviews 2009 (Hajek et al., 2009) that reassessed different randomized or quasi-randomized controlled trials of relapse prevention interventions, with a minimum follow up of six months, concluded that: (i) extended treatment with Bupropion is unlikely to have a clinically important effect; (ii) studies of extended treatment with nicotine replacement are needed and (iii) extended treatment with Varenicline may prevent relapse.

Varenicline [Systematic IUPAC name: 7,8,9,10-tetrahydro- 6,10-methano- 6H-pyrazino (2,3-h)(3) benzazepine (trade name Chantix), is an α4β2 nicotinic receptor partial agonist and an α7 full agonist. The partial agonist activity induces modest receptor stimulation that attenuates the symptoms of nicotine withdrawal and inhibits the surges of dopamine release, responsible of the reinforcement and reward associated with smoking (Coe et al.,

2005; Foulds, 2006). Consequently, Varenicline suppresses the symptoms of nicotine withdrawal and reduces the pharmacologic reward from cigarette smoking (Rollema et al., 2007).

Bupropion [Systematic IUPAC name: (±)-2-(tert-butylamino)-1-(3-chlorophenyl)propan-1-one], initially approved by the FDA as an atypical antidepressant, belongs to the chemical class of aminoketones. Although its mechanism of action in smoking cessation is not completely understood, Bupropion is an inhibitor of DA and of nor-epinephrine reuptake; but it is also a weak antagonist of nicotinic receptors (Cryan et al., 2003; Fryer & Lukas, 1999;).

6. Drugs and nAChR gene variants

Although the association of nAChR variants and ND have been extensively studied, their role in drug therapy for smoking cessation is only pioneristic. Conti et al. (2008) have identified two polymorphisms within the CHRNB2 (rs2072661 and rs2072660) having significant association with the abstinence rates, within a 6-month follow-up study on the effects of Bupropion in smoking cessation, in a placebo-controlled trial. Specifically, although a difference was found in the relapse rates at EOT (end of treatment), between carriers and non-carriers, for individuals who received Bupropion, there was a substantial increase in the relapse rates for those individuals carrying the minor allele, after they went off treatment. Follow-up analyses on the top SNP (rs2072661) indicated a role in the time to relapse within the 6-month follow-up period and an impact on withdrawal symptoms at TQD (target quit date). These two SNPs (rs2072661 and rs2072660) may be robust markers for identifying smokers most likely to relapse and those who may benefit from Bupropion therapy. In addition, these SNPs should be examined within pharmacogenetic studies of Varenicline for smoking cessation. There is evidence that smokers with a heterozygous TC genotype at SNP rs2236196 in CHRNA4 are more likely to maintain abstinence with nicotine nasal spray (Hutchison et al., 2007). Moreover, looking at rs2072661, smokers with the CHRNB2 GG genotype, could sustain more days of abstinence during the nicotine *versus* placebo patch week, compared with those with the AG or AA genotypes; regardless of patch condition, quitting on the 'target quit day' was more likely to occur in those individuals with the GG genotype versus AA/AG genotypes. Genetic associations were not observed for craving or withdrawal responses to nicotine *versus* placebo patch (Perkins et al., 2009). A recent research studied the association of the CHRNA3 gene (Tyr215Tyr or rs1051730) with quitting success in response to controlled short-term nicotine patch use in hospitalized individuals (De Ruyck et al., 2010). Point abstinence was considered, and it was found that neither this genetic polymorphisms, nor the interaction of genotype *versus* treatment group, were significantly associated with quit rates, at any of the considered time points. A recent smoking cessation pharmacogenetics study (King et al., 2012) analyzed 1476 consenting individuals (524 who take Varenicline; 440 Bupropion; 512 placebo). Among the subjects receiving Varenicline, two variants in CHRNB2 (rs3811450 and rs4262952) were significantly associated with continuous smoking abstinence. Interestingly Bupropion abstinence was associated with several SNPs within CYP2B6, one enzyme important for the metabolism of nicotine, including rs8109525.

Indeed, CYP2B6.8 (the K139E variant) is unable to metabolize Bupropion under normal turnover conditions (Zhang et al., 2011). All these data support the evidence that genetic loci contribute to smoking cessation and therapeutic response. On the other hand, the response treatment to Varenicline *versus* Bupropion is associated with different genetic signals, implying that in future research clinically useful markers shall guide treatment decisions to achieve improved smoking cessation rates and reduction in smoking occurrence.

7. Conclusions

Recognition that tobacco use is driven by the "neurobiological diseases" of "nicotine dependence" and "nicotine withdrawal", linked to specific nAChR variants, provides a rational basis for the development of drugs and treatment, as well as supporting the inclusion of pharmacotherapies for dependence and withdrawal, along with those targeting other medical disorders. In fact, the need to prevent public health and economic devastation, caused by tobacco use, supports treatment as a high priority in health care. Pharmacotherapy for tobacco dependence is also cost effective when compared to many widely supported forms of pharmacotherapy for diseases, such as hypertension and hypercholesterolemia, as well as preventive periodic screening such as mammography or Papanicolaou smears. Moreover, the nAChR SNPs examination is less expensive and less invasive that spiral-CT or PET-SCAN examination, as screening in smokers. Taken together, these data suggest that genetic susceptibility to nicotine dependence is linked to several nAChR subtype genes and variants, in each subunit gene, and that may give independent, as well as interactive, contributions to nicotine dependency at molecular level.

8. Acknowledgements

We apologize to the many contributors of this field whose work is important but that we were unable to cite here.

The painting shown in Figure 1 is the original work of Arch. Giulio Alzetta (1988, charcoal on paper) and has been included here with his permission.

Note: The Author states to disagree with the use of animals and animal models in research. As an author she is only responsible for the inclusion of the *in vitro* research and human studies reported here. She is a "conscientious objector", according to the Italian Law: "Legge n. 413 del 12 ottobre 1993" entitled "*Norme sull'obiezione di coscienza alla sperimentazione animale*" (Italian Law on "conscientious objection to animal experiments").

9. References

Amos, C.I., Gorlov, IP., Dong, Q., Wu, X., Zhang, H., Lu, EY., Scheet, P., Greisinger, A.J., Mills, G.B. & Spitz, M.R., (2010). Nicotinic acetylcholine receptor region on chromosome 15q25 and lung cancer risk among african americans: a case-control study. *J Natl Cancer Inst*, Vol. 102, No. 15, pp. 1199-1205.

Amos, C.I., Wu, X., Broderick, P., Gorlov, I.P., Gu, J., Eisen, T., Dong, Q., Zhang, Q., Gu, X., Vijayakrishnan, J., Sullivan , K, Matakidou, A., Wang, Y., Mills, G., Doheny, K., Tsai, Y.Y., Chen, W.V., Shete, S., Spitz, M.R.& Houlston, R.S. (2008). Genome-wide association scan of tag SNPs identifies a susceptibility locus for lung cancer at 15q25.1. *Nat Genet*, Vol. 40, No. 5, pp 616–622.

Benowitz ,N.L .(2010). Nicotine addiction. *N Engl J Med*, Vol. 362, No. 24, pp :2295-303.

Bierut ,L.J., Stitzel , J.A., Wang, J.C., Hinrichs, A.L., Grucza, R.A., Xuei, X., Saccone ,N.L., Saccone, S.F., Bertelsen, S., Fox, L., Horton, W.J., Breslau, N., Budde, J., Cloninger, C.R., Dick, D.M., Foroud, T., Hatsukami, D., Hesselbrock, V., Johnson, E.O., Kramer, J., Kuperman, S., Madden, P.A., Mayo, K., Nurnberger, J., Jr, Pomerleau, O., Porjesz, B., Reyes, O., Schuckit, M., Swan, G., Tischfield, J.A., Edenberg, H.J., Rice, J.P. & Goate, A.M. (2008). Variants in nicotinic receptors and risk for nicotine dependence. *Am J Psychiatry*, Vol. 165, No. 9, pp 1163–1171.

Bierut, L.J. (2010). Convergence of genetic findings for nicotine dependence and smoking related diseases with chromosome 15q24-25.*Trends Pharmacol Sci*, Vol.,31, No. 1, pp 46-51.

Breese, C.R., Adams, C., Logel, J., Drebing, C., Rollins, Y., Barnhart, M., Sullivan, B., Demasters ,B.K., Freedman, R. & Leonard, S. (1997). Comparison of the regional expression of nicotinic acetylcholine receptor alpha7 mRNA and[125I]-alphabungarotoxin binding in human post-mortem brain. *J Comp Neurol*, Vol. 387, No. 3, pp 385–398.

Brunzell, D.H., Mineur, Y.S., Neve, R.L.& Picciotto, M.R. (2009). Nucleus accumbens CREB activity is necessary for nicotine conditioned place preference. *Neuropsychopharmacology*, Vol. 34, No. 8, pp 1993-2001.

Brunzell, D.H., Boschen, K.E., Hendrick, E.S., Beardsley, P.M &, McIntosh, J.M. (2010). Alpha-conotoxin MII-sensitive nicotinic acetylcholine receptors in the nucleus accumbens shell regulate progressive ratio responding maintained by nicotine. *Neuropsychopharmacology*, Vol. 35, No. 3, pp 665– 673.

Caporaso, N., Gu, F., Chatterjee, N., Sheng-Chih, J., Yu, K., Yeager, M., Chen, C., Jacobs, K., Wheeler, W., Landi, M.T., Ziegler, R.G., Hunter, D.J., Chanock, S., Hankinson, S., Kraft, P.& Bergen, A.W. (2009). Genome-wide and candidate gene association study of cigarette smoking behaviors. *PLoS ONE* 4:e4653.

Changeux, J.P., Bertrand, D., Corringer ,P.J., Dehaene, S., Edelstein, S., Léna, C., Le Novère, N., Marubio, L., Picciotto, M. & Zoli, M. (1998) .Brain nicotinic receptors: Structure and regulation, role in learning and reinforcement. *Brain Res Brain Res Rev*, Vol. 26, No. 2-3, pp. 198–216.

Changeux, J.P. & Edelstein, S.J. (2005). Allosteric mechanisms of signal transduction. *Science*, 308, No. 5727, pp. 1424–1428.

Changeux JP (2009) Nicotinic receptors and nicotine addiction. *C R Biol*, Vol. 332, No. 5, pp. 421-425.

Coe, J.W., Brooks, P.R., Vetelino, M.G., Wirtz, M.C., Arnold, E.P., Huang, J., Sands, S.B., Davis, T.I., Lebel, L.A., Fox, C.B., Shrikhande, A., Heym, J.H., Schaeffer, E., Rollema, H., Lu, Y., Mansbach, R.S., Chambers, L.K., Rovetti, C.C., Schulz, D.W., Tingley, F.D. 3rd, O'Neill, B.T. (2005). Varenicline: An alpha4beta2 nicotinic receptor partial agonist for smoking cessation. *J Med Chem*, Vol. 48, No. 10 , pp. 3474-3477.

Conti, D.V., Lee , W., Li, D., Liu, J., Van Den Berg, D., Thomas, P.D., Bergen, A.W., Swan, G.E., Tyndale, R.F., Benowitz, N.L. & Lerman, C. (2008). Nicotinic acetylcholine receptor beta2 subunit gene implicated in a systems-based candidate gene study of smoking cessation. *Hum Mol Genet*, 17, No. 18, pp. 2834-2848.

Cryan, J.F., Bruijnzeel, A.W., Skjei, K.L.& Markou, A .(2003). Bupropion enhances brain reward function and reverses the affective and somatic aspects of nicotine withdrawal in the rat. *Psychopharmacology (Berl)*, 168, No. 3, pp. 347-358.

Dani, J.A .(2003), Roles of dopamine signaling in nicotine addiction. *Mol Psychiatry*, Vol. 8, No. 3, pp. 255-256.

Drenan ,R.M., Grady, S.R., Whiteaker, P., McClure-Begley, T., McKinney, S., Miwa, J.M., Bupp, S., Heintz, N., McIntosh, J.M., Everitt, B.J.& Robbins, T.W. (2005). Neural systems of reinforcement for drug addiction: from actions to habits to compulsion. *Nat Neurosci*, Vol. 8, No. 11, pp. 1481-1489

Exley, R. & Cragg, S.J. (2008). Presynaptic nicotinic receptors: a dynamic and diverse cholinergic filter of striatal dopamine neurotransmission. *Br J Pharmacol*, Vol. 153, Suppl 1, pp. S283-297.

Foulds, J. (2006). The neurobiological basis for partial agonist treatment of nicotine dependence: Varenicline. *Int J Clin Pract*, Vol. 60, No. 5, pp. 571-576.

Fryer, J.D.& Lukas, R.J. (1999). Noncompetitive functional inhibition at diverse, human nicotinic acetylcholine receptor subtypes by Bupropion, phencyclidine, and ibogaine. *J Pharmacol Exp Ther*, Vol. 288, No. 1, pp. 88-92.

Gahring, L.C., Vasquez-Opazo, G.A. & Rogers, S.W. (2010). Choline promotes nicotinic receptor $\alpha4+\beta2$ upregulation. *J Biol Chem*, doi:10.1074/jbc.M110.108803.

Giniatullin, R., Nistri, A. & Yakel, J.L. (2005). Desensitization of nicotinic ACh receptors: shaping cholinergic signaling. *Trends Neurosciences*, Vol. 28, No. 7, pp. 371-378.

Gotti, C. & Clementi, F. (2004). Neuronal nicotinic receptors: from structure to pathology. *Prog Neurobiol*, Vol. 74, No. 6 , pp. 363-396.

Grady, S.R., Salminen, O., Laverty, D.C., Whiteaker, P., McIntosh, J.M., Collins, A.C. & Marks, M.J. (2007). The subtypes of nicotinic acetylcholine receptors on dopaminergic terminals of mouse striatum. *Biochem Pharmacol*, Vol. 74, No. 8, pp. 1235-1246.

Hajek, P., Stead, L.F., West, R., Jarvis, M. & Lancaster, T. (2009). Relapse prevention interventions for smoking cessation. *Cochrane Database Syst Rev*, (1):CD003999.

Hurt, R.D., Ebbert, J.O., Hays, J.T.& McFadden, D.D. (2009). Treating tobacco dependence in a medical setting. *CA Cancer J Clin, Vol.* 59, No. 5 , pp. 59314-59326.

Hutchison, K.E., Allen, D.L., Filbey, F.M., Jepson, C., Lerman, C., Benowitz, N.L., Stitzel, J., Bryan, A., McGeary, J.& Haughey, H.M. (2007). CHRNA4 and tobacco dependence: from gene regulation to treatment outcome. *Arch Gen Psychiatry*, Vol. 64, No. 9, pp. 1078-1086.

Katz, B. & Thesleff, S. (1957). A study of the 'desensitization' produced by acetylcholine at the motor end-plate. *J Physiol*, Vol. 138, No. 1, pp. 63-80.

Kawai, H.& Berg, D.K. (2001). Nicotinic acetylcholine receptors containing alpha7 subunits on rat cortical neurons do not undergo long-lasting inactivation even when up-regulated by chronic nicotine exposure. *J Neurochem*,Vol. 78, No. 18, pp. 1367-1378.

King, D.P., Paciga, S., Pickering, E., Benowitz, N.L., Bierut, L.J., Conti, D.V., Kaprio, J., Lerman, C., Park, P.W. (2012) .Smoking cessation pharmacogenetics: analysis of varenicline and bupropion in placebo-controlled clinical trials. *Neuropsychopharmacol,* Vol 37, No. 3, pp. 641-650.

Koob, G.F. (2008). A role for brain stress systems in addiction. *Neuron*, 59, No. 1, pp. 11-34.

Lai, A., Parameswaran, N., Khwaja, M., Whiteaker, P., Lindstrom, J.M., Fan, H., McIntosh, J.M., Grady, S.R. & Quik, M. (2005). Long-term nicotine treatment decreases striatal alpha 6* nicotinic acetylcholine receptor sites and function in mice. *Mol Pharmacol*, Vol. 67, No. 5, pp. 1639-1647.

Li, M.D., Cheng, R., Ma, J.Z. & Swan, G.E. (2003). A meta-analysis of estimated genetic and environmental effects on smoking behavior in male and female adult twins. *Addiction*, Vol. 98, No. 1, pp. 23-31.

Livingstone, P.D., Dickinson, J.A., Srinivasan, J., Kew, J.N. & Wonnacott, S. (2010). Glutamate-dopamine crosstalk in the rat prefrontal cortex is modulated by Alpha7 nicotinic receptors and potentiated by PNU-120596. J Mol Neurosci Vol. 40, No. 1-2, pp. 172-176.

Madden, P.A., Heath, A.C., Pedersen, N.L., Kaprio, J., Koskenvuo, M.J. & Martin, N.G. (1999). The genetics of smoking persistence in men and women: a multicultural study. *Behav Genet*, Vol. 29, No. 6, pp. 423-431.

Mao, D., Perry, D.C., Yasuda, R.P., Wolfe, B.B. & Kellar, K.J .(2008). The alpha4beta2alpha5 nicotinic cholinergic receptor in rat brain is resistant to up-regulation by nicotine in vivo. *J Neurochem*, Vol. 104, No. 2, pp. 446-456.

Marks, M.J., Pauly, J.R., Gross, S.D., Deneris, E.S., Hermans-Borgmeyer, I., Heinemann, S.F. & Collins, A.C. (1992). Nicotine binding and nicotinic receptor subunit RNA after chronic nicotine treatment. *J Neurosci*, Vol. 12, No. 7, pp. 2765-84.

Marubio , L.M., Gardier, A.M., Durier, S., David, D., Klink, R., Arroyo-Jimenez, M.M., McIntosh, J.M., Rossi, F., Champtiaux, N., Zoli, M. & Changeux, J.P. (2003). Effects of nicotine in the dopaminergic system of mice lacking the alpha4 subunit of neuronal nicotinic acetylcholine receptors. *Eur J Neurosci*, Vol. 17: No. 7, pp. 1329-1337.

McCallum, S.E., Parameswaran, N., Bordia, T., Fan, H., McIntosh, J.M. & Quik, M. (2006). Differential regulation of mesolimbic alpha 3/alpha 6 beta 2 and alpha 4 beta 2 nicotinic acetylcholine receptor sites and function after long-term oral nicotine to monkeys. *J Pharmacol Exp Ther*, Vol. 318, No. 1, pp. 381-388.

Morissette, S.B., Tull, M.T., Gulliver, S.B., Kamholz, B.W. & Zimering, R.T. (2007). Anxiety, anxiety disorders, tobacco use, and nicotine: a critical review of interrelationships. *Psychol Bull*, Vol.133, No. 2, pp. 245-272.

Nashmi, R., Xiao, C., Deshpande, P., McKinney, S., Grady, S.R., Whiteaker, P., Huang, Q., McClure-Begley, T., Lindstrom, J.M., Labarca, C., Collins, A.C., Marks, M.J. & Lester, H.A. (2007). Chronic nicotine cell specifically upregulates functional alpha 4* nicotinic receptors: basis for both tolerance in midbrain and enhanced long-term potentiation in perforant path. *J Neurosci*, Vol. 27: No. 31, pp. 8202-8218.

Nestler, E.J. (2001). Molecular basis of long-term plasticity underlying addiction. *Nat Rev Neurosci*, Vol 2, No. 31, pp. 119-128.

Nestler, E.J. (2002). Common molecular and cellular substrates of addiction and memory. *Neurobiol Learn Mem*, Vol. 78, No. 3, pp. 637-647.

Pauly, J.R. (2008). Gender differences in tobacco smoking dynamics and the neuropharmacological actions of nicotine. *Front Biosci*, Vol 13, No. 1, pp. 505-516.

Perkins, K.A. (2002). Chronic tolerance to nicotine in humans and its relationship to tobacco dependence. *Nicotine Tob Res*, Vol. 4, No. 4, pp. 405-422.

Perkins, K.A., Lerman, C., Mercincavage, M., Fonte, C.A. & Briski, J.L. (2009). Nicotinic acetylcholine receptor beta2 subunit (CHRNB2) gene and short-term ability to quit smoking in response to nicotine patch. *Cancer Epidemiol Biomarkers Prev*, Vol. 18, No. 10 , pp. 2608-2612.

Perry, D.C., Mao, D., Gold, A.B., McIntosh, J.M., Pezzullo, J.C. & Kellar, K.J. (2007). Chronic nicotine differentially regulates alpha6- and beta3-containing nicotinic cholinergic receptors in rat brain. *J Pharmacol Exp Ther*, Vol. 322, No. 1 , pp. 306-315.

Picciotto, M.R., Zoli, M., Rimondini, R., Lena, C., Marubio, L.M., Pich, E.M., Fuxe, K. & Changeux, J.P. (1998). Acetylcholine receptors containing the beta2 sub- unit are involved in the reinforcing properties of nicotine. *Nature*, Vol. 391, No. 6663, pp. 173-177.

Pons, S,, Fattore, L., Cossu, G., Tolu, S., Porcu, E., McIntosh, J.M., Changeux, J.P., Maskos, U. & Fratta, W. (2008). Crucial role of $\alpha 4$ and $\alpha 6$ nicotinic acetylcholine receptor subunits from ventral tegmental area in systemic nicotine self-administration. *J Neurosci*, Vol. 28, No. 47, pp. 12318-12327.

Quik, M., Polonskaya, Y., Gillespie, A., Jakowec, M., Lloyd, G.K.& Langston, J.W. (2000). Localization of nicotinic receptor subunit mRNAs in monkey brain by in situ hybridization. *J Comp Neurol*, Vol. 425, No..1, pp. 58-69.

Quick, M.W. & Lester, R.A. (2002). Desensitization of neuronal nicotinic receptors. *J Neurobiol*, Vol. 53, No. 1, pp. 457-478.

Rasmussen, B.A. & Perry, D.C .(2006). An autoradiographic analysis of [125I]alpha-bungarotoxin binding in rat brain after chronic nicotine exposure. *Neurosci Lett*, Vol. 404, No. 1-2, pp. 9-14.

Rollema, H., Coe, J.W., Chambers, L.K., Hurst, R.S., Stahl, S.M. & Williams, K.E. (2007.) Rationale, pharmacology and clinical efficacy of partial agonists of a4b2 nACh receptors for smoking cessation. *Trends Pharmacol Sci*, Vol. 28, No. 7, pp. 316-325.

Russo, P., Catassi , A., Cesario, A. & Servent, D. (2006). Development of novel therapeutic strategies for lung cancer: targeting the cholinergic system. *Curr Med Chem*, 13, No. 29, pp. 3493-3512.

Russo, P., Cesario, A., Rotella, S., Veronesi, G., Spaggiari, L., Galetta, D., Margaritora, S., Granone, P.& Greenberg, D.S. (2011). Curr Med Chem, Vol. 18, No. 1, pp. 91-112.

Russo, P., Nastrucci, C., Alzetta, G. & Szalai, C. (2011). Tobacco habit: Historical, cultural, neurobiological and genetical features of people's relationship with an addictive drug. *Perspectives Biol Med*, Vol. 54, No. 4, pp. 557-577.

Saccone, N.L., Culverhouse, R.C., Schwantes-An, T.H., Cannon, D.S., Chen, X., Cichon, S., Giegling, I., Han, S., Han, Y., Keskitalo-Vuokko, K., Kong, X., Landi, M.T., Ma, J.Z., Short, S.E., Stephens, S.H., Stevens, V.L., Sun, L., Wang, Y., Wenzlaff, A.S., Aggen, S.H., Breslau,. N., Broderick, P., Chatterjee, N., Chen, J., Heath, A.C., Heliövaara, M., Hoft, N.R., Hunter, D.J., Jensen, M.K., Martin, N.G., Montgomery, G.W., Niu, T., Payne, T.J., Peltonen, L., Pergadia, M.L., Rice, J.P., Sherva, R., Spitz, M.R., Sun, J., Wang, J.C., Weiss, R.B., Wheeler, W., Witt, S.H., Yang, B.Z., Caporaso, N.E., Ehringer, M.A., Eisen, T., Gapstur, S.M., Gelernter, J., Houlston, R., Kaprio, J., Kendler, K.S., Kraft, P., Leppert, M.F., Li, M.D., Madden, P.A., Nöthen, M.M., Pillai, S., Rietschel, M., Rujescu, D., Schwartz, A., Amos, C.I. & Bierut, L.J. (2010). Multiple Independent Loci at Chromosome 15q25.1 Affect Smoking Quantity: a Meta-Analysis and Comparison with Lung Cancer and COPD. *PLoS Genet*, Vol. 6, No.8, pii: e1001053.

Saccone, S.F., Hinrichs, A.L., Saccone, N.L., Chase, G.A., Konvicka, K., Madden, P.A., Breslau, N., Johnson, E.O., Hatsukami, D., Pomerleau, O., Swan, G.E., Goate, A.M., Rutter, J., Bertelsen, S., Fox, L., Fugman, D., Martin, N.G., Montgomery, G.W., Wang, J.C., Ballinger, D.G., Rice, J.P.& Bierut, L.J. (2007). Cholinergic nicotinic receptor genes implicated in a nicotine dependence association study targeting 348 candidate genes with 3713 SNPs. *Hum Mol Genet*, Vol. 16, No. 1, pp. 36-49.

Salas,, R., Cook, K.D., Bassetto, L., De Biasi, M. (2004). The α3 and β4 acetylcholine receptor subunits are necessary for nicotine-induced seizures and hypolocomotion in mice. *Neuropharmacology*, Vol. 47, No. 3, pp. 401-407.

Shiffman, S., West, R., Gilbert, D., Trials, S.W. (2004). Recommendation for the assessment of tobacco craving and withdrawal in smoking cessation trials. *Nicotine Tob Res*, Vol. 6, No. 4, pp. 599-614.

Soderpalm, B., Ericson, M., Olausson, P., Blomqvist, O. & Engel, J.A. (2000). Nicotinic mechanisms involved in the dopamine activating and reinforcing properties of ethanol. *Behav Brain Res*, Vol. 113, No. 1-2, pp. 85-96.

Spitz, M.R., Amos, C.I., Dong, Q., Lin, J.& Wu, X. (2008). The CHRNA5-A3 region on chromosome 15q24-25.1 is a risk factor both for nicotine dependence and for lung cancer. *J Natl Cancer Inst*, Vol. 100, No. 21, pp. 1552-1556.

Taly, A., Corringer, P., Guedin, D., Lestage, P. & Changeux, J. (2009). Nicotinic receptors: allosteric transitions and therapeutic targets in the nervous system. *Nat Rev Drug Discov*, Vol. 8, No. 9 , pp. 733-750.

Tapper, A.R., McKinney, S.L., Nashmi, R., Schwarz, J., Deshpande, P., Labarca, C., Whiteaker, P., Marks, M.J., Collins, A.C. & Lester, H.A. (2004) Nicotine activation of alpha4* receptors: sufficient for reward, tolerance, and sensitization. *Science*, Vol. 306, No. 5698, pp. 1029-1032.

Thorgeirsson, T.E., Geller, F., Sulem, P., Rafnar, T., Wiste, A., Magnusson, K.P., Manolescu, A., Thorleifsson, G., Stefansson, H., Ingason , A., Stacey, S.N., Bergthorsson, J.T., Thorlacius, S., Gudmundsson, J., Jonsson, T., Jakobsdottir, M., Saemundsdottir, J., Olafsdottir, O., Gudmundsson, L.J., Bjornsdottir, G., Kristjansson, K., Skuladottir, H., Isaksson, H.J., Gudbjartsson, T., Jones, G.T., Mueller, T., Gottsater, A., Flex, A., Aben, K.K., de Vegt, F., Mulders, P.F., Isla, D., Vidal, M.J., Asin, L., Saez, B., Murillo, L., Blondal, T., Kolbeinsson, H., Stefansson, J.G., Hansdottir, I., Runarsdottir, V., Pola, R., Lindblad , B., van Rij, A.M., Dieplinger, B., Haltmayer, M., Mayordomo, J.I., Kiemeney, L.A., Matthiasson, S.E., Oskarsson, H., Tyrfingsson, T., Gudbjartsson, D.F., Gulcher, J.R., Jonsson, S., Thorsteinsdottir, U., Kong, A. & Stefansson, K. (2008). A variant associated with nicotine dependence, lung cancer and peripheral arterial disease. *Nature*, Vol. 452, No. 7187 , pp. 638-642.

U.S. Surgeon General. 1988. The health consequences of smoking: Nicotine addiction. A report of the Surgeon General. http://profiles.nlm.nih.gov/NN/B/B/Z/D/.

Vallejo, Y.F., Buisson, B., Bertrand, D. & Green, W.N. (2005). Chronic nicotine exposure upregulates nicotinic receptors by a novel mechanism. *J Neurosci*, Vol. 25, No. 23, pp. 5563-5572.

Wonnacott, S., Sidhpura, N, & Balfour, D.J. (2005). Nicotine: from molecular mechanisms to behaviour. *Curr Opin Pharmacol*, Vol. 51, No. 1, pp. 53-59.

Wu, H., Zhou, Y.& Xiong, Z.Q. (2007). Transducer of regulated CREB and late phase long-term synaptic potentiation. *FEBS J*, Vol. 274, No. 13, pp. 3218-3223.

Zhang, H., Sridar, C., Kenaan, C., Amunugama, H., Ballou, D.P,, Hollenberg, P.F. (2011). Polymorphic variants of cytochrome P450 2B6 (CYP2B6.4-CYP2B6.9) exhibit altered rates of metabolism for bupropion and efavirenz: a charge-reversal mutation in the K139E variant (CYP2B6.8) impairs formation of a functional cytochrome p450-reductase complex. *J Pharmacol Exp Ther, Vol.* 338, No. 3, pp. 803-809.

Zoli, M., Moretti, M., Zanardi, A., McIntosh, J.M., Clementi, F. & Gotti, C. (2002). Identification of the nicotinic receptor subtypes expressed on dopaminergic terminals in the rat striatum. *J Neurosci*, Vol. 22, No. 20, pp. 8785-8789.

5

Psychiatric Drugs in Medical Practice

María-José Martín-Vázquez
University Hospital "Infanta Sofía", Deparment of Psychiatry,
San Sebastián de los Reyes, Madrid
Spain

1. Introduction

Psychiatric symptoms are very frequent in medical practice, up to 40% of the people that have physical problems present anxiety or depressive symptoms associated to physical illness. Due to this, psychiatric liaison is an important part of hospital attention and many people usually have psychiatric drugs associated to other treatments.

Psychiatric drugs usually are classified into six great families depending on their principal focus of action or their use in the main psychiatric disorders:

- Antidepressants: these drugs act on depressive illness through the action on various neurotransmitter systems: serotonine, noradrenaline and dopamine. The most used of these are SSRI (serotonine selective reuptake inhibitors), because of their efficacy and good profile of side effects.
- Antipsychotics: they are used in the control of psychotic symptoms and as major tranquilizers. Antipsychotics are classified on first generation and second generation. The first of them act upon dopamine receptors and the second ones upon serotonine and dopamine receptors to have antipsychotic effects. This second generation substances have less side effects and a different profile of action.
- Anxiolytics: the most widely used are benzodiacepines, which act upon a specific GABA receptor. This family of drugs has a very quick effect, but they aren't recommended for a long time use because they can produce dependence and their effects are limited. They are also used like anticonvulsivants.
- Antiepileptics: This group of drugs is used in psychiatry for the maintenance and control of bipolar disorders, and they are useful too like antiaggressive drugs. The therapeutic drug monitoring is necessary when some of these substances are administrated because of their potential toxicity and the pharmacological interactions with other treatments.
- Lithium: it is a salt used for control of manic symptoms and maintenance of bipolar disorders. Its action mechanism is unknown, despite its usefulness and generalized utilization. It's necessary to control its plasmatic level into a tight range to avoid toxicity and to achieve its function.
- Other drugs widely used in psychiatric disorders: methadone, anticholinesterases, stimulants, alcohol aversives are also important due to their side effects and their pharmacologic interactions.

2. Antidepressants

First antidepressant drugs were a casual finding and they affect to various neurotransmitters systems. Usually these old drugs produce many secondary effects. Afterwards, some hypotheses have emerged about the neurotransmission implicated in depression (monoamines: serotonin, noradrenalin and dopamine). Drug development progresses in parallel to this investigation so more selective drugs appeared as Selective Serotonin Reuptake Inhibitors, (from now on SSRIs), ameliorating secondary effects.

Antidepressant classification depends on the assumption of their action mechanism. Following that schema, there are eight different pharmacological mechanisms at least. The most of the antidepressants block monoamine reuptake, but others block alpha-2 receptors or monoamineoxidase enzyme.

2.1 Monoamine reuptake inhibitors

2.1.1 Tricyclic and tetracyclic antidepressants (TCA)

The tricyclic and tetracyclic branch of antidepressants has a demonstrated and high efficacy, only limited by their sedative and anticholinergic effects. They act on a huge number of receptors, and are cardiotoxic in case of overdoses, as anticholinergic toxicity and convulsions.

Pharmacological actions: A significant part is absorbed totally after oral administration. They have a significant metabolism by first-pass. Maximum plasmatic concentration is reached in 2-48 hours but equilibrium appears after 5-7 days. Their long half-life allows them to be used once in a day. Clearance of tricyclics is dependent primarily on hepatic cytochrome P450 (CYP) oxidative enzymes.

Effects on organs and special systems: Significant effects on the cardiovascular system appear at therapeutic dose: they are classified as anti-arrhythmic type IA, since they interrupt the ventricular fibrillation and can increase the collateral blood flow of ischemic heart. In overdose they are highly cardiotoxic and cause a decrease in contractility, increased irritability myocardial, hypotension and tachycardia.

2.1.2 Main therapeutic indications

Depression: treatment of one major depressive episode and prophylaxis of one major depressive episode (main directions); depression in Bipolar type I disorder (in resistant cases, with many precautions to prevent swinging: associated with anticonvulsivants or lithium); one depressive episode with psychotic manifestations almost always requires the simultaneous administration of an antipsychotic drug and an antidepressant; Disorder mood due to a general medical disease with depressive features

- Panic disorder.
- Generalized anxiety disorder.
- Obsessive-compulsive disorder: clomipramin especially. None of the others seems so effective.
- Others: Alimentary conduct disorder and pain disorder.

2.1.3 Precautions and adverse reactions

- Psychopathological effects: possibility of inducing a manic episode, especially in patients with a history of Bipolar disorder. It has been also described that the tricyclic antidepressants can exacerbate or precipitate psychotic symptoms in vulnerable patients.
- Anticholinergic effects: They consist of dry mouth, constipation, blurred vision, urinary retention, closed angle glaucoma
- Sedation.
- Effects on the autonomous nervous system: orthostatic hypotension, profuse sweating, palpitations, and increased blood pressure.
- Effects on the cardiovascular system: tachycardia, QT prolongation, flattening of T wave, ST depression, etc.
- Neurological effects: Delirium (cholinergic effects). Psychomotor stimulation. Parkinsonism, dyskinesia, akathisia, and inclusive by dopaminergic blockade: neuroleptic malignant syndrome. Finally there is a relatively small risk of induce convulsions, so in risky patients is encouraged to use lower doses.
- Allergic and haematological effects: rash, and much less frequently jaundice, agranulocytosis, leukocytosis, leukopenia, and eosinophilia.
- Other: frequent weight gain, sexual dysfunction, digestive discomfort (nausea, vomiting) and much more rarely syndrome of inappropriate secretion of antidiuretic hormone.
- Avoid in pregnancy and lactation. Use with caution in patients with kidney or liver disease. Increased risk of cardiac adverse effects if it is associated to electroconvulsive therapy. If there is a history of heart disease the TCA administration must start with low-dose, gradually increasing while maintaining a surveillance of cardiac functions. Their administration must be suspended the prior days to a surgical intervention, due to the risk of hypertensive episodes. Prior to starting treatment with any TCA basal EKG should be made. Try to avoid in patients with closed glaucoma, if necessary you may need to manage at the same time pilocarpine eye drops.

2.2 Serotonin Selective Reuptake Inhibitors (SSRIS)

Serotonin is a neurotransmitter especially relevant in neurobiological basis in affective disorders, compulsive-obsessive disorder, and aggressive behavior.

SSRIs block the serotonin reuptake bombs action, augmenting serotonin concentration in synapsis and postsynapsis receptors' occupation. Though this effect appears early during treatment, clinical effects delay 3-6 weeks.

They are metabolized at liver, present a low affinity except for serotonin receptors, are enough sure in overdoses, change sleep structure (reduce latency and total amount of REM sleep) and might be avoid used with MAOIs, due to the risk of serotoninergic syndrome.

Therapeutic indications: Depression; Anxiety disorders, including Obsessive-Compulsive Disorder; Bulimia nervosa; Psychosomatic disorders

Precautions and adverse reactions: Sexual dysfunction, digestive discomfort, weight gain, headache, serotoninergic syndrome, anticholinergic effects, and other: hematological effects, alterations in electrolytes and glucose, allergic and endocrine reactions, galactorrea, and abrupt suspension discontinuation syndrome.

2.3 Noradrenalin selective reuptake inhibitors (reboxetine)

It selectively inhibits the reuptake of norepinephrine, but it has little effect on the reuptake of serotonin or dopamine. It is structurally related to fluoxetine. It has little affinity for muscarinic receptors or cholinergic and does not interact with the alfa1, alpha2, adrenergic beta, serotonergic, dopaminergic or histaminergic receptors. Therefore, SSRIs and reboxetine have some complementarity effects and are used together in the clinic in some resistant depressions.

Reboxetine has a rapid absorption; food does not affect the speed of it. It is metabolized in liver, mainly through the 3A4 isozyme of cytochrome P450 and it is excreted by kidney.

Medical indications: depressive disorders and social phobia. Adverse reactions: the most common are: faltering urination, headache, constipation, nasal congestion, sweating, dizziness, dry mouth, decreased libido, insomnia. Hypertension and tachycardia can appear at high doses, as well as psychomotor retardation if it is taken with alcohol. The syndrome of inappropriate secretion of antidiuretic hormone is exceptional. Precautions: contraindicated in pregnancy and breastfeeding. The doses must be reduced in elderly patients and serious renal impairment.

2.4 Inhibitors of the reuptake of serotonin and norepinephrine

2.4.1 Venlafaxine

It is a potent inhibitor of the reuptake of serotonin, at higher doses inhibits the reuptake of noradrenaline and slightly inhibits the reuptake of dopamine.

The absorption is good at digestive level and suffer important hepatic metabolism, by CYP 2D6 isoenzyme, so some SSRIs isozyme inhibitor drugs may increase plasma levels of venlafaxine, giving effects at low doses which are resolved once the inhibitor drug is withdrawn.

Therapeutic indications: depression, generalized anxiety disorder. Venlafaxine can be effective in: OCD, panic disorder, agoraphobia, social phobia, Attention Deficit and Hiperactivity Disorder (ADHD) and treatment of chronic pain. The most frequent side effects are nausea (less frequent with the retard formulation), drowsiness, dry mouth, dizziness, anxiety, constipation, asthenia, sweating, anxiety, anorexia, blurred vision, sexual dysfunction. A syndrome of discontinuation can appear if it stopped suddenly (nausea, drowsiness and insomnia...), so it should be reduced gradually. At high doses can precipitate high blood pressure.

It should be used cautiously in patients with pre-existing hypertension, administering lower doses, avoid its use in pregnancy and lactation and in children has not established safety or efficacy. In major liver or kidney function deterioration doses must be reduced. Venlafaxine overdosage may be more serious than with SSRIs and similar to tricyclic. It may be appropriate to avoid prescribing venlafaxine to patients who have high risk of poisoning.

2.4.2 Duloxetine

Like venlafaxine, it inhibits the reuptake of both serotonin and norepinephrine, Duloxetine has a minimal affinity for dopamine and histamine receptors.

It has significant hepatic metabolism, with many metabolites. It's a moderate inhibitor of CYP 2D6. Its excretion is renal.

Clinical indications: depression, Treatment of diabetic peripheral neuropathic pain. Contraindications: it must never be administered in patients with liver failure and it's not recommended in patients with terminal stage renal disease. Secondary gastrointestinal effects are common: nausea, dry mouth and constipation. Diarrhea and vomiting are less frequent. Insomnia, dizziness, somnolence and sweating are also common. Sexual dysfunction appears less frequently than with SSRIs, particularly in women.

2.4.3 Inhibitors of the reuptake of norepinephrine and dopamine (bupropion)

It is usually more effective on symptoms of depression than anxiety and quite useful in combination with SSRIs. It has some dopaminergic effects and therefore can induce mild psychostimulant effects. The mechanism of action is not known with accuracy. It seems that weakly inhibits the reuptake of dopamine, raising levels of it in the nucleus accumbens. This increase in dopamine levels in the "area of reward" of the brain may be responsible for the use of bupropion in the cessation. Some data indicate that it exerts its antidepressant effects increasing the functional efficiency of the noradrenergic systems. Apparently it has no effect on the serotonin system, so it is not effective to block panic attacks.

Pharmacokinetics: Good absorption at digestive tract; extensively metabolized in the liver. It seems to inhibit the isozyme CYP 2D6. It is also important to note that drugs that inhibit the isozyme will increase levels of bupropion, raising the risk of seizures.

Indications: depression: because of its stimulating effect, is used in depressive patients with fatigue and lack of concentration. The improvement of the sleep at the beginning of the treatment is less common than with other antidepressants, but does not alter sleep architecture. It is useful for abandonment of tobacco, in combination with conduct programs. It has also proposed its use in disorders attention deficit and on substance abuse (seems to decrease the craving in cocaine addiction).

Contraindications: Bulimia and anorexia, history of seizures or epilepsy, alcohol consumption, recent discontinuation of benzodiazepines, organic brain disease, cranial traumatism or EEG discharges. It isn't recommended in pregnancy or lactation.

The most common side effects are high respiratory discomfort, nausea, headache and insomnia. There may also be anxiety, agitation and irritability. It's the antidepressant with less inhibition of sexual function and it is more likely to reduce the weight than to increase it. The retard formulation is associated with an incidence of seizures of 0.1% at usual doses. Exceptionally it could cause psychotic hallucinations, delusions, catatonia symptoms, as well as delirium (by enhancing dopamine). It can increase blood pressure in previously hypertensive patients. There is no indication of significant effects on the heart, kidney or liver function.

2.5 Blockers of presynaptic autorreceptors: Mirtazapine

Its unique mechanism of action is blocking the receptors Alpha2 pre and post synaptic, as well as the serotonergic 5HT2 and 5HT3 receptors. In contrast to the TCA, mirtazapine has low affinity receptors alfa1 blocking. It has little interaction with receptors for acetylcholine, but blocks histamine receptors in a powerful way.

It is proposed that the antagonism of the presynaptic Alpha2 receptors leads to a significant increase in noradrenergic neurotransmission. This augmentation produced by mirtazapine increases the release of serotonin, producing the antidepressant effect.

Pharmacokinetics: rapid and complete absorption in the digestive tract; plasma clearance: up to 30% slower if there is impaired liver function, up to 50% slower if there is deterioration of kidney function. It has hepatic metabolism, by CYP 1A2, 3A4, 2D6 and CYP2C9.

Side effects: drowsiness (50% of treated patients). Managing at bedtime can be reduced. It appears more at low doses. It causes weight gain, increase in appetite, dry mouth, dizziness and lower risk of sexual dysfunction than with other antidepressants.

Precautions: it can increase levels of cholesterol and triglycerides, increase transaminases, reduce of the absolute count of neutrophils to 500/mm3 or below (some of the patients had symptomatic infections), it is a reversible alteration and is more likely to occur if there are other risk factors for neutropenia. In elderly individuals, kidney or liver failure can be necessary to use lower doses.

2.6 Serotoninergic modulators: Trazodone

Its mechanism of action is the modulation of serotonergic neurotransmission; it is a relatively specific inhibitor of the reuptake of serotonin. It does not cause any anticholinergic effects. It has Alfa1 adrenergic antagonism and antihistaminergic activity, so has more sedative effects than other antidepressants. The sedative effects appear to one hour after administration and antidepressant effects at 2-4 weeks.

Indications: Depression (especially effective in regulating the quality of sleep). Also it has been proposed for use in anxiety disorder, disorder panic, obsessive-compulsive disorder, insomnia, severe agitation in older people (50 mg/day), post-traumatic stress disorder (PTSD) and as coadjuvant in schizophrenia

Most common side effects: sedation (it is often used at low doses: 50 - 100 mg/day to induce sleep or treat insomnia due to SSRI); nausea, postural hypotension, priapism (rare, but dangerous).

Special situations: it has been rarely associated with cardiac arrhythmias and it should be used cautiously in patients with cardiac disease. It is contraindicated in pregnancy and lactation. It should be used cautiously in patients with kidney or liver disease.

2.7 Monoamine Oxidase Inhibitors (MAOIs)

They inhibit the enzyme MAO, who is responsible for the oxidative deamination of neurotransmitters such as serotonin, norepinephrine, or dopamine.

There are two ways for MAO enzyme: MAOa and MAOb. The MAOa metabolizes the monoaminergic neurotransmitters more closely associated with depression (norepinephrine and serotonin). The MAOb acts upon some aminergic substrates, called protoxins, toxins that can cause neural damage. Therefore the inhibition of the MAOa is associated both hypertensive effects and therapeutic effects. Inhibition of the MAOb is associated with the prevention of neurodegenerative disorders, such as Parkinson's disease processes.

The MAO is widely distributed in the body. The blockade of the MAOa in the gastrointestinal tract is responsible for the "cheese effect". It consists of a severe hypertensive crisis that occurs in patients who are taking MAOIs and ingest food containing tyramine. Tyramine is usually metabolized in the digestive tract but the blocking of the MAOa allowed their passage into general circulation. So, patients in treatment with IMAOs must follow a tyramine-restricted diet.

They exert their effects primarily in the CNS. They act on the mood, decreased sleep and insomnia and daytime sleepiness. They are characterized by a significant reduction of REM sleep. The MAOIs are not considered antidepressants in frontline due to restrictions in the diet, its pharmacological interactions and its broad side effect profile.

Medical indications: depression, Panic disorder, PTSD, eating disorders, social phobia and pain disorder.

Side effects: the most frequent: orthostatic hypotension, insomnia, weight gain, dry mouth, headache, edema, and sexual dysfunction. Rare: spontaneous hypertensive crisis. Rarely: paresthesias, myoclonus, and muscle ache. Confusion or drunkenness (it is necessary to reduce doses). They have few liver toxic effects and less cardiac effects than the tryciclic antidepressants.

RIMA (reversible monoamine oxidasa inhibitor: moclobemide) can produce dizziness, nausea and insomnia. It has less gastrointestinal effects than SSRIs and no sexual effect.

Special situations: caution in patients with renal, cardiovascular disease or hyperthyroidism. In diabetes they can reduce blood glucose, so physician can be forced to change the dose of hypoglycaemic drugs. They have been associated to manic induction in individuals in depressive phase of a Bipolar disorder type I and psychotic decompensation in patients with schizophrenia. They are contraindicated in pregnancy and lactation. In elderly: the MAO activity increases with age, so the dose of MAOIs to elderly people and young adults are the same. Phenelzine and isocarboxazid have been associated with significant risk of hepatotoxicity.

Drug interactions: can be serious and even fatal. They can never be administered with drugs that increase the concentrations at the synaptic level of biogenic amines: most antidepressants. There is risk of trigger a serotonin syndrome. They enhance alcohol and barbiturates, and other CNS depressants sedative effects. It is important to make a washing period when changing treatment.

Rich in tyramine foods must be avoided during treatment with a MAOIs: cheeses, cured meats, sausages, bananas, avocados, dried figs, smoked fish, chocolate, alcoholic beverages.

3. Classic and second generation antipsychotics

3.1 Classic antipsychotics

Among classis antipsychotics (AP) there is no one that has a clear superiority over the others, so choice must be made depending on previous response or side effects profile.

The AP are well absorbed orally, although their bioavailability is altered with the intake of certain foods, coffee, calcium antacids and excessive consumption of nicotine, which can reduce the absorption from the intestinal tract. They have great solubility and easily cross the blood-brain barrier.

Classic antipsychotics include: Clorpromacine, levomepromacine, flufenacine, perfenacine, trifluoperacine, haloperidol, zuclopentixol, molindone, and pimocide.

The AP show a great affinity for plasma proteins (85-90%), which involves risk of toxicity when other drugs that also bind to proteins are running simultaneously. On the other hand, given that they pass easily through the blood-brain barrier, concentrations achieved in CNS doubles those that are quantified in the peripheral circulation. They also cross the placental barrier, reaching to the fetus during pregnancy. Due to their lipophilic properties, antipsychotics are stored in the peripheral fat, so dialysis is ineffective in cases of overdose.

Traditional antipsychotic drugs are metabolized in the liver via hydroxylation and demethylation in cytochrome P450 processes. Some, such as haloperidol, suffer an additional glucuronidation and remain active as dopamine antagonists. Major isozymes in the metabolism of these drugs are the 2D6 and the 3A4. It is estimated that between 5 and 10% of individuals in white, and one much higher proportion of black individuals are slow track metabolizers of cytochrome P450 2D6, so it is predictable that submit side effects with a greater frequency and severity.

The AP are removed primarily by urine and feces, through bile, but also by the saliva, tears, sweat, and breast milk. The elimination half-life varies between 18 and 40 hours. In the elderly, who often have impaired kidney function to a greater or lesser extent, physician should proportionally reduce the dose.

3.1.1 Clinical Indications

The AP have been the most commonly used drugs in the treatment of acute episodes and as therapy for schizophrenia maintenance. Its mechanism of action is basically attributed to the blockade of receptors D2 between five types of recipient described dopamine. The blocking dopamine at mesolimbic track is responsible for the therapeutic effect, with reduction of delusions and hallucinations. For its part, the nigroestriada via controls movement, and so its blockade produces akathisia and dystonia and parkinsonism. The dopaminergic mesocortical via seems involved in the mediation of negative and cognitive symptoms of schizophrenia, and last but not least, the tubero-infundibular that controls the secretion of prolactin, blocked by antipsychotic medication stimulates production with galactorrhea.

The usefulness of antipsychotics in the treatment of affective disorders that have psychotic symptoms, as well as the acute control Mania and severe bipolar disorder is well known.

Antipsychotics are used as antiemetics and in the palliative treatment of some movement disorders as Huntington and other chorea disorders. Tics that characterised the Tourette's syndrome also respond well to dopamine antagonists.

The more sedative action and lower incidence of extrapyramidal side effects with some AP are particularly indicated for the treatment of great psychomotor agitation, especially in situations of urgency and in a timely manner.

3.1.2 Side effects

The low-power typical antipsychotics, those that require higher doses to produce therapeutic benefits, tend to have more sedative, anticholinergic, and antihypertensive effects than the most powerful drugs. At the same time the latter tend to cause more extrapyramidal symptoms because of the antagonistic effect of dopamine on the dopaminergic nigroestriatal via.

The anticholinergic effects of less incisive drugs, or incisive at high doses, cause sometimes problems in elderly and heavily dependent patients, which may present difficulties in concentration, decreased performance, confusion and delirium. These effects are more intense in the early stages of treatment and generate some tolerance over time. On the other hand, the less powerful drugs have idiosyncratic reactions more often. For example, chlorpromazine can cause hypersensitivity to light or greyish skin patches requiring the preventive use of sunscreens.

Extrapiramidalism: Akathisia, a subjective sensation of motor restlessness and associated psychological discomfort, is the most common extrapyramidal adverse effect. It can appear at any time, being most common at the beginning of the treatment. Akathisia can improve decreasing the dose of the antipsychotic or associating with it a β-Blocker such as propranolol or a long-life benzodiazepine.

Acute dystonia is a short, sharp and painful muscle spasm that usually affects the face muscles, neck (retrocolis spasm), back (opisthotonos) and the extraocular muscles. This side effect usually affects young males who had not received prior treatment with antipsychotic medication. Dystonia is much more prevalent, the greater is the power of the drug. Symptoms usually improve managing anticholinergic drugs.

Tardive dyskinesia is a persistent syndrome in patients that keep treatment with antipsychotic drugs for prolonged periods. It is characterized by involuntary and repetitive abnormal choreoatethosic movements of the head, trunk and extremities.

Neuroleptic Malignant Syndrome is a very serious idiosyncratic reaction that appears hours or days after the initiation or augmentation of treatment with antipsychotic drugs. There are elevation of transaminases and lactate dehydrogenase (LDH). This syndrome involves a mortality approaching 30% being the most common causes of death, cardiac arrhythmias, secondary respiratory failure, aspiration pneumonia and renal failure for rhabdomyolysis. Bromocriptine has traditionally been used for mild cases and dantrolene intravenous for more serious cases

Cardiac effects: due to the action of the AP on the adrenergic α1 receptors in the initial stages of the treatment may appear hypotension postural and tachycardia that tend to improve progressively with the time. The low-power APs may cause arrhythmia with widening of the QRS or QTc interval, polymorphous ventricular tachycardia and ventricular fibrillation.

Gastrointestinal side effects: due to the anticholinergic activity it appears dryness of mouth, nausea, vomiting and especially constipation that can even evolve towards ileus.

Endocrine effects of hyperprolactinemia: galactorrhea, menstrual disturbances, delays of ovulation and infertility, early reduction of bone density and osteoporosis, erectile dysfunction and decreased libido. They can precipitate increase in weight and intolerance to the carbohydrates and diabetes

Genitourinary effects: urinary retention and difficulty in starting urination, secondary urinary tract infections.

Hematological effects: leukopenia, (in general, it is temporal and it is not severe), thrombocytopenic Purpura, hemolytic anemia and pancytopenia

3.2 Atypical or Second Generation Antipsychotics (SGA)

Clozapine produces a total blockade of D2 receptors, so it does not cause extrapyramidal symptoms. Properties of clozapine are due to the combination of a low affinity for the D2 receptors along with strong affinity to serotonergic 5HT2A and 5HT1C, adrenergic and cholinergic receptors. Clozapine joins less intensely this receiver, which is displaced by endogenous dopamine. This property is present in many SGA, not only clozapine, so these drugs cause fewer movement disorders as side effects

The indication of clozapine is the treatment of schizophrenia in patients who do not respond (after at least two months of treatment at appropriate doses) or that they do not tolerate the AP, although occasionally prescribed for other purposes such as the treatment of psychosis by L-DOPA in Parkinson's disease patients with mania. It can produce leukopenia, so it's important to control it weekly during the first six months of treatment and every fifteen days from then. However, it should be noted that this risk is low, less than 1%. Other adverse effects are: orthostatic hypotension and tachycardia, increased sedation, and the decline of the seizure threshold with the consequent risk of convulsions in 5-10% of cases. Some patients develop a symptomatic complex called metabolic syndrome which consists of weight gain, increased insulin resistance, increased risk of diabetes type 2, and elevation of plasma lipids. Clozapine may increase plasma levels of enzymes such as transaminases GOT and GPT (alanino aminotransferase and aspartate aminotransferase), alkaline phosphatase, gamma glutamiltranspeptidasa (GGT) and lactate dehydrogenase.

Risperidone: Its mechanism of action is mediated by its high affinity for D2 receptors, 5HT2A receptors and the adrenergic $\alpha 1$ and $\alpha 2$ receptors. Unlike haloperidol shows a low affinity for muscarinic receptors for which leads to fewer anticholinergic effects. With a similar effectiveness or even something greater than haloperidol, involves a greater tolerance, although risperidone at high doses can also cause extrapyramidal symptoms.

It is considered a SGA first line in the treatment of psychoses with particular effectiveness in the prevention of recurrences. It has been used in child psychiatry in the treatment of aggressive and serious behaviour disorders.

There is an increase in brain-vascular accidents in connection with the use of risperidone and olanzapine in elderly patients with dementia, a complication which advised the prescription of this drug with much caution in such patients.

There is a long-acting form of risperidone that can be used twice a month in injection for maintenance treatment.

Adverse reactions that occur more frequently with therapeutic doses of risperidone are sedation, orthostatic hypotension, tachycardia, increase in weight and erectile dysfunction, hyperprolactinemia. At high doses anticholinergic effects such as dry mouth, constipation, changes in vision, and urinary retention may appear.

No significant pharmacological interaction with risperidone has been described what can be a great advantage in patients with a lot of pharmacological treatment, particularly in the framework of liaison psychiatry.

Olanzapine: its main indication has been the treatment of schizophrenia, acute episodes of mania and maintenance of bipolar affective disorder. Its structure is similar to clozapine and its mechanism of action is unknown, although it has a stronger affinity for the receptor 5HT2A than by the dopamine receptor D2. Olanzapine also acts at various levels, interacting with D1 and D2 dopaminergic, 5HT2A serotoninergic, H1 histaminergic, and muscarinic receptors.

Among his include anorexia nervosa, post-traumatic stress disorder and borderline personality disorder where, at low doses, it seems to improve objectives such as aggression and impulsiveness parameters.

Olanzapine is metabolized in the liver by oxidation and glucuronidation by cytochrome P450 isoenzyme 1A2. In smokers it must be important to adjust the dose, since the consumption of cigarettes induce 1A2 isozyme and increases drug elimination.

The main adverse effect that occurs in patients in treatment with olanzapine is weight gain, so, an important risk that must be taken into account in relation to this and other drugs which produce significant weight gain is the metabolic syndrome. Other side effects of olanzapine are: sedation, elevation of prolactin, leukopenia (without agranulocytosis), and decrease the seizure threshold. Olanzapine carries a lower risk of episodes of Parkinsonism, dystonia and tardive dyskinesia.

Quetiapine has clozapine similar profile, with a moderate affinity to D2 receptors and moderate-intense to 5HT2 serotoninergic repceptors. It is a partial agonist of 5HT1A receptors, which increase dopamine concentrations in mesocortical area, improving cognitive and negative schizophrenics symptoms.

It produces few extrapyramidal symptoms and risk of tardive dyskinesia. These features make it the choice for the treatment of disorders of behavior in Parkinson's patients and patients treated within the framework of liaison psychiatry. Undesirable side effects are sedation and weight gain with alteration of glucose and lipid metabolism. However, it does not produce a significant increase in prolactin levels

Quetiapine is metabolized in the liver by the cytochrome P450 3A4 enzyme, so drugs that produce a large inhibition of the isozyme (such as erythromycin) may increase their serum levels. Carbamazepine and phenytoin reduce levels of quetiapine as behave as enzyme inducers forcing adjust the dose to avoid possible relapse in patients who are simultaneously being treated with these drugs.

Ziprasidone has high antagonism of 5HT2A, 5HT1D, 5HT2C serotoninergic and D2 dopaminergic receptors. It has a low tendency to cause extrapyramidal effects because their high ratio 5HT2A / D2 and its low affinity for adrenergic, muscarinic and histaminergic receptors.

Ziprasidone is metabolized in the liver by isoenzymes 3A4 of the P450, through a process of reduction effect of aldehyde oxidase. Its bioavailability increase when ziprasidone is administrated along with food. This compound intensely joins proteins and has not been shown to see displaced by other drugs with similar affinity.

In addition to the indication in the acute treatment and maintenance of schizophrenia, given that it exists in injectable presentation, you can use in patients who do not collaborate in the taking of oral medication and in emergency situations characterized by agitation or serious behavior disorders.

It is the antipsychotic with a lesser influence upon weight. The most frequent adverse effects are drowsiness, insomnia, constipation and nausea. Normally these effects tend to be temporary and, in general, ziprasidone is well tolerated.

Amisulpiride: While it has no affinity for subtypes D1, D4 and D5 presents affinity on the D2 and D3 of the dopamine receptor subtypes. Unlike other AP, it has no affinity for serotonergic, adrenergic, cholinergic and H1 histaminergic receptors.

An important feature that distinguishes it from other antipsychotic group is its low liver metabolism which must be taken into account within the framework of the psychiatric consultations when treating patients with liver failure that you do not need to adjust the dose. Their degree of plasma protein binding is low (around 16%). The drug is eliminated through the kidneys in 90% during the first 24 hours. In patients with severe kidney disease dosages should be reduced.

Adverse reactions that occur most often are: insomnia, anxiety and even turmoil psychomotor, which can appear at the beginning of treatment and declining thereafter. As with other antipsychotics the amisulpiride can reduce the seizure threshold, which requires a control of treatment in patients with a history of seizures. A reversible increase of plasma levels of prolactin can be seen. No drug interactions with this compound have been described so far.

Aripiprazol: This is a partial agonist of dopamine receptor D2, D3 and serotonergic 5HT1A and works as a 5HT2A serotonin receptor antagonist.

In some situations aripiprazole would act as an antagonist and in others as agonist. That way there would be a self-regulation of dopamine, so the drug would act as antidopamine at the mesolimbic via and as prodopamine at the mesocortical via, without significantly affecting the nigroestriada or the tuberoinfundibular paths.

Its theoretical advantages would be improvement in cognitive aspects and motor effects in the long term such as tardive dyskinesia. It is metabolized in the liver by isoenzymes of the cytochrome P450 3A4, and 2D6 so that compounds which interact at this level (carbamazepine, quinidine, ketoconazole, fluoxetine and paroxetine) could alter the plasma concentrations of aripiprazole. It is a well tolerated drug that does not affect significantly the weight or the levels of prolactin for patients, or metabolism of glucose and lipids. The most frequent side effect is drowsiness.

Paliperidone: It is an active metabolite of risperidone. It presents a great affinity for 5HT2A receptors and moderated by the D2 receptors, with a lower lipophilicity than risperidone. The pharmacological activity of this compound is similar to other high power

SGA. The receptor binding profile is similar to risperidone and ziprasidone, though unlike risperidone and other SGA it has a low rate of hepatic metabolism. Its adverse effects are similar to the risperidone although they produce a greater increase in the rate of hyperprolactinemia.

4. Lithium and anticonvulsants

Although there is no agreed definition, stabilizer of the mood would be the drug with the potential to be used as monotherapy in acute bipolar disorder (BD) phases and its prophylaxis.

Lithium: Its mechanism of action is not clearly established, although it competes with other monovalent cations, such as sodium, altering metabolism and the action of certain neurotransmitters such as serotonin and Catecholamines.

Indications: bipolar and recurrent major depressive disorders. It has a narrow therapeutic range (between 0,60 and 1.5 mEq/L).

Contraindications Leukemia for possible reactivation.

Side effects: are frequent, could be severe and usually related to doses. Initial symptoms are nausea, diarrhea, abdominal pain, dizziness, muscle weakness, fine trembling hands. It can precipitate a rhenal Diabetes Insipidus (polyuria and polydipsia), which can lead to dehydration and increased toxicity. Hypothyroidism has benn described in prolonged treatments, it is recommended to carry out periodic checks on the thyroid function. Other: increase in weight, swelling, leukocytosis, hypercalcemia due to hyperparathyroidism, hipermagnesemia.

Interactions: the thiazides may reduce renal excretion of lithium and may increase its toxicity. NSAIDs: reduce renal excretion of lithium and increase the risk of toxicity, particularly indomethacin. The analgesic of choice if needed would be ASA and acetaminophen. Carbamazepine: have described cases of serious neurotoxicity. ACE Inhibitors: can decrease renal excretion of lithium in patients of advanced age, renal failure or hypovolemia. Selective serotonin reuptake inhibitors: risk of serotonin syndrome.

Valproate: It facilitates the action of GABA, a neural inhibitor neurotransmitter, and as a result decreases neuronal excitability.

Indications Epilepsy, Infantile febrile convulsions, Bipolar disorder

It is postulated that there is a good correlation between the pharmacological effect and the plasma concentration, with a margin of optimal concentration of 50-150 mg/l. Some patients respond to concentrations outside this interval. Valproic acid is hepatotoxic.

Side effects are relatively frequent and usually transient or dose-related adverse effects. Gastrointestinal: nausea and vomiting, polyphagia with weight gain; rarely pancreatitis; increase of liver enzymes, hepatitis and hepatic encephalopathy syndrome (Reye in children), has described particularly in the first months of treatment. Nervous system: tremor and headache (usually the first sign of overdose), drowsiness, ataxia, confusion, dementia. Hematological: idiosyncratic depression of the bone marrow with thrombocytopenia, leukopenia and agranulocytosis, not related to the dose in nature. Skin: idiosyncratic character.

Special situations

- Liver function: recommended a special control of high-risk patients, including the epilepsy with combination therapy, and evaluate the liver function before treatment and for at least every six.
- Discontinuation of treatment: the sudden suspension of the drug should be avoided because of the risk of seizures.
- Pregnancy: category D of the FDA. Isolated cases of defects of the neural tube in newborn infants, especially in women with combination therapy have been described. It has been observed that the incidence is higher than with other antiepileptic drugs. It is recommended to assess each case carefully, because the risk of the treatment is lower than the derivative of precipitate seizures. In any case, it is recommended to take supplements of folic acid before conception and during pregnancy to prevent these defects.
- Lactation: it is excreted in breast milk in a proportion that does not seem to pose risk to the infant. It is compatible, although some cases of thrombocytopenia associated with valproic in an infant has been described.

Interactions Carbamazepine, phenytoin, and Phenobarbital: the interaction is complex and unpredictable. Polytherapy recommends adjusting the dosage on plasma levels and the patient's clinical status. Lamotrigine: valproic increases lamotrigine plasma levels by inhibiting its metabolism. In addition, severe toxic reactions (rash, tremors) have been described. It is recommended halving the dose of lamotrigine.

Carbamazepine: It inhibits the voltage-dependent sodium channels of the CNS neurons, reducing neuronal excitability of the epileptic focus. It also has analgesic and antimaniac properties.

Indications: Epilepsy, Trigeminal neuralgia, Bipolar disorder and potential use in impulsive disorder, addiction and personality disorders.

Hematological, hepatic, renal and cardiac functions and electrolytes should be explored before starting treatment. Plasma levels are: optimum plasma concentration 6 - 12 mg/L in monotherapy and 4 - 8 mg/L in combination therapy.

Contraindications: A history of depression of the bone marrow, Atrioventricular conduction disturbances, Porphyria due to risk of exacerbation of disease.

Adverse effects are relatively frequent (up to 50% of patients) and generally related to the dose.

- Nervous system: drowsiness, dizziness, headache, blurred vision and dyplopia, nausea and vomiting, confusion and agitation (in older people).
- Hematological: idiosyncratic character, unrelated with the dose. Leukopenia, thrombocytopenia, agranulocytosis, and rare cases of fatal aplastic anemia has been occasionally described.
- Skin: idiosyncratic character. Regard rash, rarely Stevens-Johnson Syndrome.
- Other: hyponatremia, urinary retention, impotence, proteinuria, glycosuria, peripheral neuropathy, paresthesias, tinnitus, alopecia.

Precautions

- Liver failure: increases the risk of toxicity because the drug is eliminated mostly by this route. It is recommended to carry out periodic checks on the liver function.
- Renal insufficiency: increases the risk of toxicity because the active metabolite is eliminated through the kidneys. It should adjust the dose according to the functional level.
- Heart failure: can worsen and cause arrhythmia and fluid retention.
- Blood disorders: increases the risk of aplastic anemia or agranulocytosis. It is recommended to carry out periodic checks on hemogram.
- Alcohol: it should be avoided because it induces hepatic metabolism of the drug and is epileptogenic
- Suspension of the treatment: the sudden suspension should be avoided because there is a risk of seizure.
- Pregnancy: category C of the FDA. Although isolated cases of abnormalities in newborns have been described, it is recommended not to suspend the antiepileptic treatment unless the risk of seizures is low, because the risk of the treatment is lower than the derivate of precipitate seizures.
- Breastfeeding: it is excreted in breast milk in a proportion that does not seem to pose risk to the infant. It is compatible, although at high doses there is risk of liver disease in infant.
- Geriatrics: it is recommended to use lower initial doses, usually half of it and adjust according to plasma level.

Interactions: With Phenytoin, valproic acid the interaction is complex, because both can induce the metabolism of the other. Occasionally neurotoxicity can appear with lithium.

Oxcarbazepine: It is a carbamazepine analog, and its indications are partial seizures with or without secondary generalization, bipolar disorder and other potential uses in psychiatry as carbamazepine.

Side effects:

- Nervous system: frequently, drowsiness, headache, and dizziness. Also nystagmus, Vertigo. Occasionally ataxia, agitation, difficulty in concentration.
- Gastrointestinal: frequently, nausea and vomiting. Occasional constipation, diarrhea, and abdominal pain. Occasionally increase in liver transaminases
- Skin: rash, acne, alopecia.
- Eye: frequently diplopia, blurred vision.
- Hyponatremia: it can be severe, especially for elderly, renal failure or treatment with diuretics.

Special situations:

- Suspension of the treatment: the sudden suspension should be avoided because it can cause seizures.
- Pregnancy: category C of the FDA. Malformations in animals have been described but there is no information in humans.
- Breastfeeding: Oxcarbazepine and its active metabolite are largely excreted in breast milk. Although the effects on the infant are unknown, its use is not recommended.

- Renal insufficiency: half of the initial dose is recommended in case of serious failure and then adjust the dose more slowly

Lamotrigine: It reduces the excitability of neuronal inhibitor dependent sodium channels and blocks the release of glutamate. Its indications are epilepsy, Lennox-Gastaut syndrome and bipolar disorder

Side effects: They are relatively common, while in most cases these effects are minimized if the dose is gradually increased. It can produce headache, dizziness and drowsiness; nausea and vomiting, and abdominal pain; dyplopia, nystagmus, arthralgia, sore back, depression of the bone marrow (anemia, leukopenia, thrombocytopenia and associated infections) and dysmenorrhoea.

Special situations:

- Liver failure: increases the risk of toxicity because the drug is eliminated mostly by this route. Initial and maintenance doses should be reduced typically in moderate failure to 50% and 75% in the event of serious failure.
- Pregnancy: cat.C of the FDA. There has been an increase in the risk of oral fissure.
- Lactation: excreted in milk, can reach therapeutic concentrations in the infant.

Gabapentine: It is structurally similar to GABA with antiepileptic and analgesic action. It facilitates neural inhibitory action of this neurotransmitter, and consequently decreases the epileptic crises responsible of neuronal excitability. It is eliminated by renal excretion with a half-life of 5-7 hours, unlike traditional antiepileptic, eliminated by hepatic metabolism.

Special situations:

- Renal insufficiency: due to it is removed by this way, it is important to adjust the dose to the functional level.
- Special activities: the onset of drowsiness and dizziness before driving or operate dangerous machinery must be controlled.
- Pregnancy: category C of the FDA.
- Lactation: it is excreted in breast milk but unknown effects on the infant. Caution is advised.

Topiramate: It inhibits the voltage sodium dependent channels implicated in the spread of the epileptic focus, it reduces the excitatory action of glutamate. It is eliminated by renal excretion with a half-life of 20-24 hours.

Indications: Epilepsy in adults and children (monotherapy or combination therapy), Lennox-Gastaut syndrome, in combination therapy. Migraine prophylaxis in patients. Bulimia with overweight and alcoholism, binge disorder and bipolar disorder

Side effects: are frequent but generally moderate. They can be minimized by gradually increasing the dose and usually resolve spontaneously over treatment or when the dose is reduced. Nervous system: 10-30% of patients can suffer from fatigue and sleepiness and paresthesias at the beginning of treatment, although they are not usually serious. It also produces ataxia, nervousness, confusion, loss of concentration, anxiety, depression, cognitive disturbances. Visual: the first month of treatment may be acute nearsightedness, diplopia and/or nystagmus, not related to the dose, which can lead to glaucoma.

Gastrointestinal: abdominal pain, nausea, anorexia, taste alterations, gingivitis. Other: anorexia and weight loss associated with a diuretic effect (very common) and nephrolithiasis.

Special situations: there is risk of formation of nephrolithiasis in patients with antecedents. It is necessary to maintain adequate hydration during the treatment. As it is excreted through the kidneys, in renal failure doses must be reduced up to 50%.

Pregabaline: It is structurally similar to GABA, with antiepileptic, anxiolytic and analgesic action. It facilitates neural inhibitory action of this neurotransmitter and consequently decreases the epileptic crises.

Indications: Treatment of adult central and peripheral neuropathic pain. Epilepsy in adults: combined treatment of partial seizures with or without secondary generalization. Anxiety disorders in adults.

5. Benzodiacepines

Benzodiacepines (BZD) are CNS depressors with anxiolytic and hypnotic-sedative properties, and antiepileptic and muscle relaxing effects. They are more secure in overdoses than barbiturates and other sedative drugs. They have similar action mechanism and side effects, and differ in onset time and activity duration, which is relevant in treatment and indications.

Absorption in the gastrointestinal tract is very good, especially on an empty stomach, so that the oral via is the choice for these agents. Diazepam and clorazepate are absorbed more quickly than the others. Other routes of administration are less recommended and should be reserved only for cases of urgency: the intramuscular absorption is erratic and intravenous absorption can be dangerous. The BZD are lipophilic agents, so cross the blood-brain barrier well, exerting their action at the level of the central nervous system quickly. They also cross the placental barrier and are excreted through breast milk. Furthermore, their solubility makes that most of them are accumulated, gradually, in body fat resulting in a high volume of distribution, which directly influences the duration of the action.

The biotransformation is at hepatic level through a process of oxidation and conjugation. Some BZD (such as the diacepam or cloracepato) have pharmacologically active metabolites which, sometimes, even have longer life than the active ingredient.

In addition, should take into account that in the healthy elderly these processes are altered, so you have to choose BZD not metabolized by microsomal liver enzymes and without active metabolites as oxazepam or lorazepam. They are eliminated on a majority basis through the kidneys (70-90%), after their hepatic metabolism. The rest are eliminated through the stool or bile.

All BZD's action is at CNS, by their ability to enhance the inhibitory actions of GABA, stimulating the GABA-A receptor. It is believed that their anxiolytic action is due to the inhibitory action on neurons in the limbic system, including the amygdala, and serotonergic and noradrenergic neurons of the CNS. The fact that ethanol, barbiturates, and BZD have similar actions on the same receptor explains their drug synergy (and therefore the danger of the combined overdose) and its cross tolerance. This last property is used in the detoxification of alcoholics with BZD.

5.1 Other hypnotics/anxiolytics agents

Zolpidem, zopiclone and zaleplon: Three non-benzodiacepinic preparations that interact with a smaller subset of receptor GABA-A (type 1), therefore presenting crossed reactivity with these to some extent. It seems that by their more selective binding, they are effective for short-term insomnia treatment, but they lack significant muscle relaxing, anti-epileptic and anti-anxiety effects. They have lower risk of dependence and abstinence than BZD.

Buspirone: It is believed that it exerts anxiolytic effect acting as a partial agonist of the 5-HT1A receptors (of serotonin). Its advantages include the absence of induced physical dependence and withdrawal, does not interact with alcohol or other CNS depressants, has no sedative effect and amnesiante, does not diminish the psychomotor performance and not depressed respiration (being useful in the elderly and patients with respiratory problems). Its main drawback is the delay in the onset of the anxiolytic effect (up to 2 weeks) and its ineffectiveness in patients previously treated with BZD.

5.2 Adverse effects and contraindications

The most frequent adverse effects are: drowsiness, sedation and psychomotor performance. Anterograde amnesia is associated with the use of more powerful BZD. Very rarely allergic reactions or a paradoxical increase in aggressiveness have been described. They can produce respiratory deficiency in patients with chronic obstructive pulmonary disease or sleep apnea. They should be administered with caution in patients with substance abuse, liver disease, kidney disease, Porphyria, depression from CNS or myasthenia gravis. Despite being one of the tools most often used in cases of suicidal ideation, Benzodiazepines alone are relatively safe in overdose (especially as compared with other sedatives like barbiturates). In addition, the fact of having selective antagonists of the benzodiacepinic receptor, such as Flumazenil, limited the dangerousness of these poisonings. The most dangerous effects occur when administered concomitantly with other sedatives such as alcohol (in these cases can occur excessive sleepiness, disinhibition and respiratory depression, as well as severe cognitive deficits).

Buspirone, zolpidem, zopiclone and zaleplon can produce nausea, dizziness and headaches, and except the first, others can also produce drowsiness and certain anterograde amnesia.

There are few absolute contraindications for BZD: allergic reactions to the drug and angle closure glaucoma. Other related are: severe apnea sleep, first trimester of pregnancy, respiratory failure and cognitive disorders.

5.3 Tolerance and dependence

All BZD may exhibit properties of tolerance and dependence. However, there is to be noted that they do not constitute a group of drugs of addictive nature, as with the characteristics of drugs of abuse have no place tolerance is defined as the increasingly low intense effects production, maintaining the same dose of drugs. The use of BZD at long term can cause a phenomenon of tolerance to their pharmacological effects, it is clearer to the hypnotic, sedative effect and impaired psychomotor performance (1-2 weeks tolerance). On the other hand, tolerance to the anxiolytic effects and mnesic is very unlikely, and when it appears, at very late onset.

Most antianxiety agents give after their sudden suspension, a series of symptoms of withdrawal or "deletion syndrome" which usually correspond to the image in mirror of its therapeutic effects

5.4 Clinical indications

Anxiety, insomnia, depression, alcohol deshabituation. Although Benzodiazepines are marketed for other indications (such as fluracepam, temacepam or triazolam for insomnia, or diazepam for anxiety) is likely all drugs of this class to share most of their therapeutic properties. The indications for which they are adopted reflect many times commercial decisions rather than a rational therapeutic. It is best to choose the drug based on differences in pharmacokinetic and power.

5.5 Special situations

Pregnancy and breastfeeding: BZD cross the placental barrier and GABA is involved in the reorganization of the massif of the palate. There are studies in which there has been an increase of teratogenia in pregnant women treated with chlordiazepoxide during the first quarter and retrospective studies and cases in which noted an increase in risk of cleft palate and cleft lip associated with the use of BZD by the mother.

- Syndrome of the hypotonic newborn: depression of the CNS, with hypotonia, lethargy, weak suction and respiratory depression.
- Neonatal abstinence syndrome: hyperactivity, irritability, and hypertonia.

BZD are excreted in breast milk. Infants metabolize them slowly, so it is possible the accumulation and toxicity, with lethargy, feeding difficulty and weight loss as well as withdrawal symptoms in the infant. For this reason, and despite the fact that the plasma/milk proportions are low in some BZD is necessary the evaluation of risk-benefit from the establishment of breastfeeding. In case of need for treatment BZD in postpartum period, as a general rule will be necessary to resort to artificial feeding.

Elderly: There is the need of a special caution in the treatment with BZD in this population due to there is increased sensitivity to the pharmacological action, there are deficiencies in the hepatic metabolization (reducing the reactions of phase I: oxidation) and possible decreases in renal elimination, increase in the amount of free medication for decrease in plasma proteins, increase in the volume of distribution with the possibility of accumulation. These cause an increase in side effects in this population: sedation, cognitive alterations and decline of the alert. There is an increase in the risk of falls and fractures and an increased risk of suffering from delirium, especially in treatments with long half life BZD. It is recommended a reduction of 30 to 50% of the doses, and the use of short half life BZD that are metabolized in phase II (glucuronidation) as oxazepam and lorazepam.

Children and adolescents: There are few studies of effectiveness/security in concrete disorders, and there is risk of abuse/dependence and paradoxical reactions.

Liver insuficience: Liver failure affects mainly the metabolic processes involving the cytochrome P450. So, there have been significant increases in the half-life of diazepam, chlordiazepoxide and its metabolites. Also, the metabolism of alprazolam, clobazam and diazepam and midazolam is affected significantly in cirrhosis, it would be advisable to drop doses in these BZD. BZD who suffer processes of glucuronidation (lorazepam, oxazepam and temazepam) are little affected in liver failure, being at low doses the choice treatment. Patients with liver failure are more sensitive to the sedative effects of BZD, and these may precipitate hepatic encephalopathy, so they are contraindicated in cases of serious-preencefalopatic liver failure and hepatic encephalopathy.

Renal failure: When treating with BZD patients with renal failure is necessary to take into account: the degree of renal failure, the existence of active metabolites, whose clearance may be diminished and binding to plasma proteins. To avoid this risk, is preferable to the use of BZD without active metabolites in low doses.

Respiratory failure: The BZDs, due to its CNS depressant effect, can reduce ventilatory response to hypoxia, so they must be used with caution in patients with COPD and are contraindicated in sleep apnea.

Porphyria: The hepatic metabolism of BZD may enhance the synthesis of ALAsintetasa, giving rise to an increase of Porphyrin with exhacerbación of the disease.

Dementia and delirium: Action on the CNS of BZD has been linked to cognitive impairment and their use in patients with dementia can precipitate delirium, so, as far as possible, it's better to avoid their use, being preferable to the use of antipsychotics in low doses. In delirium, except for the secondary to abstinence from alcohol or benzodiazepines, it is necessary to avoid the use of BZD, especially those of long half life, as they may aggravate the confusional syndrome.

Interactions: The main pharmacodynamic of BZD interactions occur with central nervous system depressant drugs (opioids, barbiturates, anticonvulsants, anesthetics, tricyclic antidepressants, central antihistamines, MAOIs, antipsychotic drugs and alcohol). In combination with these drugs, there is a strengthening of the depression of the CNS, which increased sedation, impaired psychomotor and respiratory depression.

Pharmacokinetic interactions are those related to the absorption, fixation to plasma proteins, metabolism and excretion. BZD requiring metabolization by reactions of phase I are influenced by processes of inhibition and metabolic induction, unlike BZD who suffer glucoronización are hardly influenced.

6. Drugs used in opioid addiction: Methadone

Methadone is an opioid analgesic with an outstanding action on the mu receptor. In cases of opioid dependence methadone is useful for treatment of detoxification, maintenance, and harm reduction.

Side effects: The most frequent are nausea, vomiting, constipation, sweating, sedation, euphoria, dependency and respiratory depression. In addition, it has a special impact effects on sexual function (decreased libido, decrease of serum levels of testosterone in men) and endocrine (deficit of production of ACTH and subsequent secondary hyposuprarrenalism cases). Other less common but important side effects are: urinary retention, agitation, drowsiness, headache, disturbance of sleep, confusion and psychotic symptoms.

Special situations: Opioid analgesics are generally contraindicated in acute respiratory depression, obstructive respiratory processes and patients in treatment with opioid antagonists (naltrexone). They are also contraindicated or should be used with great caution in alcoholism, seizure disorders, head injuries and processes that have increased intracranial pressure. They must not be administered to patients in a coma. In patients with biliary disorders it's usually recommended to avoid the use of opiates. Opioid analgesics should be administered with caution or dosage reduced in patients with: hypothyroidism, adrenocortical insufficiency, asthma, or decreased respiratory reserve, kidney or liver failure, prostate hyperplasia, hypotension, shock, inflammatory or obstructive intestinal disorders and myasthenia gravis. The dose should be reduced in elderly or debilitated patients. Methadone can prolong cardiac QT interval, increasing the risk of torsades de pointes, which implies risk of sudden death.

7. Stimulants

It is a group of drugs that in addition to its use in hyperactivity (ADHD) and attention deficit disorder have been used in the treatment of resistant depression, and narcolepsy.

Amphetamine is a sympathomimetic which facilitates the release of NA and dopamine. It has a strong stimulatory effect on the central nervous system (CNS), particularly with regard to the cerebral cortex

Side effects: The most frequent are anxiety, agitation, and decrease in sleep. Sometimes, dry mouth, anorexia, colic and other gastrointestinal discomfort. They can also lead to headaches, dizziness, tremors, sweating, tachycardia, palpitations and elevation (sometimes decrease) of blood pressure. Serious adverse effects such as psychosis, arrhythmias, hyperthermia, rhabdomyolysis, and seizures, especially with toxic doses that in some cases are not necessarily high are described. There is reasonable evidence that stimulant medication, especially at high doses, inhibits growth moderately. There are indications of that part of the growth is recovered when the treatment is interrupted.

Special situations: It is contraindicated in patients with cardiovascular disease, including hypertension moderate to severe, and in patients with hyperthyroidism, glaucoma, psychosis, or states of agitation. It is more likely abusive consumption in patients with a history of alcoholism or drug addiction. Amphetamines can trigger symptoms in patients with tics or Gilles de la Tourette syndrome.

Methylphenidate: Methylphenidate is a stimulant of the central nervous system and an indirect sympathomimetic (inhibits the reuptake of norepinephrine and dopamine) with the same indications as dexamfetamine. It is indicated in Narcolepsy, ADHD and Treatment-resistant depression. The most frequent adverse effects are similar to amphetamines.

Modafinil is a "wakefulness Enhancer compound". It selectively activates the hypothalamus areas that regulate the vigilia-sueño cycle, although the exact mechanism of action is not known. It is indicated in narcolepsy, excessive daytime sleepiness adults, in ADHD improves attention and impulse control. Adverse effects on the CNS may give rise to nervousness, excitement, irritability, insomnia and anorexia, which rarely require the removal of the treatment. Also it has been associated with gastrointestinal disorders, such as nausea and abdominal pain, dry mouth, headache, and cardiovascular effects such as hypertension, palpitations and tachycardia. Modafinil is contraindicated in patients with hypertension of moderate to severe cardiac arrhythmias, it is not recommended in patients with a history of left ventricular hypertrophy or coronary alterations of the EKG, chest pain and prolapse of the mitral valve.

8. Non-stimulant treatment of ADHD

Atomoxetine is a selective inhibitor of the reuptake of norepinephrine used in the treatment of the attention deficit and hyperactivity disorder in adolescents and children from 6 years.

Adverse effects described in patients in treatment with Atomoxetine include dyspepsia and other gastrointestinal disorders, anorexia and weight loss, fatigue, disturbances of sleep, irritability, and mood swings. Also hypertension, tachycardia, dizziness, cough, sinusitis or runny nose, bed wetting or urinary retention, decrease of libido and sexual dysfunction, rash, increased sweating and hot flashes. Rarely, hypersensitivity reactions occur. There have been some reports of serious hepatotoxicity. Atomoxetine is contraindicated in patients with glaucoma. It should be used with caution in patients with hypertension, tachycardia, or cerebrovascular or cardiovascular disease. Treatment with Atomoxetine should start with caution in patients with a history of seizures. There is a potential risk of seizures with Atomoxetine.

9. Special situations

9.1 Psychiatric drugs in pregnancy and lactation

All psychotropic so far studied cross the placenta, most reach the amniotic fluid and almost all are eliminated through breast milk. 3-5% of the newborns have genetic malformations; 65-70% by unknown factors, hereditary factors 12-25%, 10% by environmental factors (drugs, infections, diseases...) and 3% by direct exposure to drugs. Most studies suggest that the psychotropic drugs are not associated with a significantly increased risk of organic disgenesias. Congenital anomalies are not more frequent in a group of regular consumers of drugs compared with a control group. Perinatal mortality was similar in both groups (0.8% and 0.9%). It is essential to inform the patient of the potential risks of medication, obtain the informed consent of the patient, taking into account the ability and desire to tolerate the symptoms without drugs.

Absortion	**Metabolism**
Decrease in the rate of gastric emptying. Reduction of intestinal motility.	Increase in cardiac output. Changes in the activity of various liver enzymes
Distribution	Elimination
Increase of blood flow in the tissues. Increase in plasma volume. Increase in the extracellular fluid volume. Increase in adipose tissue (nearly all psychotropic are highly fat-soluble). Changes in the concentration of some plasma proteins.	Increase in the renal blood flow. Increased glomerular filtration rate.

Table 1. Changes in drug metabolism during pregnancy

The prescription of psychoactive drugs only must be made if the benefit (to mother) is greater than the risk (to the fetus). If possible, avoid all drugs (especially during the first trimester of pregnancy) and managing the minimum effective dose. It is preferable to use drugs already tested with good safety profile, than new drugs, with a theoretical more secure profile but not tested. Smaller than 1,500 molecular weight drugs can cross the placental barrier and potentially affect the fetus, but few have demonstrated teratogenic effects. It is important to provide contraceptive information to women in chronic treatment and review the treatment early in the pregnancy.

Due to changes in pharmacokinetic and pharmacodynamic factors during pregnancy, often different doses are needed (may be higher or lower) than in normal conditions to treat the symptoms properly.

The intensity of fetal exposure to the psychotropic also depends on the placental transference: Type I or complete transference: the concentrations are quickly balanced between maternal and fetal compartments; Type II or excessive transference: Fetal drug concentrations are higher than the maternal ones; Type III or incomplete transference: Fetal concentrations are lower than the maternal ones.

9.2 Elderly

General elderly people have a health more fragile than other stages of life. They suffer from various diseases and receive different treatments, which leads to higher risk of adverse reactions. As a result of this overlap pharmacokinetics and pharmacodynamics changes in this age group and responses to treatments are different. Variations in therapeutic response and side effects and interactions, which are more frequent and more serious, result in more yatrogenia and worst compliance.

Interactions in the elderly, drug interactions are between 3 and 5 times more frequent than in other stages of life. The elderly modifies the absorption process. Esophageal motility is reduced. The aclorhydria increases with age. Gastric motility and intestinal irrigation are reduced. But, in general, all these changes in the absorption are not very relevant from a clinical point of view.

The majority of psychoactive drugs, except lithium, are lipophilic and go preferably to fatty tissue, including the brain. With age, albumin decreases and increases the proportion of free drug, increases the fat mass generally between 25-40%, it's reduced lean mass and the proportion of body water, especially with relative increase in the extracellular intracellular water, which increases the volume of distribution of soluble drugs and decreases of the water-soluble. Clinically the relevance is moderate but it can extend drugs half-life.

Old age significantly modifies the metabolism by loss of hepatic mass, decreased blood flow, lower microsomial enzyme activity and tendency to prolong the half-life. From the age of 65, hepatic perfusion is reduced in about one-third.

With age, glomerular filtration and hepatic metabolism are reduced which leads to increase drug concentration and, consequently, increasing the therapeutic and toxic effect. It can be compensated reducing the dose or spacing this. Drugs with long half life tend to accumulate.

Elders suffer almost always several concomitant pathologies so they receive the respective treatments. The majority of clinical trials have been developed in younger people. Receiving different products makes pharmacokinetic and pharmacodynamics interactions more frequent. It is common that an older is receives at least 6-8 drugs a day, each with its corresponding mechanism of action, side effects that join or therapeutic effects to be antagonized. In addition, it's not exceptional self-medication through acquaintances or relatives, with increased risk.

The frequency of adverse reactions is doubled in the elderly with respect to those that occur among adults and its severity is much greater. The greater is the number of drugs receives, higher is the risk. In elderly the most frequent adverse reactions are acute confusional states, psychomotor agitation, instability and falls, extrapyramidal symptoms, constipation or incontinence, anticholinergic symptoms, orthostatic hypotension or impaired heart function. If these factors are not taken into account, the yatrogenia among the old can be high and with unpredictable consequences.

9.3 Psychopharmacology in children and adolescents

The decision to use a pharmacological treatment in a child or adolescent with psychiatric disease should be based on a clear clinical need. Prepubescent children often metabolize drugs rapidly and tolerate doses of drugs per unit weight slightly higher than the adult. After puberty, metabolism seems to young adults. In general if a drug is safe in adults, it will be also in children. The period of maximum drug vulnerability is in the intrauterine stage. The majority of psychoactive drugs have not been approved by the FDA for use in children and adolescents, mainly because there are no studies to support it.

1. Psychiatric diagnosis must be made before the prescription of psychotropic drugs.
2. Define clearly target symptoms and the goals of treatment for the use of psychotropics
3. The doctor should carefully consider the possible side effects, including those which are rare but potentially serious, and assess the overall benefits from the risk of pharmacological treatment except in cases of urgency.
4. Informed consent must be obtained before starting medication psychotropic
5. Monotherapy wherever possible
6. Doses must be, in general, low and when it's necessary to increase, do it carefully.
7. The frequency of doctor-patient follow-up should be appropriate according to the severity of the pathology and must comply with to control the response.
8. In the treatment of depression, it's important to assess the possibility of that emerge suicidal tendencies during the treatment, especially at the beginning.
9. If who carries out the prescription is not a child psychiatrist, the patient must be sent for consultation specializing in child and adolescent mental health.
10. Before adding other psychotropic medications, it should be evaluated the proper adherence to treatment, the accuracy of the diagnosis, the emergence of comorbid disorders, and the influence of psychosocial stressors.
11. If a drug is being used for a symptom not associated to a diagnosis of psychotic disorder in DSM IV, and this symptom has been in remission for six months, it should be considered seriously to initiate the reduction and subsequent suspension of the drug. If you decide to continue with treatment, the need of it should be evaluated at least every six months.
12. The clinician must clearly document the care provided in the medical record, including medical history, mental status evaluation, physical findings (when appropriate), the diagnostic impressions, a proper follow-up of laboratory tests to rule out use of substances and the potential known risks, response to medication, presence or absence of side effects, treatment plan and prescripted medications.

10. Hepatic failure

With the notable exception of the lithium the liver is the responsible for the clearance of the majority of psychoactive drugs, as they are generally lipophilic and therefore need to be transformed into water-soluble compounds so that they can be filtered and eliminated by the kidney. This transformation takes place largely in the liver, but also occurs to a lesser extent in other tissues. The inactivation is carried out by the large number of enzymes available in hepatocytes, which are responsible for reducing the size of the molecules or to add components to turn them into more hydrosoluble, with the final result of an easier elimination.

Due to the anatomical arrangement of the blood circulation of the gastrointestinal tract, absorbed drugs cross the liver before entering the general circulatory system. On some occasions, originated substance is an active metabolite, although the level of activity can vary widely. This effect called "first step" at times is very significant. This phenomenon also helps explain why parenteral medications are often more powerful than the oral equivalent. For example, antipsychotic drug intramuscular administration has approximately twice the power of those administered by mouth, although this varies widely from patient to patient.

The greater the degree of liver failure, greater degree of alteration of metabolism, and therefore, higher risk of toxicity from drugs. As a result, it is convenient to use possible smaller start dose, gradually setting it up to a maximum dose as low as possible. Patients are going to suffer more readily predictable or frequent adverse effects. Liver function tests do not necessarily correlate well with the deterioration of the metabolism, although they can serve as a reasonable approximation. It is important to be very careful with drugs with a high first pass metabolism, which in case of liver disease will be a minor inactivation during transport from the intestine to the circulatory system and therefore will be far higher plasma levels. As a general rule, avoid drugs that have marked effects like constipation and sedation in patients with severe liver disease. Monitor - wherever possible - the plasma levels of the drugs used

11. Renal failure and psychoactive drugs

If the drug is dialyzable, such as lithium, it will experience a sharp decline in its blood levels after dialysis, so post-dialytic of such drugs levels should be obtained to determine what amount is provided after the process. Certain drugs that are metabolized / eliminated by the kidney will accumulate, with the risk of toxicity, despite not using high doses of these, so that such drugs should be avoided or give at lower doses.

In general, the doses to be used will be two-thirds of the usual doses of the drug, except drugs with primarily renal elimination, in which will have to evaluate the clearance of creatinine (ClCr) as an indicator of renal function and the dose to use of the drug. Plasma levels of the drug in question must be controlled, at least once a month, and immediately after the initial dose of medication must provide wherever possible.

In renal failure protein binding is lower than in healthy individuals, so usually there is a greater amount of free drug in plasma, with higher therapeutic and side effects. The higher protein binding, the lesser dialyzable is the drug, what it's important to prescribe lower doses. In general, the most of the psychotropic substances aren't dialyzable, except lithium, gabapentine, pregabaline and others.

12. Cardiopathy and arterial hypertension

Antidepressant in cardiac illness must be used in therapeutical efficient doses, not lower doses, because metabolism is not affected if there is no hepatic afectation. Tryciclic antidepressants have severe cardiac side effects, so they have to be avoided if there is not a clear indication, monitoring EKG frequently. Venlafaxine can increase arterial tension in high doses. SSRIs, bupropion and mirtazapine are secure in cardiac patients. Stimulants have to be avoided due to cardiac effects.

Lithium can produce sinodal nodus dysfunction and can be altered if there are rapid alterations of electrolite equilibrium. Carbamacepine has quinidin-like effects.

Antipsychotic drugs can prolong QT interval and produce orthostatic hypotension, and new substances can induce diabetes mellitus type II and weight gain.

13. Pneumology

Main pharmacologic interactions in patients with respiratory illness are those that appear between rifampicine and theophiline, and psychotropic drugs.

Benzodiacepines produce relaxation on respiratory vias and reduce the air pass, so they are contraindicated in sleep obstructive apnea and in chronic restrictive pulmonary illness. Zolpidem is the hipnotic drug with less effect on respiration.

There are some drugs used in pneumologic illness that have been related to psychiatric syndromes, as corticoides, diuretics, beta-blockers or central action antihypertensives.

14. Obesity and diabetes

When treating a patient suffering from morbid obesity, diabetes or organic pathology which could be descomensated with weight gain, the drug must have little effect on weight. It is recommended to use SSRIs or noradrenergic with little effect on weight and watch for possible hipoglucemias that could need adjusting antidiabetic drug. Avoid MAOIs and heterociclic antidepressants. Clozapine and olanzapine promove weight gain and can precipitate diabetes. Risperidone and quetiapine produce lower weight gain and ocasionally diabetes. Aripripazol and ziprasidone don't alter weight and don't produce metabolic syndrome. When a patient with overweight, obesity, prediabetes, diabetes or diabets risk factors is receiving any psychoactive drug, it's important to monitorize laboratory analysis, arterial tension, and weight, at least basal, every three months the first year and then yearly.

15. Oncology

In the treatment of patients suffering from cancer or in a final stage of the illness, the pharmacological prescription has to be accurate to physical state secondary not only to symptomatology related to cancer but to treatment too. In general, it's better to use drugs without active metabolites, without hepatic metabolism, well know drugs, without anticholinergic side effects (due to adition to cancer treatment ones) and with a good side effects profile. Though these considerations, psychiatric symptoms must be treated when appear in association to opioid analgesia if there is pain. In many cases the treatment with stimulants and antidepressants if there is depression is more efficacy than antidepressants alone, with a low risk of dependence. Zolpidem and zopiclone can produce metallic taste, so they must be avoid in cancer patients.

16. AIDS

There is risk of a poor tolerance, especially with high potence antipsychotics in the final stages of AIDS, due to extrapiramidal effects. Risperidone seems to have low interactions profile with drugs used for the infection. Agranulocytosis risk can be increased in treatment with clozapine. To treat depression it is recommended the use of citalopram, escitalopram and sertralina due to the lower risk of interactions (especially with ritonavir), though a serotoninergic síndrome can appear. There are sparse and poor evidence of interactions with other antidepressants. Oxazepam, lorazepam and temazepam are anxiolytic choice treatment, due to their short half life, their metabolism and low profile or interactions. Lithium provokes frequently side effects. When using anticonvulsivants as mood stabilizers, it's important to monitorize liver function. Stimulants can be used with a good profile of secureness and tolerance in patients with cognitive deterioration and depression.

Many drugs used in HIV infection treatment precipitate psychiatric symptoms (depression, anxiety, and insomnia). It is frequent the use of illegal drugs that interfere with treatment and can produce symptoms too.

17. Delirium

Treatment of delirium may complicate evolution of it, so it's important to select drugs with little sedative and anticholinergic effect, if possible one only drug, starting at low doses and during a short time, maintaining non-pharmacological measures (soft light, orientation, treatment of basal physical state…). The treatment is based in the use of antipsychotics, except in alcohol abstinence, where benzodiacepines must be used. Haloperidol is the choice drug, though there is little evidence about the usefulness of atypical antipsychotics. Benzodiacepines must be avoided because can cause a paradoxical effect with an increase of agitation.

18. References

Abuin y cols. Guia clinica de la insuficiencia renal en atenci6n primaria. Comisi6n mixta SEMERGEN-SEMFYC. Nefrología. Vol XXI, supl.5.2001.

Alan F. Schatzberg, Charles B. Nemeroff. Essentials of Clinical Psychopharmacology. Washington: American Psychiatric Publishing; 2006

Altshuler, L.L.; Cohen, L.; Szuba, M.P.; Burt, V.K.; Gitlin, M.; Mintz, J. "Pharmacologic management of psychiatric illness during pregnancy: dilemmas and guidelines" Am. J. Psychiatry, 153 (5): 592-606, 1996

American Diabetes Association, American Psychiatric Association, American Association of Clinical Endocrinologist and North American Association for Study of Obesity. Consensus Development Conference on Antipsychotic Drugs and Obesity and Diabetes. Obesity Research 2004; 12(2):362-68.

American Psychiatric Association. Guías clínicas para el tratamiento de los trastornos psiquiátricos. Compendio 2006. Ars Medica. Barcelona. 2006.

American Psychiatric Association. Practice guidelines for the treatment of patients with delirium. Washington DC. American Psychiatric Association. 1999

Angelino, AF, Treisman, GJ. CI Management of psychiatric disorders in patients infected with human inmunodeficiency virus. Clin Infect Dis 2001 Sep 15; 33(6): 847-56.

Arana G.W., Rosembaum J.F. Drogas psiquiátricas. 4ª Edición. Marbán. 2002.
Azanza J. R. Guía práctica de farmacología del sistema nervioso central., 2006.
Azanza JR, Marcellán T, Francés I. Avances farmacológicos en el tratamiento de la depresión. El médico 2004; 10: 27-50.
Bacire, S. Psychotropic drug directory 2003-2004. Fivepin Publishing Limited. 2003
Baptista T, Elfakih Y, Uzcátegui E, Sandia I, Tálamo E, Araujo de Baptista E, Beaulieu S. Pharmacological management of atypical antipsychotic-induced weight gain. CNS Drugs. 2008; 22(6):477-95.
Baxter, K. Stockley. Interacciones farmacológicas. 2ª edición. Pharma editores, S.L. 2007.
Bazire, S. "Directorio de fármacos psicotrópicos, 2000. Manual del profesional". Ed. Quay Books, Snow Hill, UK, 1999.
Bennett, W. M., et al., Drug prescribing in Renal Failure: Dosing Guidelines for Adults, American College of Physicians, Philadelphia, 1987.
Blumenthal JA, Lett HS, Babyak MA et al: Depression as a risk factor for mortality after coronary artery bypass surgery. Lancet 2003; 362: 604-609.
Bobes J; Casas M y Gutierrez M. Manual de evaluación y tratamiento de drogodependencias. Ars Medica. Barcelona. 2003.
Breitbart W, Marotta R, Platt MM, Weisman H, Derevenco M, Grau C, et al. A double blind trial of haloperidol, chlorpromazine and loracepam in the treatment of delirium in hospitalised AIDS patients. Am J Psychiatry 1996; 153: 231-237
Breitbart, W.; Cohen, K.R. Delirium. en Psycho-oncology. Editor: Jimmie C. Holland. Oxford University Press, New York, 1998, pag 564-675
Breitbart, W.; Wein, S.E. Metabolic disorders and neuropsychiatric symptoms. en Psycho-oncology. Editor: Jimmie C. Holland. Oxford University Press, New York, 1998, pag 639-649
Breitbert, W.; Jaramillo, J.R.; Chichinov, H.M. Palliative and terminal care. en Psycho-oncology. Editor: Jimmie C. Holland. Oxford University Press, New York, 1998, pag 437-449
Brown ThE Trastorno por déficit de atención y comorbilidades en niños, adolescentes y adultos. Ed masson. Madrid 2003.
Brown TM, Stoudemire A. Cardiovascular agents in psychiatric side effects of prescripcion and over the counter drugs. Washington DC. American Psychiatric Press 1998: 209-238.
Caballero; Nahata. Use of selective serotonin-reuptake inhibitors in the treatment of depression in adults with HIV. Ann Pharmacother. 2005 Jan; 39(1): 141-5.
Casas M; Collazos F; Ramos-Quiroga JA; Roncero C (coordinadores). Psicofarmacología de las drogodependencias. Fundación Promedic. Barcelona. 2002
Christensen DD. Rational antidepressant selection in the elderly. Geriatrics 1995; 50 (suppl 1): 41-50.
Christos AB, Dwight LE, Dinges DF. Psicoestimulantes en psiquiatría. En Schatzberg AF y Nemeroff CB, Tratado de Psicofarmacología. Masson. Barcelona, pp 735-750. 2006.
Ciraulo D, Shader R, Greenblatt D, Creelamn W. Drug interactions in psychiatry. Baltimore: Williams & Wilkinson, 1995.
Cirera Costa, E.; Salamero Bravo, M.; Estapé Medinabeitia, T. Neoplasias. En Interconsulta Psiquiátrica. Ed. Rojo Rodes, J.E. y Cirera Costa, E. Ed. Biblio stm, Masson, Barcelona. Pag 395-410, 1997

Coccaro E.F. and I. J. Silver, Second Generation Antidepressants: A Comparative Review, Journal of Clinical Pharmacology, 25, pp. 241-260, 1985.

Coffman K. Psychiatric issues in pulmonary disease. Psychiatr Clin North Am. 2002 Mar;25(1):89-127.

Cohen, L.S.; Rosenbaum, J.F. "Psychotropic drug use during pregnancy: weighing the risks" J. Clin. Psychiatry, 59 (suppl 2): 18-28, 1998

Cole MG, Primeau FJ, Elie LM. Delirium: Prevention, treatment, and outcome studies. J Geriatr Psychiatry Neurol. 1998; 11: 126-137

Consejo General de Colegios Oficiales de Farmacéuticos. Catálogo de medicamentos 2007. Colección Consejo Plus.

Cozza KL; Armstrong SC; Oesterheld JR. Principios de interacción farmacológica para la práctica médica. Ars Medica. Barcelona. 2006.

Crockcroft DW, Gault MH. Prediction of creatinine clearment from serum creatinine. Nephron; 16: 31-41. 1976

David Taylor, Carol Paton, Robert Kerwin. The Maudsley Prescribing Guidelines. London: Informa Healthcare; 2007

De la Serna de Pedro, I de la. Psicofármacos en geriatría. Barcelona: Ars médica, 2006.

De la Serna de Pedro, I de la. Utilización de psicofármacos en el anciano. Interacciones y efectos secundarios. Rev Psiq Fac Med Barcelona 2000; 27: 292-296.

De Vane CL, Nemeroff CB. 2002 guide to psychotropic drug interactions. Primary Psychiatry 2002; 9: 28-57.

Derijks HJ, Meyboom RH, Heerdink ER, De Koning FH, Janknegt R, Lindquist M, Egberts AC. The association between antidepressant use and disturbance in glucose homeostasis: evidence from spontaneus reports. Eur J Clin Pharmacol 2008; 64(5): 531-8.

Diaz M. Presente y futuro del tratamiento farmacológico de la obesidad. Rev Argent Cardiol 2005; 73:137-44.

Fava M. Weight gain and antidepressants. J Clin Psychiatry 2000; 61(suppl 11):37-41.

First MB, Frances A, Pincus HA. DSM-IV-TR Guía de uso. Edición española. Barcelona: Masson; 2005.

Fleischman, S.B.; Kalash, G.R. Chemotherapic agents and neuropsychiatric side effects. en Psycho-oncology. Editor: Jimmie C. Holland. Oxford University Press, New York, 1998, pag 630-638

Frager, G.; Shapiro, B. Paediatric palliative care and pain management. en Psycho-oncology. Editor: Jimmie C. Holland. Oxford University Press, New York, 1998, pag 907-922

García Esteve, L; Cardona Lluria, X.; Cuesta Serramiá, L.; Grau Morillo, M.; Pantinat Giné, L.; Usall Rodie, J. Recomendaciones en el embarazo y la lactancia en "RTM-II. Recomendaciones terapéuticas en los trastornos mentales". Comité de Consenso de Catalunya en Terapéutica de los Trastornos Mentales, Cood. Soler Insa, P.A.; Gascón Barrachina, J. 2ª edición. Ed. Masson, Barcelona, 1999.

García, E; Mendieta, S; Cervera G; Fernández Hermida JR (coordinadores). Manual SET de alcoholismo. Sociedad Española de Toxicomanías. Ed. Médica Panamericana. Madrid. 2003.

Gentile, S. Clinical utilization of atypical antipsychotics in pregnancy and lactation. Annals Pharmacother, 38 (7-8): 1265-71, 2004

Genuth S, Alberti KG, Bennett P, Buse J, Knowler WC, Lebovitz H, Lernmark A, Nathan D, Palmer J, Rizza R, Saudek C, Shaw J, Steffes M, Stern M, Tuomilehto P. Expert Committee on the Diagnosis and Classification of Diabetes Mellitus: Follow-up report on the diagnosis of diabetes mellitus. Diabetes Care 2003; 26:3160-67.

George CF. Perspectives on the management of insomnia in patients with chronic respiratory disorders. Sleep, 2000; 23 Supl. 1: S31-5.

Gold, L.H. "Treatment of depression during pregnancy" J. Women Health Gend. Med., 8 (5): 601-607, 1999

Goldberg JF. What constitutes evidence-based pharmacotherapy for bipolar disorder? Part 1: first-line treatments. J Clin Psychiatry. 2007 Dec;68(12):1982-3

Gretchen A. Anxiety and Chronic Obstructive Pulmonary Disease: Prevalence, Impact, and Treatment. Psychosomatic Medicine 2003, 65:963–970.

Insensé Pons B. Interconsulta Psiquiátrica, Pfizer, capítulo 12, Sistema renal y urinario, 1998, pags. 289-310.

Jacobson SA, Pies RW, Greenblatt DJ. Handbook of geriatric psychopharmacology. Washington: American Psychiatric Publishing, 2002.

Joy CB, Adams CE, Lawrie SM. Haloperidol versus placebo for schizophrenia. Cochrane Database Syst Rev. Oct 18;(4):CD003082. 2006.

Julio Vallejo, Carmen Leal. Tratado de Psiquiatría. Barcelona: Ars Medica; 2005

Kaplan & Sadock's Comprehensive Textbook of Psychiatry. Philadelphia: Lippincott Williams & Wilkins; 2005

Koda-Kimble, M.A.; Young, L.Y. Applied Therapeutc. Tihe clinical use of drug. Pippincott Williams &Wilkins 2001.

Koren, G.; Cohn, T.; Chitayat, D.; Kapur, B.; Remington, G.; Reid, D.M.; Zipurski, R.B. Use of atypical antipsychotics during pregnancy and the risk of neural tube defects in infants. Am. J. Psychiatry 159 (1): 136-7, 2002

Kuller, J.A.; Katz, V.L.; MacMahon, M.J.; Wells, S.R.; Bashford, R.A. "Pharmacologic treatment of psychiatric disease in pregnancy and lactation: fetal and neonatal effects" Obstretics and Gynecology, 87 (5): 789-794 (1996)

Lamberg, L. "Safety of antidepressant use in pregnant and nursing women" JAMA, July, 1999, pag 222-223

Larivaara, P.; Hartikaimen, A.L.; Rantakallio, P. "Use of psychotropic drugs and pregnancy outcome" J. Clin. Epidemiol., 4 (11), 1309-1313, 1996

Levi, N.B., Psychopharmacology in Patients with Renal Failure, Intl. J. Psychiatry in Medicine, vol.20 (4) 325-334, 1990.

Levi, N.B., Use of Psychotropics in Patients with Kidney Failure, Psychosomatics, 26, 699-709, 1985.

Littrell, K.H. Johnson, C.G. Peabody, C.D. Hilligoss, N. Antipsychotics during pregnancy. Am. J. Psychiatry 157(8): 1342, 2000

Lonergan E, Britton AM, Luxenberg J, Wyller T. Antipsychotics for delirium. Cochrane Database of Systematic Reviews 2007, Issue 2. Art. No.: CD005594

Lozano, M.; Ramos, J.A. . Utilización de psicofármacos en psiquiatría de enlace. Masson 2002.

Martín-Vázquez, M.J. Tratamiento psicofarmacológico en embarazo y lactancia. en Psicofarmacología y otras terapias biológicas. Ed. Guindeo, J. y Ríos, B. Ed. Lilly, 2004, pag 244-260

Martín-Vázquez, M.J.; Crespo, M.D. Embarazo, parto, aborto, infertilidad y nuevas técnicas de reproducción. En Trastornos depresivos en la mujer, coordinado por C. Leal, Ed Masson, Barcelona, 1999, Pag 75-90

Massie, M.J.; Popkin, M.K. Depressive disorders. en Psycho-oncology. Editor: Jimmie C. Holland. Oxford University Press, New York, 1998, pag 518-540

Medimecum, Guía de terapia farmacológica, Adis international Ltd., 2005.

Michael G. Wise, James R. Rundell. The American Psychiatric Press Textbook of Consultation-Liaison Psychiatry: Psychiatry in the Medically Ill. Washington: American Psychiatric Publishing Inc; 2002

Newcomer JW. Metabolic considerations in the use of antipsychotic medications: A review of recent evidence. J Clin Psychiatry 2007; 86(1):20-27.

Newport, D.J.; Fisher, A.; Graybeal, S.; Stowe, Z.N. Psicofarmacología durante el embarazo y la lactancia. En Tratado de psicofarmacología. Ed. Schatzberg, A.F y Nemeroff, C.B. Ed. Masson, Barcelona, capítulo 64, pag 1237-77, 2006.

Noyes, R.; Holt, C.S.; Massie, M.J. Anxiety disorders. en Psycho-oncology. Editor: Jimmie C. Holland. Oxford University Press, New York, 1998, pag 548-563

Passik, S.D.; Rickett, P.L. Central Nervous System Tumors en Psycho-oncology. Editor: Jimmie C. Holland. Oxford University Press, New York, 1998, pag 303-313

Rubio G., Huidobro A. Guía para el uso racional de las benzodiacepinas. Grupo Editorial Entheos. 2003.

Sadock BJ, Sadock V (eds): Comprehensive Textbook of Psychopharmacology. Philadelphia, PA, Lippincott Williams & Wilkins, 2000

Sadock, B.J.; Sadock, V.A. . Kaplan - Sadock . Sinopsis de Psiquiatría. Ciencias de la conducta/Psiquiatría clínica. 9ª edición. Waverly Hispánica. 2004.

Salazar M, Peralta C, Pastor J. Tratado de psicofarmacología. Bases y aplicación clínica.Madrid: Editorial Panamericana; 2005

San Sebastián FJ. Psiquiatría infanto-juvenil de enlace. Monografías de psiquiatría. Año XIV. Nº1. Ene-Feb 2002. Aula médica ediciones.

Schatzberg A, Nemeroff C. Tratado de Psicofarmacología. Barcelona. Masson; 2006.

Schatzberg AF, Cole JO, DeBattista Ch. Manual de psicofarmacología clínica 2008. Luzán 5, S.A. ediciones.

Scicutella A. Delirium. En Manual de Medicina para Psiquiatras. Manu P, Suarez RE, Barnett BJ. (Eds.) 1ª Ed. Barcelona. Elsevier-Doyma. 2007

Seitz DP, Gill SS, Van Zyl LT. Antipsychotics in the treatment of delirium: A systematic review. Journal of Clinical Psychiatry. 2007; 68(1): 11-21

Seymour RM, Routledge PA. Important drug-drug interaction in the elderly. Drugs Aging 1998; 12: 285-294

Singh D, Goodkin K. Psychopharmacologic treatment response of HIV-infected patients to antipsychotic medications. J Clin Psychiatry. 2007 Apr; 68(4): 631-2.

Stahl SM. Psicofarmacología esencial. Bases neurocientíficas y aplicaciones clínicas.2ª ed Barcelona. Editorial Ariel, S. A; 2002

Stege G, Sleep, hypnotics and chronic obstructive pulmonary disease. Respir Med. 2008, 102(6):801-14.

Stephen Bazire. Psychotropic Drug Directory 2009. Aberdeen: HealthComm UK Limited; 2008

Stockley IH. Interacciones farmacológicas. Barcelona: Pharma Editores; 2004.

Strain, J.J. Adjustment disorders en Psycho-oncology. Editor: Jimmie C. Holland. Oxford University Press, New York, 1998, pag 509-517

Thompson, A.; Silverman, B., Dzeng, L.; Treisman, G. Psychotropic Medications in HIV. Clin Infect Dis 2006 May 1; (42): 1305-1310

Vallejo, J; Leal, C. Tratado de Psiquiatría. Ars Médica 2005.

Wise MG, Hilty DM, Cerda GM et al: Delirium (confusional states). En: American Psychiatric Publishing Textbook of Consultation-Liaison Psychiatry: Psychiatry in the Medically Ill, 2nd Edition. Wise MG, Rundell JR (Eds.). Washington DC. American Psychiatriuc Publishing, 2002, pp 257-272.

Woods JE, Winger G. Abuse and therapeutic use of benzodiazepines and benzodiazepines-like drugs. In Psychopharmacology: the fourth generation of progress. Edited by Floyd e Blomm and David J Kupfer. Raven Press Ltd. New York, 1995.

Yan LL, Liu K, Mattheus KA. Psychosocial factors and risk of hypertension: the coronary artery risk development in young adult (CARDIA) study. JAMA 2003; 290:2138-2148.

Yonkers, K.; Wisner, K.; Stowe, Z.; Leibenluft, E.; Cohen, L.; Miller, L. et al. Management of bipolar disorder during pregnancy and the postpartum period. Am. J. Psychiatry 161 (4): 608-20, 2004

Yoshida, K.; Smith, B.; Kumar, R. "Psychotropic drugs in mother's milk: a comprehensive review of assay methods, pharmacokinetics and of safety of breast-feeding" J. Psychopharmacology, 13 (1): 64-80, 1999

Section 4

Up-to-Date in Anti-Inflammatory Therapy

6

State of the Art of Anti-Inflammatory Drugs

Túlio Ricardo Couto de Lima Souza, Graziella Silvestre Marques,
Amanda Carla Quintas de Medeiros Vieira
and Juliano Carlo Rufino de Freitas
Universidade Federal de Pernambuco
Brazil

1. Introduction

The steroidal and non-steroidal anti-inflammatory drugs are known to be among the most commercialized drugs worldwide, however several discussions have been raised about its side effects, caused especially in the chronic use. In this context, the discovery of new prototypes with improved anti-inflammatory activity and therapeutic safety is one of the targets in the area of research, development and innovation of the pharmaceutical industry.

The intensive search for new anti-inflammatory therapeutic options with effective therapies and fewer adverse effects resulted in the development of non-steroidal anti-inflammatory drugs (NSAIDs) with selective inhibition of cyclooxygenase-2 (coxibs). This new generation of drugs came to market due to their greater efficiency and minor capacity to damage gastric and renal sites compared to non-selective NSAIDs. This advantage would be pharmacodynamically explained by its ability to selectively inactivate the inducible cyclooxygenase-2 (COX-2), the enzyme that induces prostaglandin synthesis at the inflammation site, preserving the constitutive cyclooxygenase-1 (COX-1) responsible for physiological protection carried by prostaglandins in those sites. Despite the therapeutic efficiency, some of the developed coxibs has been removed from the market by causing significant cardiovascular effects.

Thus, efforts are still underway to discover new anti-inflammatory chemical entities. Several studies have been conducted with synthetic agonists (thiazolidinodiones) of a biological anti-inflammatory target discovered in the nineties, the peroxisome proliferator activated receptor γ (PPARγ). The research of drugs with anti-inflammatory activity carried out by different mechanisms of action from the conventional ones is extremely important in an attempt to expand the therapeutic options for patients who have restrictions on the use of the available anti-inflammatory drugs.

1.1 History

The hability to treat fever and inflammation dates back to 2500 years ago (400 B.C.) to a time when the Greek physician Hippocrates prescribed an extract from willow bark and leaves (Rao & Knaus, 2008). Later, in 1860, with the discovery of the active ingredient of willow bark salicin in Europe, the Kolbe company in Germany started mass producing salicylic acid. Acetysalicylic acid (Aspirin®), the more palatable form of salicylic acid was introduced into the market by Bayer in 1899 (Vane, 2000).

In the 1930s and 1940s, numerous developed studies allowed the recognition of the effects of adrenocortical hormones on electrolyte balance (mineralocorticoids effects) and carbohydrate metabolism (glucocorticoids effects). In 1946, cortisol was synthesized, and in 1948, first used by Hench in patients with rheumatoid arthritis. In the 1950s, changes in the structure of cortisol resulted in new drugs such as prednisone and prednisolone. Later, the side effects related to the use of these therapies have been recognized, adding limitations to the therapeutic use of glucocorticosteroids.

In 1946 was brought to the market phenylbutazone, the first drug other than Aspirin® of the category of what are now known as the NSAIDs, followed by indomethacin in the 1960's (by Merck & Co). In the 1950-1960's Ibuprofen was developed by Boots (UK), and it was the first NSAID (other than Aspirin®) to be approved for non-prescription use in the UK (1963), then USA (1964), and later in many other countries worldwide. Just after the advent of Ibuprofen, in the seventies John Vane discovered the mechanism of action of Aspirin® and other NSAIDs: the inhibition of cyclooxygenase (COX) enzyme (Vane, 1971). After that, a large number of pharmaceutical companies undertook the discovery and development of many other NSAIDs.

In the early 90's there was reported the presence of an inducible isoform of the COX enzyme, later identified as COX-2 (Kujubu & Herschman, 1992). This discovery led to the hipothesis that the non-inflammatory prostaglandins were produced by the constitutive COX-1 and pro-inflammatory prostaglandins by the non-constitutive COX-2 (Meade et al., 1993). The conventional anti-inflammatory drugs were known to inhibit both isoforms of the enzyme. The COX-1 inhibition would explain the gastrointestinal adverse effects caused by the NSAIDs. In an attempt to research new therapeutic agents with fewer adverse effects, the pharmaceutical companies focused their efforts on the design of selective COX-2 inhibitors. In 1999, G.D. Searle and Pfizer (now Pfizer Inc) launched the first selective COX-2 inhibitor, celecoxib (Celebrex®) (Rao & Knaus, 2008). This was followed by the launch of Merck's rofecoxib (Vioxx®) and other coxibs (Prasit, 1999).

The research and development of new therapies to treat inflammation, pain and arthritis is still a constant in the pharmaceutical industry. Between 1999 and 2010, at least 12 arthritis and inflammation related new chemical and biological entities were released, 5 of them anti-inflammatory agents. However, rofecoxib (Vioxx®) and valdecoxib (Bextra®) were still withdrawn from the market due to the high cardiovascular risk related to its use (United States Food and Drug Administration [FDA], 2011).

1.2 Anti-Inflammatory use and market

The anti-inflammatory class of drugs is among the most widely prescribed groups of medicines in clinical practice worldwide. The global market for treatment of pain in 2009 amounted to US$ 50 billion, of which 27 billion in the seven largest economies (USA, Japan, France, Germany, Italy, Spain and UK). Of these US$ 27 billion, NSAIDs constitute 28% NSAIDs and selective COX-2 inhibitors 7% (Melnikova, 2010). Other data that brings the high use of anti-inflammatory drugs reveal that 40 thousand tons of acetyl-salicylic acid are ingested every year around the world (Menezes et al., 2009), besides the large number of

NSAIDs available for purchase in the market, many of them obtained without prescription. This fact can explain the high cash income derived from the NSAIDs prescription.

Recently, a study carried out in six European countries showed an increase in the use of anti-inflammatory drugs during the 2002-2007 period. It is important to emphasize that during this period the use of conventional NSAIDs increased by 2.07%, while the stronger COX-2 inhibitors use increased by 325% (Inotai et al., 2010).

The numbers regarding the use of corticosteroids as anti-inflammatory therapy in the U.S. shows that each year approximately 67 million prescriptions are written, despite their multiple side effects. In 2007, the combined annual sales for corticosteroids totaled about US$ 7.4 billion, not including generics (Hollis-Eden Pharmaceuticals, 2007).

Associated with these high values regarding anti-inflammatory therapies, there are other ones related to its adverse effects. Some studies developed at the US showed that, for each dollar spent on NSAIDs, from U$0.66 to U$1.25 may be spent due to gastrointestinal adverse effects. Aditionally, almost 1/3 of the medical costs in arthritis patients may be related with gastrointestinal effects (Laine et al., 2010).

1.3 Physiopathology

Acute inflammation may be triggered by a variety of stimuli and is characterized by the rapid host response to the sites of infection or tissue injury, with the delivery of leukocytes and plasma proteins, such as antibodies, to the referred site. Chronic inflammation may develop following acute inflammation and may last for weeks or months, and in some instances for years.

During both acute and chronic inflammatory processes, a number of soluble factors are involved in leukocyte recruitment through increased expression of cellular adhesion molecules and chemoattraction. Through this mechanism, many soluble mediators regulate the activation of resident cells, such as endothelial cells, fibroblasts, tissue macrophages and mast cells, as well as newly recruited inflammatory cells such as monocytes, lymphocytes, neutrophils and eosinophils. Some of these mediators result in the systemic inflammatory responses, as fever, hypotension, the synthesis of acute phase proteins, leukocytosis and cachexia (Feghali & Wright, 1997).

Some transcription factors play a significant role in the inflammatory process. In this context, an important one is Nuclear Factor-kappa B (NF-κB), which controls the transcription of DNA (Gilmore, 2006). Activation of the NF-κB transcription family, by nuclear translocation of cytoplasmic complexes, plays a central role in inflammation through its ability to induce transcription of proinflammatory genes and consequently mediators like cytokines and chemokines, matrix metalloproteinases (MMPs), COX-2, and inducible nitric oxide (iNOS) (Baldwin, 1996). NF-κB activation also increases expression of the adhesion molecules E-selectin, vascular cell adhesion molecule 1 (VCAM-1), and intercellular adhesion molecule 1 (ICAM-1), while inhibition reduces leukocyte adhesion and transmigration (Chen et al., 1995). The activity of NF-kB is tightly regulated by interaction with inhibitory IkB proteins (Gilmore, 2006).

The mediators that act in the inflammatory process can be divided in cell-derived and plasma protein-derived. These include:

- Cell-derived: Histamin, Serotonin, Prostaglandins, Leukotrienes, Platelet-activating factor, Reactive oxygen species, Nitric oxide, Cytokines (tumor necrosis factor - TNF, interleukin-1 - IL-1), Chemokines;
- Plasma-protein derived: Complement products (C3a, C4a, C5a), Kinins, Proteases activated during coagulation.

Among the mediators of inflammation many are derived from the arachidonic acid. The scheme below shows the biochemical cascade that leads to some of them (Figure 1):

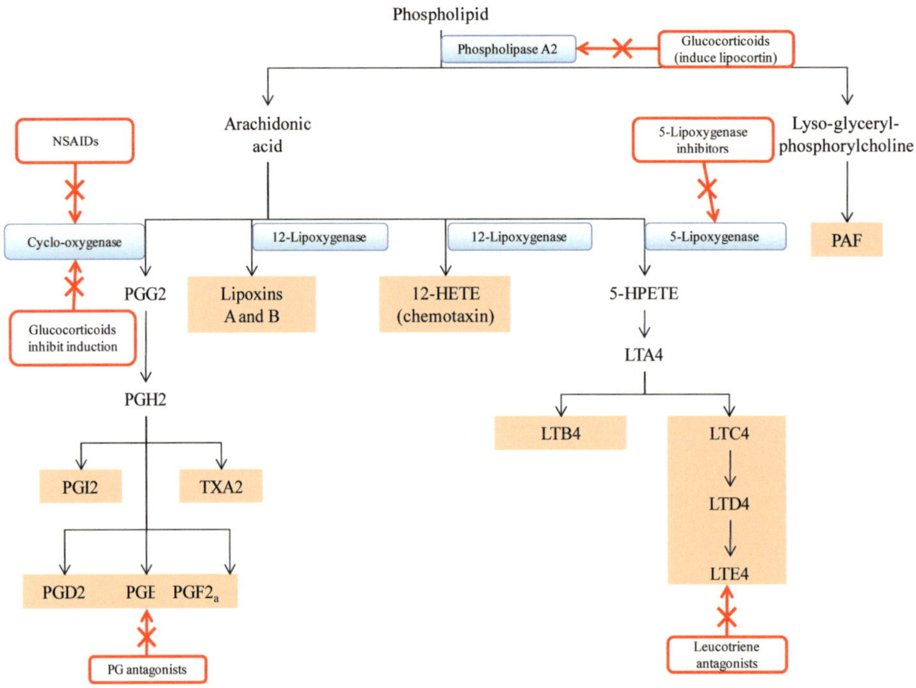

Fig. 1. The arachidonic acid cascade leads to a number of mediators of inflammation. As indicated in red, many steps of this cascade are potential anti-inflammatory targets, such as enzymes and eicosanoids receptors. In this chapter, will be discussed the NSAIDs and glucocorticosteroids. PAF, platelet-activating factor; PG, prostaglandin; 12-HETE, 12-hydroxyeicosatetraenoate; 5-HPETE, 5-hydroperoxyeicosatetraenoate; TXA2, thromboxane A2; LT, leukotriene.

The classic anti-inflammatory therapies are based on the inhibition of the cyclooxygenase enzymes (NSAIDs) and cyclooxygenase 2 expression (glucocorticosteroids), thus preventing the prostanoids to be generated and on the phospholipase A2 enzyme expression inhibition (glucocorticosteroids), inhibiting the whole arachidonic acid cascade. Moreover, corticosteroids induce key anti-inflammatory genes and selectively repress specific inflammatory genes that encode a number of other mediators of inflammation, consequently inhibiting the inflammatory response. The anti-inflammatory response of these medicines can be explained by the reduction of the inflammatory response of such mediators, once its generation is decreased by the action of the medicines. Many side effects experienced by these drugs users can be explained by the absent physiological role of these mediators (Table 1).

PGI_2	PGD_2 & $PGF_{2\alpha}$	PGE_2	TXA_2
Platelets: Inhibits platelet aggregation and disaggregates preformed clumps. Limits platelet activation by TxA_2, reducing the thrombotic response to vascular injury. **Kidneys**: Maintain renal blood flow and salt excretion. PGI2 promotes renin release and natriuresis via effects on tubular reabsorption of Na^+.	**Vascular smooth muscle ($PGF_{2\alpha}$)**: Vasoconstriction; **Uterus**: Relaxation (PGD_2) and contraction ($PGF_{2\alpha}$).	**Pregnancy**: COX-2-derived PGE_2 maintains the ductus arteriosus patent until birth. Reduced PGE_2 levels permit closure. Stimulates contraction of the pregnant human uterus; **Kidneys**: Maintain renal blood flow and salt excretion; **Gastric and intestinal secretions**: Contributes to increased mucus secretion (*cytoprotection*), inhibition of gastric acid secretion, and reduced pepsin content. Inhibits gastric damage caused by a variety of ulcerogenic agents and promote healing of duodenal and gastric ulcers; **Bones**: Stimulates bone formation by increasing osteoblastogenesis. Bone resorption also is mediated via PGE_2, through activation of osteoclasts	**Platelets**: Induces platelet aggregation; Vascular tone: Causes vasoconstriction; Parturition: Important in the final stages of parturition.
Inflammation: Increases local blood flow, vascular permeability, and leukocyte infiltration **Pain**: Reduces the threshold to stimulation of nociceptors, causing *peripheral sensitization*.	**Inflammation (PGD_2)**: Contributes to inflammation in allergic responses. Increases perfusion and vascular permeability and promotes T_H2 cell differentiation. PGD_2 also can activate mature T_H2 cells and eosinophils via its DP_2 receptor.	**Inflammation**: Increases local blood flow, vascular permeability, and leukocyte infiltration **Pain**: Reduces the threshold to stimulation of nociceptors, causing *peripheral sensitization* **Fever**: PGE_2 can cross the blood-brain barrier and acts on EP_3 and perhaps EP_1 receptors on thermosensitive neurons. This triggers the hypothalamus to elevate body temperature by promoting an increase in heat generation and a decrease in heat loss.	**Inflammation**: Increases platelet–leukocyte interaction.

Table 1. The diverse activities of prostaglandins are reflected by their involvement in both normal homeostasis (blue) and pathophysiology (red). Many of the NSAIDs side effects can be explained by the absent physiological role of prostanoids (renal, cardiovascular, gastrointestinal) due to the COX inhibition (Goodman et al., 2010).

Among the soluble factors that mediate inflammation, a group of secreted polypeptides known as cytokines play essential roles in orchestrating the process. They can be divided into two groups: those involved in acute inflammation and those responsible for chronic inflammation (See Figure 2 and Table 2).

The most important cytokines involved in inflammatory reactions are listed. In this context, TNF-α and IL-1 are important in developing the acute and sustaining the chronic inflammatory process (O'Neill, 2008). Working in concert with each other and various cytokines and growth factors (such as IL-6, IL-8 and granulocyte-macrophage colony-stimulating factor [GM-CSF]), they induce gene expression and protein synthesis (including expression of COX-2, adhesion molecules, and acute-phase proteins) in a range of cells to mediate and promote inflammation. Other cytokines may play lesser roles in inflammation.

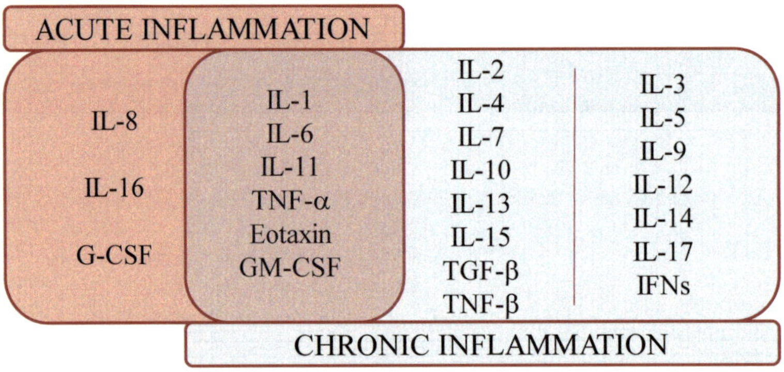

Fig. 2. Cytokines involved in acute and chronic inflammatory responses. IL, interleukin; TNF, tumor necrosis factor; GM-CSF, Granulocyte-colony stimulating factor; TGF, Transforming growth factor; IFN, interferon.

Principal cytokines	Principal sources	Principal actions in inflammation
TNF	Mast Cells, Macrophages, T lymphocytes	Stimulates expression of endothelial adhesion molecules and secretion of other cytokines; systemic effects
IL-1	Macrophages, endothelial cells	Similar to TNF; greater role in fever
IL-6	Macrophages, other cells	Systemic effects
IL-12	Dendritic cells, macrophages	Increased production of IFN-γ
IL-17	T-Lymphocytes	Recruitment of neutrophils and monocytes
Chemokines	Macrophages, endothelial cells, T lymphocytes, mast cells, other cell types	Recruitment of leukocytes to sites of inflammation; migration of cells to normal tissues
IFN-γ	T lymphocytes, NK cells	Activation of macrophages (increased ability to kill microbes and tumor cells)

Table 2. Principal cytokines in inflammation (Robbins et al., 2010). NK, natural killer.

The extravasion of leukocytes is controlled by the expression of cell surface adhesion molecules on both the circulating cells and on the vascular endothelium. The TNF-α signaling pathway, mediated by NF-κB, is responsible for the expression of adhesion molecules such as VCAM-1 and ICAM-1 in the endothelium (Collins et al., 1995). TNF-α was previously shown to induce ICAM-1 expression (Fingar et al., 1997). These adhesion molecules allow the attachment of leukocytes to the endothelium and may permit their subsequent transmigration into peripheral tissue. At the same time, microvascular permeability is increased (Frank & Lisanti, 2008).

2. Non-Steroidal Anti-Inflammatory Drugs (NSAIDs)

The NSAIDs are a heterogeneous group of molecules that share certain therapeutic actions and side effects. The first drug belonging this class, Aspirin®, was introduced to the market in 1899. After that, several other anti-inflammatory drugs were introduced over the years, until the discovery of selective inhibitors of COX-2, called coxibs. Both traditional NSAIDs and the recent coxibs are effective anti-inflammatory agents and analgesics. However, in recent years it has been questioned the safety associated with the use of these drugs in clinical practice, due to the range of side effects caused due to consumption of these drugs, many times inappropriately.

2.1 Mechanism of action

The anti-inflammatory action of NSAIDs can be explained by the effect of inhibiting the enzyme COX, which is responsible for the synthesis of prostaglandins, mediators with a great ability to induce inflammation (Tanaka et al., 2009). COX has two isoforms: COX-1 and COX-2. The first is constitutively expressed in a wide variety of cells, promoting physiological functions, such as gastric mucosal protection, control of renal blood flow, hemostasis, autoimmune responses, lungs, central nervous system, cardiovascular system and reproductive functions (Grosser et al., 2006).

On the other hand, COX-2 is an inductive enzyme, which is expressed significantly due to various stimuli such as cytokines, endotoxins and growth factors. COX-2 originates inducing prostaglandins, which contribute to the development of the four cardinal signs of inflammation: pain, heat, redness and swelling (Fitzgerald, 2004), thus being considered as the main target for the anti-inflammatory action. In this context, the recently developed coxibs act through selective inhibition of COX-2. However, although inductive, this COX isoform is also expressed in normal vascular endothelial cells, synthesizing prostacyclin, an important substance in maintaining the prothrombotic/antithrombotic blood balance (Antman et al., 2007), which can trigger severe cardio-vascular problems.

2.2 Therapeutic uses

The effects of inhibiting the COX enzyme explain the clinical uses of the NSAIDs (including selective COX-2 inhibitors), mainly as antipyretics, analgesics and anti-inflammatory agents.

- **Inflammation:** As anti-inflammatory agents, are used to treat muscle injuries, tendinitis, bursitis and in relieving postoperative pain, in addition to its indication for chronic rheumatic diseases such as rheumatoid arthritis, osteoarthritis, gouty arthritis and ankylosing spondylitis (Pountos et al., 2011). In the latter cases, NSAIDs are often associated with disease modifying anti-rheumatic drugs (DMARDs), so that in addition to reducing pain and discomfort of the patient, also promote the regression of the disease.
- **Pain:** Its use as analgesic is indicated for relieving mild to moderate pain. They are particularly effective when inflammation has caused peripheral and/or central sensitization of pain perception. Thus, postoperative pain or pain arising from inflammation, such as arthritic pain, is controlled well by NSAIDs, whereas pain arising from the hollow viscera usually is not relieved (Goodman et al., 2010).
- **Fever:** NSAIDs are thought to be antipyretic largely through inhibition of prostaglandin production in the hypothalamus. They can reduce fever in most situations, but not the circadian variation in temperature or the rise in response to exercise or increased ambient temperature. McAdam et al. (1999), in a comparative study of the impact of non-selective NSAIDs and selective COX-2 inhibitors, suggested that COX-2 is the main source of PGs that mediate the rise in temperature caused by bacterial lipopolysaccharide (LPS) administration.

- **Cardioprotection:** The suppression of platelet TxA2 formation promotes the cardioprotective effect of aspirin. It is used as an antiplatelet drug, in the management of the myocardial infarction and in angina, reducing the risk of serious vascular events in high-risk patients (e.g., those with previous myocardial infarction) by 20-25%. Low-dose (<100 mg/day) aspirin, is as effective as higher doses (e.g., 325 mg/day) but is associated with a lower risk for gastrointestinal adverse events (Goodman et al., 2010).
- **Cancer Chemoprevention:** Studies of patients with familial adenomatous polyposis and Gardner's syndrome (Waddell et al., 1983, 1989) introduced the idea that NSAIDs may inhibit cancer progression. Cha & Raymond (2007) found that in colorectal cancers the same occurs because COX-2 is selectively upregulated, which was subsequently found to be elevated in other epithelial tumors including breast, stomach, pancreas, bladder, lung and prostate cancers. Since the NSAID action is inhibition of the enzymatic activities of COX-1 and COX-2, it was hypothesized that the beneficial effect of NSAIDs was due, in part, to inhibition of COX-2 in the tumor microenvironment. Additionally, recent clinical trials clearly demonstrate that celecoxib is very effective in reducing polyp recurrence in patients who have undergone a polypectomy (Arber et al.; Bertagnolli et al., 2006). This drug is particularly effective in reducing recurrence of very large polyps, which are more likely to progress into cancer. Recently, a new group of NSAIDs have been explored for their effectiveness in several diseases, such as cardiovascular, rheumatological and lung diseases, Alzheimer's disease, and cancer: the Nitric oxide-donating nonsteroidal antiinflammatory drugs (NO-NSAIDs). These drugs consist of a traditional NSAID to which a NO releasing moiety is covalently attached, and may have an important role in colon cancer prevention and/or treatment (Yeh et al., 2004).
- **Alzheimer's Disease:** Observational studies have suggested that NSAID use, in particular ibuprofen, is associated with lower risk of developing Alzheimer's disease. The same was not observed when a randomized, controlled clinical trial comparing celecoxib, naproxen, and placebo (ADAPT Research Group, 2008) was performed, where the researchers did not find a significant reduction in Alzheimer's dementia with the use of NSAIDs.
- **Other Clinical Uses:** In patients with systemic mastocytosis, PGD2, released from mast cells in large amounts, has been found to be the major mediator of severe episodes of flushing, vasodilation, and hypotension. The addition of aspirin or ketoprofen has provided relief (Worobec, 2000). Large doses of niacin (nicotinic acid), effectively used to lower serum cholesterol levels, reduce low-density lipoprotein, and raise high-density lipoprotein, can induce intense facial flushing. This flushing is mediated largely by release of PGD2 from the skin, which can be inhibited by treatment with aspirin (Jungnickel et al., 1997). Bartter syndrome includes a series of rare disorders characterized by hypokalemic, hypochloremic metabolic alkalosis with normal blood pressure and hyperplasia of the juxtaglomerular apparatus. Renal COX-2 is induced, and biosynthesis of PGE2 is increased. Treatment with indomethacin, combined with potassium repletion and spironolactone, is associated with improvement in the biochemical derangements and symptoms. Selective COX-2 inhibitors also have been used (Guay-Woodford, 1998).

2.3 Side effects

The use of NSAIDs has been associated with a high number of side effects. Thus, the prescription of these drugs should be made through a previous study of the individual patient, taking into account the required dosage and the use of other drugs, in order to understand the patient risk-benefit relation. The most prominent side effects are described below:

- **Gastrointestinal effects:** Several prostanoids, especially prostacyclin and PGE 2, are crucial to protect the gastric mucosa from the corrosive effects of stomach acid, as well as to maintain the naturally healthy condition of the gastric mucosa (Antman, 2007). Therefore, the consequences of inhibition of COX-1 may lead to the triggering of various side effects ranging from nausea to bleeding ulcers, which can lead the user to death (Pountus et al., 2011). The use of high doses or the prolonged consumption of NSAIDs, along with its administration with corticosteroids and/or anticoagulant drugs, smoking and/or alcohol, increases the probability of experiencing these effects. However, some in vitro studies reported that there is a relationship between the besides the NSAIDs and COX adversities stomach: Some drugs shown to have direct cytotoxic action on cells of the gastric mucosa, may also be the reason of such effects (Siew & Francis, 2010).
- **Cardiovascular effects and the coxibs:** Some prostaglandins and other substances produced by COX regulates complex interactions between platelets and the blood vessel walls. In this context, prostacyclin, a substance produced by COX-2, antagonizes the action of platelet aggregation by interacting with its receptor IP. However, platelets contain only one isoform of COX, able to convert a large quantity of arachidonic acid to a potent aggregating agent, thromboxane A2 (TXA2). Therefore, with the administration of selective COX-2 drugs (coxibs), an imbalance can occur in the production of prostacyclin and TXA2, reflecting in a prothrombotic/antithrombotic blood imbalance and a consequent increase in risk of thrombotic events (Topol, 2004; Antman et al., 2005). In this context, the studies of Grahamm and coworkers (2005) showed an increase of 1.49 times in the risk of acute myocardial infarction patients for consuming rofecoxib at a dose of 25mg/day (maximum dose chronic allowed) in a three years period. Additionally, the author noticed an increase of 3.58 times in this risk with the consumption of doses greater than 25mg/day of celecoxib. A number of other studies reported a significant increase in the risk of developing acute myocardial infarction associated with the use of such medicines (Bresalier et al., 2005). Given these results, the Food and Drug Administration (FDA) has formalized the limited use of these drugs. Two of them (rofecoxib and valdecoxib) were still withdrawn from the market (United States Food and Drug Administration [FDA], 2011).
- **Erectile dysfunction:** Inhibition of prostaglandin synthesis and TXA2 by NSAIDs may interfere with the physiological process of penile erection through nitric oxide, which is an essential physiological signal for penile erection (Shiri et al., 2006). According to the study of Shiri and coworkers, 2006, Erectile dysfunction is related to the used therapy, regardless the incident disease. The author of the study showed that the onset of the erectile dysfunction in patients with arthritis treated with NSAIDs was lower than expected in the use of the drug in the absence of a disease, indicating a negative function between the use of NSAIDs in arthritis and the risk of developing the disorder. In addition, the study concluded that it is a reversible process, with enhanced sexual performance when the drug is discontinued.
- **Nephrotoxicity:** Inhibition of COX-1 results in declining levels of renal vasodilatory prostaglandins, which among other effects, maintains renal blood flow and glomerular filtration rates. This effect is mainly exerted by them relaxing preglomerular resistance

and acting as angiotensin II and norepinephrine antagonists. Aditionally, they cause an increase in organ perfusion and reduction in the release of noradrenaline. In this context, the inhibition of such mechanisms tends to decrease the total renal perfusion and redistribute blood flow to the cortex, especially when there is stimulation of the renin-angiotensin-aldosterone system and/or stimulation of the sympathetic nervous system. Such processes may result in acute renal vasoconstriction, medullar ischemia, and under certain conditions, acute renal failure. Therefore, the use of NSAIDs may result in varying degrees of renal dysfunction, ranging from the reversible commitment of glomerular filtration rate to irreversible renal damage (Winkelmayer et al. 2008; Pountos, 2011).

2.4 Contra-indications

The contraindications for NSAIDs are quite understandable and are closely related to its adverse effects. The FDA proposes the contraindications for hypertensive patients, patients with chronic renal, cardiovascular and gastroesophageal diseases (Keenan et al., 2011).

Additionally, there is not a clear dividing line for the clinical use of NSAIDs and their toxicology, where it is necessary the cautious interpretation of clinical risk factors. Such factors may increase the likelihood of developing these side effects, and are described in Table 3 (Holdgate & Pollock, 2004; Berenbaum, 2004).

Risk factors related to the consumption of NSAIDs	
Patient	Older than 65 years, consumption of alcohol and/or smoke.
Clinical History	Gastrointestinal (GI) events or ulcers, prior induction of GI events by NSAIDs consumption, comorbid conditions, poor functional status.
Drug	Chronic use, high doses, concomitant use with other NSAIDs.

Table 3. Risk factors related to the use of NSAIDs (Pountos et al., 2011).

Several studies include pregnant and lactating women in the clinical contraindicated profile, which culminated in a warning issued by the Adverse Drug Reactions Advisory Committee (ADRAC) in 1991. It emphasized the congestive heart failure and poor prognosis risks related to the use of NSAIDs during pregnancy (Hofstadler et al., 1996), reporting cases of premature closure or constriction of the ductus arteriosus in women with diclofenac, indomethacin and mefenamic acid treatment due to low back pain, premature labor and polyhydramnios, respectively.

2.5 Drug interactions

Some studies report that the administration of traditional NSAIDs concomitantly with Aspirin® may antagonize its antiplatelet action, compromising its cardioprotective function (Kurth et al., 2003). Additionally, the combination of NSAIDs and coxibs with low-dose Aspirin® significantly increases the likelihood of gastroinestinais adverse events compared with the isolated use of any NSAID (Gladding et al., 2008).

The combined therapy of these drugs with angiotensin-converting enzyme (ACE) inhibitors can cause renal failure (Seeling et al., 1990), commonly seen in elderly patients. The same results from the attenuation of the effectiveness of ACE inhibitors due to the blocked production of vasodilator and natriuretic prostaglandins by NSAIDs. The drug interaction also occurs with thiazide diuretics, which can cause impaired renal function and electrolyte imbalance (Secoli, 2010).

Although they are often used to treat rheumatoid arthritis and cancer, the concomitant use of NSAIDs and methotrexate leads to drug interaction, increasing the blood concentration and time of excretion of methotrexate. According to Maeda et al., 2008, there is a competition for the renal transporter, the main route of elimination of methotrexate.

NSAIDs also present interactions with alcohol. Studies have demonstrated that this interaction causes the prolongation of the bleeding mediated by Aspirin® when administered concomitantly. This mechanism is not yet well understood, but some in vitro studies show that this relationship arises from the increase in the inhibiting power of prostacyclin on platelet aggregation (Jakubowski et al., 1988).

2.6 Main categories of NSAIDs

- **Salicylates:** Aspirin® is the pioneer of this class of anti-inflammatory drugs. It is often used for prophylaxis of cardiovascular events at a dosage of 40 to 80 mg/day. Additionally, it has analgesic action and antipyretic in the dosage of 325 to 650mg every 4 to 6 hours. At a dosage of 1g every 4 to 6 hours is indicated for the treatment of rheumatic fever. The dosage for children is changed, being 10mg/kg every 4 to 6 hours. Diflunisal® (difluorophenyl) has about 4 to 5 times more analgesic and anti-inflammatory power than Aspirin®. However, its antipyretic effect is reduced. The administration of diflunisal is performed at doses of 250 to 500mg every 8 to 12 hours. It presents fewer side effects on platelets and the gastrointestinal tract. Its excretion can be achieved through breast milk, being contraindicated for pregnant women.
- **Para-aminophenol derivatives:** Acetaminophen or Paracetamol has effective analgesic and antipyretic activity, but its anti-inflammatory activity is insufficient. It is used at a dosage of 10 to 15 mg/kg every 4 hours, not exceeding the maximum of 5 doses every 24 hours. High doses of acetaminophen cause the production of toxic metabolites and hepatic necrosis.
- **Acetic acid derivatives:** Indomethacin is 10 to 40 times more potent than salicylic acid. Its peak blood concentration is reached 1-2 hours after administration. It is used at a dosage of 25 mg 2-3 times/day or 75 to 100 mg/night. Its side effects affect 30 to 50% of users, characterized by frontal headache, neutropenia and thrombocytopenia. About 20% of patients discontinue the therapy. Fenamates have similar effectiveness compared to acetylsalicylic acid, but isolated cases of hemolytic anemia have been reported. Its side effects can reach about 25% of users. Tolmetin, a heteroaryl acetate derivative, also has similar effectiveness compared to Aspirin®. It is used at a dose of 400 to 600mg, three times a day, and 20mg/kg/day for children, in 3 to 4 fractionated doses. The absorption of Tolmetin is delayed and decreased in the presence of food. The interruption of therapy occurs in 5-10% of patients. Diclofenac, a phenylacetate derivative, is administered in doses of 50mg three times daily or 75mg, 2 times a day. It is more potent than Aspirin®, but 20% of patients develop side effects, 2% discontinue the use and 15% develop elevation of liver enzymes.
- **Propionic acid derivates:** In general, they are better tolerated than Aspirin®, with equivalent to or higher power than the same. Ibuprofen is widely used in clinical practice, and presents a large potential to cause renal toxicity. About 10 to 15% of users

discontinue treatment due to adverse effects. It is administered at a dose of 200 to 400mg every 4 to 6 hours for analgesia, whereas for anti-inflammatory the dosage is 300mg every 6-8h or 400 to 800mg three to four times a day. The dosage for anti-inflammatory for children decreases to 5 to 10mg/kg every 6h, with the maximum dose of 40 mg/kg/day. In children, anti-inflammatory action is achieved with dosages of 20 to 40 mg/kg/day in 3 to 4 fractionated doses. Naproxen has a long half-life of 14 hours, and can provide cardioprotection in some patients. It is used in the maximum daily dose of 1000 mg being 250 mg 4 times daily or 500 mg two times a day. For children, anti-inflammatory dosage is reduced to 5mg/kg, two times a day. In elderly patients, the drug has lower protein binding and delayed excretion, increasing the likelihood of toxicity in these patients. In the case of fenoprofen, the dosage is 200mg 4-6 times a day. About 15% of users experience side effects, but few discontinue use. Drugs with high half-life, as oxaprozin (40 to 60h) allows administration once daily. However, it is indicated for fever or acute analgesia because the onset of action is slow. Oxaprozin is used in dosage from 600 to 1800 mg/day.

- **Enolic acid derivates:** This class is constituted by piroxicam, meloxicam and nabumetone. Both meloxicam and nabumetone have relative selectivity for COX-2. Piroxicam has equivalent power to Aspirin® and is better tolerated. However, it can inhibit the activation of neutrophils and the activity of collagenase and proteoglycanase. This drug is administered in daily doses of 20mg. About 20% of users develop side effects, while 5% discontinue the treatment. Nabumetone has fewer side effects than many NSAIDs. Its administration is performed at doses of 500 to 1000mg, 1 to 2 times a day. Meloxicam dosage is 7.5 to 15 mg/day (Goodman et al., 2010).

3. Glucocorticosteroids (GCs)

Glucocorticosteroids (GCs) (glucocorticoids; also known as corticosteroids or steroids) are steroid hormones derived from cholesterol metabolism. Their basic molecular structure is the cyclopentanoperhydrophenanthrene, derived from cholesterol.

The natural GC representative is the cortisol or hydrocortisone. They are effective anti-inflammatory and immunosuppressive agents, produced naturally in the adrenal gland after stimulation of the hypothalamic-pituitary-adrenal (HPA) (Fernandes et al., 2008; Barnes & Adcock, 2009). Since the availability of cortisone in the late 1950s, several synthetic GC agonists have been developed, such as prednisone, dexamethasone and betamethasone (Löwenberg et al., 2008). The synthetic GCs are obtained from folic acid (taken from cattle) or some plants of the families *Liliaceae* and *Dioscoreaceae* (Timóteo & Dos Santos, 2008). For decades, they have been among the most commonly prescribed classes of immunomodulatory and anti-inflammatory drugs, being widely used as treatment of choice for several autoimmune and inflammatory diseases, including asthma, rheumatoid arthritis, inflammatory bowel disease and polymyalgia rheumatica. However, serious side effects, such as osteoporosis, skin atrophy, cushingoid appearance, diabetes and glaucoma, frequently accompany GC therapy, which place limitations on the use of higher dosages and long-term use of GCs (Flammer & Rogatsky, 2008; Löwenberg et al., 2008). Moreover, nowadays, various side effects of glucocorticoids are well-known and physicians often anticipate on these side effects (De Nijs, 2008).

3.1 Molecular actions of glucocorticosteroids

GCs act through many molecular mechanisms. One of them occurs through traditional glucocorticoid receptor mediated pathways to directly regulate gene expression. In this mechanism, the CGs freely diffuses across the cell membrane and act by binding to and activating specific cytosolic glucocorticoid receptors (GR). In its inactive state, the GR exists as a cytosolic protein bound to two heat shock protein 90 chaperonin molecules. The binding to the GC ligand results in a conformational change that allows dissociation of the GR from the protein complex, and a quick translocation into the cell nucleus where they can modulate gene transcription either by stimulation or inhibition (De Paiva & Pflugfelder, 2008; Barnes & Adcock, 2009). The glucocorticoid-receptor complex can either induce key anti-inflammatory genes that encode anti-inflammatory molecules (e.g. lipocortin-1, IL-10, IL-1Rα6, TGF-β and inhibitory IkB proteins) following direct association with glucocorticoid response elements (GREs) in the promoter regions of these genes, or selectively repress specific inflammatory genes that encode cytokines (e.g. IL-1, IL-6, IL-8, TNF-α), chemokines, adhesion molecules (e.g. adhesion molecules E-selectin, ICAM-1, VCAM-1), inflammation-associated enzymes (e.g. phospholipase A2, COX-2, iNOS), lipid mediators of inflammation (e.g. prostaglandins) and receptors by protein-to-protein interaction with transcription factors such as the nuclear factor (NF)-κB and activator protein 1 (AP-1), which interact with transcriptional coactivator molecules to activate gene transcription (Derendorf & Meltzer, 2008; Fernandes et al., 2008). Multiple mechanisms are involved in GC-mediated anti-inflammatory activity in addition to direct GR/NF-κB interaction, such as GC-induced up-regulation of IκB and glucocorticoid-induced leucine zipper (GILZ), two proteins able to bind and inhibit NF-κB activation (Cuzzocrea et al., 2008).

Furthermore, it has been reported that peroxisome proliferator activated receptor-α (PPAR-α) can contribute to the anti-inflammatory activity of GCs. PPAR-α is an intracellular transcription factor activated by fatty acids that plays a role in inflammation. Previous studies indicate that PPAR-α expression is induced by GCs and can mediate some of the GC effects, such as modulation of insulin sensitivity and resistance, and can contribute to GC-induced hyperglycemia and blood pressure increase. Moreover, it has been reported that PPAR-α activation can result in inhibition of NF-κB activation and inflammatory gene expression (Cuzzocrea et al., 2008).

3.2 Therapeutic uses

- **Skin diseases:** Several skin diseases are typically treated with systemic or topical GCs. The main indications are psoriasis, contact dermatitis, atopic dermatitis, exfoliative erythroderma, pemphigus vulgaris, pemphigus foliaceus, bullous pemphigoid, cicatricial pemphigoid, gestational herpes, acquired epidermolysis bullosa, linear IgA bullous dermatosis, Stevens Johnson syndrome, toxic epidermal necrolysis, erythema multiforme minor, lupus erythematosus, dermatomyositis, vasculitis, pyoderma gangrenosum, sweet's syndrome, behcet's disease, lichen planus, sarcoidosis and chronic urticaria (Pereira et al., 2007; Akama et al., 2009). In pediatric dermatology, long-term systemic steroids may be used for the treatment of erythroderma due to atopic eczema, pustular psoriasis, childhood pemphigus, chronic bullous dermatosis of childhood, systemic lupus erythematosus, pyoderma gangrenosum or complicated hemangiomas (Deshmukh, 2007).

- **Respiratory tract diseases:** Intranasal GCs are effective treatments for allergic rhinitis, rhinosinusitis, and nasal polyposis. They are the most common treatment for patients with nasal polyposis and have been designated as the treatment of choice for allergic rhinitis (Derendorf & Meltzer, 2008; Zele et al., 2010). The systemic GCs are effective in treating allergic rhinitis, but the high risk of serious toxicity with long-term administration has hindered their usefulness. The first successful use of GC as a pressurized aerosol with no apparent evidence of systemic toxicity was the beclomethasone in 1972. In the following years, corticosteroid molecules have been refined to create more potent agents with lower bioavailability and enhanced safety profiles. Nowadays, various compounds are approved for the management of allergic rhinitis in the United States: triamcinolone acetonide, flunisolide, budesonide, beclomethasone dipropionate, ciclesonide, fluticasone propionate, mometasone furoate, fluticasone furoate (Derendorf & Meltzer, 2008; Zele et al., 2010). Likewise, GCs are the most effective and widely used anti-inflammatory drugs for the treatment of asthma (Maneechotesuwan et al., 2010; Hagan et al., 2011). The introduction of GCs, in the form of cortisone, for the treatment of asthma more than 60 years ago resulted in pronounced clinical effects. Today, inhaled GCs are considered to be the most effective anti-inflammatory treatment, safe in appropriate doses when given to asthmatic children and adults who need regular therapy to control symptoms or prevent exacerbations owing to reduced systemic absorption and risk of systemic side-effects (Rottier & Duiverman, 2009). Moreover, about 40-50% of patients with chronic obstructive pulmonary disease are being treated with inhaled GCs (Löwenberg et al., 2008).
- **Rheumatologic diseases:** Long-term therapy with GCs is often necessary to control the symptoms of rheumatoid arthritis and other rheumatic conditions (Neeck et al., 2002; Paul-Clark et al., 2002). It has been reported that up to 60% of patients with rheumatoid arthritis are treated more or less continuously with GCs (Löwenberg et al., 2008). Polymyalgia rheumatica is also a common indication for long-term glucocorticoid therapy and has a favorable prognosis. However there is considerable heterogeneity in patients' clinical course and response to this therapy. In addition, the patients are usually maintained on the lowest possible dose to control disease symptoms and to minimize GCs complications (Salvarani et al., 2002; Kremers et al., 2007).
- **Gastrointestinal inflammatory diseases:** Glucocorticoids are an effective treatment for inflammatory bowel disease such as ulcerative colitis and Crohn's disease (Löwenberg et al., 2008). Crohn's disease is a chronic inflammatory disorder of the bowel whose cause is unknown. During the acute phase of the disease, glucocorticoids such as prednisolone and prednisone are commonly used (Thomsem et al., 1998). In ulcerative colitis prednisolone was found to induce remission of symptoms concomitantly with reduction of endoscopically viewed colonic inflammation (Olaison et al., 1990). However, failure to respond, acutely or chronically, to GC therapy is a common indication for surgery in inflammatory bowel disease, with as many as 20% of patients with ulcerative colitis and approximately 50% of patients with Crohn's disease requiring surgery in their lifetime as a result of poor response to medical therapy (Farrell & Kelleher, 2003).
- **Other therapeutic uses:** GCs have been successfully used in the management of patients with renal diseases, allergic reactions, thrombocytopenia, corneal epithelial disease in dry eye and Graves' ophthalmopathy (De Paiva & Pflugfelder, 2008). In addition, these agents play an important role in the treatment of immune disorders,

including reducing the immune response in autoimmune diseases and organ transplantation (Grbović; Radenković, 2005). In short term, high dose suppressive GC therapy is also indicated in the treatment of medical emergencies such as necrotising vasculitis, status asthmaticus and anaphylactic shock (Swartz; Dluhy, 1978).

3.3 Side effects and contraindications

The physiologic effects of GCs are numerous and widespread. They influence electrolyte and water balance, carbohydrate metabolism, protein metabolism, lipid metabolism, cardiovascular system, skeletal muscle, central nervous system (CNS), formed elements of blood and affect other organs and tissues in a wide variety of ways (Chaney, 2002). The effect on fluid and electrolytes is due to their mineralocorticoid effect. It causes salt and water retention leading to edema, weight gain and hypertension. The potassium loss leading to hypokalemia can cause severe weakness (Deshmukh, 2007). Hyperglycemia is a known complication of GC therapy caused mainly by increased hepatic capacity for gluconeogenesis and reduced sensitivity to insulin. This increase in blood sugar levels can be a negative prognostic factor for ill patients (Davenport et al., 2010). Furthermore, GCs also increase lipid levels because of increased lipid production in liver and due to lipolysis from adipose tissue; and cause redistribution of carbohydrate, fat and protein reserves. This along with the increase in appetite can lead to the Cushingoid habitus (moon facies, buffalo hump and central obesity) (Deshmukh, 2007).

Due to these effects in the body, GC therapy is frequently hampered by severe side effects, especially when used in high doses for prolonged durations. The adverse effects of corticosteroids seen during short-term therapy include increased appetite, weight gain, fluid retention, gastritis, headache, mood swings, increase in blood sugar, hypertension and glaucoma. Adverse effects seen when therapy is given for longer duration include suppressed immunity, increased susceptibility to infections, increased cholesterol levels, weight gain, osteoporosis, deposition of body fat, thinning of skin, cataracts, stunting and hypothalamopituitary axis suppression (Löwenberg et al., 2008). Bone loss is one of the most important side effects of GC use. It starts promptly after initiation and mainly takes place in the first six months of treatment. Several studies and reports show a decrease in bone mineral density and an increased risk of fractures during GC use. The main effect of GC on bone is inhibition of osteoblast function, leading to a decrease in bone formation (De Nijs, 2008).

These side effects are responsible for several contraindications and limit the use of higher dosages and long-term use of GCs (Niedner, 2001; Löwenberg et al., 2008) The most important contraindications for the therapy of systemic GCs are uncontrolled hypertension, glaucoma, uncontrolled diabetes mellitus, osteoporosis, acute viral infections, bacterial infections, systemic fungal infections, parasitic diseases and psychiatric history (Niedner, 2001). Thus, the clinician must carefully consider in each case the presence of contraindications and the gains that can reasonably be expected from GC therapy versus the inevitable undesirable side effects of prolonged therapy (Niedner, 2001). The risk of glucocorticoid-induced osteoporosis can be reduced, for example, by general measurements like prescribing GCs in a low dose and for a short period of time. Furthermore, calcium and plain vitamin D3 supplementation and pharmacological intervention with bisphosphonates are considered as important support for prevention and treatment of glucocorticoid-induced osteoporosis (De Nijs, 2008).

3.4 Glucocorticosteroid resistance in inflammatory diseases

GCs resistance or insensitivity is a major barrier to the treatment of several common inflammatory diseases, including chronic obstructive pulmonary disease and acute respiratory distress syndrome; it is also an issue for some patients with asthma, rheumatoid arthritis, and inflammatory bowel disease. The resistance to the anti-inflammatory effects of GCs can be induced by several mechanisms that may differ between patients. These mechanisms include reduced GR expression, altered affinity of the ligand for GR, reduced ability of the GR to bind to DNA, increased expression of inflammatory transcription factors (eg, NF-κB, AP-1), raised macrophage migration inhibitory factor, and increased P-glycoprotein-mediated drug efflux. Patients with GC resistance can be treated with alternative broad-spectrum anti-inflammatory treatments, such as calcineurin inhibitors and other immunomodulators, or novel anti-inflammatory treatments, such as inhibitors of phosphodiesterase 4 or NF-κB (Barnes & Adcock, 2009).

3.5 Main glucocorticoid drugs

Several synthetic GC agonists have been developed since the availability of cortisone in the late 1950s (Löwenberg et al., 2008). The pharmacologic differences among various GCs derivatives result from structural alterations of the basic steroid nucleus and its side groups (Cevc & Blume, 2004). The main representatives of this class drugs and their peculiarities are described below.

- **Hydrocortisone:** A steroid hormone secreted by the adrenal cortex, is a short-acting GC (biological half-life of 8–12 hours) available in drug forms as unchanged hormone either different salts thereof (acetate, cypionate, sodium phosphate, butyrate, valerate, and sodium succinate). The hydrocortisone is used orally, in combination with fludrocortisone, for replacement therapy in adrenal insufficiency (Deshmukh, 2007). The effect of this agent on the milk is not known (Damiani et al., 2001). Hydrocortisone sodium succinate, the water-soluble derivative, is administered parenterally for a quicker effect in emergencies (Deshmukh, 2007);
- **Prednisone:** An intermediate-acting GC (biological half-life of 12–36 hours), is four to five times more potent than hydrocortisone (Zoorob; Cender, 2000). This GC is a prodrug, converted in normal circumstances in the body to prednisolone. It's widely used orally in the acute and long-term management of various disorders and for anti-inflammatory and immunosuppressant effects (Deshmukh, 2007). The use of prednisone can be done in nursing mothers (Damiani et al., 2001);
- **Methylprednisolone:** An intermediate-acting GC, is four to five times more potent than hydrocortisone as well as prednisone (Zoorob; Cender, 2000). It has less mineralocorticoid activity than prednisone/prednisolone while having a similar duration of action and may be preferred when mineralocorticoid effect is particularly undesirable. An alternate day regimen should be considered during long-term therapy (Deshmukh, 2007). The use of methylprednisolone can be done in nursing mothers, only in low dose (less than 8 mg/day) and the child should be breastfed after 4 hours of taking the GC (Damiani et al., 2001);
- **Triamcinolone:** An intermediate-acting GC, five times more potent than hydrocortisone can be done in nursing mothers (Damiani et al., 2001);

- **Dexamethasone:** Is a long-acting GC (biological half-life of 36–72 hours) highly potent, available as oral, parenteral, topical (spray), and ophthalmic dosage forms (Cevc; Blume, 2004). Its potency is about 25 times greater than the short-acting products (Zoorob; Cender, 2000). This GC has minimal mineralocorticoid activity and is used most often in the management of acute disorders because prolonged treatment is associated with severe suppression of the HPA axis. Furthermore it's not suitable for alternate day regimens where the aim is to maintain the responsiveness of the HPA axis (Deshmukh, 2007);
- **Betamethasone:** Similar to dexamethasone, is unsuitable for long-term alternate-day therapy due to its long duration of action (Deshmukh, 2007).

The therapeutic dosing regimen of these agents is very wide and depends on the indication for treatment. The basis for the use of different dosages in different clinical conditions is essentially empirical. Thus, the appropriate dose for a specific therapeutic effect should be determined by trial and error as well as should be reassessed periodically, particularly when complications arise during a therapy (Buttgereit et al., 2002)

3.6 Drug Interactions

GCs are known substrates and inducers of cytochrome P450 3A (CYP3A), enzymes which constitute the major phase one drug-metabolizing enzyme family in humans (Anglicheau et al., 2003). Thus, drugs that inhibit CYP 3A4, such as erythromycin, clarithromycin, ketoconazole, itraconazole, act to reduce serum levels of GC, consequently increasing the incidence and severity of side effects of GCs. On the other hand, drugs that induce CYP 3A4, such as barbiturates, phenytoin, rifampin, act to reduce serum levels, consequently decreasing the activity of several systemic GCs (Pereira et al., 2007).

These agents are also known substrates and inducers of P-glycoprotein (P-gp), product of the multidrugresistance gene responsible for the transmembrane efflux of many drugs. P-gp reduces the intracellular concentration of various xenobiotics. The high dose steroid therapy was recently shown to lower tacrolimus blood levels in the rat, as a result of the induction of P-gp and CYP3A in the intestine and liver (Anglicheau et al., 2003).

Other drug interactions, which involve other mechanisms, are described below (Table 4):

Drug	Mechanism of drug interaction	Consequence
Estrogens	↑ half-life and ↓ clearance of GCs	↑ action of GCs
Antacids	↓ absorption of GCs	↓ action of GCs
Cholestyramine	↓ absorption of GCs	↓ action of GCs
Ephedrine	↓ half-life and increased clearance of GCs, particularly of dexamethasone	↓ action of GCs
Cyclosporine	Inhibition of metabolism of cyclosporine by prednisolone	↑ action of cyclosporine
Isoniazid	↓ level serum of isoniazid by GCs	↓ action of isoniazid
Salicylates	↑ clearance of salicylates by GCs	↓ action of salicylates
Digitalics	GC-induced hypokalemia may ↑ serum concentration of digitalics	↑ action of digitalics

Table 4. GC interactions and clinical consequences (Pereira et al., 2007; Anti et al., 2008)

4. New anti-inflammatory agents

Nowadays, the increasing research developments in the fields of chemistry, pharmacology and molecular modeling, among others, share a common purpose: the pursuit and design of new agents and therapeutic targets. In this context, one area has raised interest in the field of therapeutic innovation: the treatment of inflammatory diseases.

Although its high therapeutic power, the anti-inflammatory therapies on the market have a high incidence of side effects resulting from its use (especially chronic), making unfavorable the risk/benefit ratio of these medications in many patients. Given this context, it becomes necessary to introduce new therapeutic options with more effective, specific and with fewer adverse effects actives. Currently, several targets and agents are being tested for their anti-inflammatory activity, such as:

- Components of signal transduction (e.g. NF-κB and mitogen-activated protein kinase such as p38 kinase and c-Jun N-terminal kinases - JNKs): Some of small molecules that inhibit p38 kinase are in the final stages of clinical trials (Kulkarni et al., 2006);
- Dual inhibitiors of COX-2 and 5-lipoxygenase (5-LOX): Various structural families of dual inhibitors have been designed and several compounds are currently undergoing pre-clinical or clinical development. By preventing the biosynthesis of both prostanoids and LTs, they are potent anti-inflammatory agents (Charlier & Michaux, 2003);
- Proinflammatory cytokines: Given their central role in the regulation of inflammatory responses, cytokines are clearly appealing targets for therapeutic intervention. Emphasis has been placed on cytokines that are produced early in the inflammatory cascade such as TNF-α and IL-6. Therapeutics neutralizing these cytokines or their receptors are already on the market or in late-phase development (Kopf et al., 2010).

Recently, a new biological target for anti-inflammatory therapy has been identified: the peroxisome proliferator-activated receptors (PPAR). PPARs are ligand-activated transcription factors belonging to the nuclear receptor superfamily. This superfamily includes steroidal transcription factors, non-steroidal receptors, PPARs and liver X receptor (LXR).

Three major subtypes of the receptor have been identified: PPAR-α, PPAR-β and PPAR-γ.

Originally, the PPAR activity was thought to be limited to lipid metabolism and glucose homeostasis, being the PPAR-γ agonists (known as thiazolidinediones) commonly prescribed for the treatment of diabetes. Later studies showed that PPAR activation regulates other biological functions such as cell proliferation, differentiation and apoptosis (Moraes et al, 2006).

Several studies have showed that PPAR-α and PPAR-γ inhibit the expression of inflammatory genes. All available data indicate that the activation of PPAR-α and PPAR-γ modulates oxidative stress-sensitive pathways, NF-κB, AP-1, and signal transducers and activators of transcription (STAT). These findings strongly indicate the potential as therapeutic target sites of PPAR-α and PPAR-γ in controlling the inflammatory process and age-related inflammatory diseases. In support of evidence on the role of PPAR-α in the suppression of NF-κB activity, PPAR-α agonists are shown to decrease production of pro-inflammatory mediators such as IL-6, IL-12, IL-1a, iNOS, and COX-2, which are associated with the decrease in NF-κB activation.

Apart from its role as a transcription factor, PPAR-γ also acts as a trans-repressor of macrophage inflammatory genes. Ligand-independent activation of PPAR-β/δ can suppress bowel disease by down regulation of inflammatory signaling (Chung et al., 2008).

During inflammatory responses, PPARs can be activated by eicosanoids. Ligands for PPAR-γ include leukotriene B4, 8(S)-hydroxyecosatetraenoic acid (HETE), 15-deoxy-D-12,14-prostaglandin J2, 15-HETE and 13-hydroxyoctadecadienoic acid. Nuclear receptors can regulate macrophage gene expression in response to changes in cellular lipids and arachidonic acid metabolites that occur during inflammatory responses (Rizzo & Fiorucci, 2006).

PPAR-γ protein was identified in the antigen presenting cells, monocytes and macrophages and synthetic PPAR-γ agonists including pioglitazone, troglitazone and rosiglitazone were shown to suppress production of inflammatory cytokines by these cells (Jiang et al., 1998; Ricote et al., 1998). Subsequently, PPAR-γ was identified in dendritic cells. The same thiazolidinedione compounds were demonstrated to decrease dendritic cell secretion of IL-12, a potent TH1-type inflammatory cytokine (Martin, 2010).

In this context, PPAR-γ agonists have been investigated for their anti-inflammatory effects. Beneficial effects of the PPAR-γ activator, rosiglitazone, were reported in two recent clinical trials for the treatment of Ulcerative Colitis (Lewis et al., 2008; Liang & Ouyang, 2008). Animal models of inflammation are now being used to explore the utility of PPAR-γ agonists in other inflammatory diseases.

5. Conclusion

The steroidal and non-steroidal anti-inflammatory drugs provide efficient therapies for the treatment of inflammatory diseases. However, several adverse effects related to acute and especially cronic use of such drugs limit its use in some patients. Thus, the clinician should take into account the risks and benefits of treatment for the patient before starting the therapy.

Recent searches for new targets and anti-inflammatory agents aim to attend the demand for new secure and equally efficient therapies for the treatment of inflammation. In this context, PPAR-γ agonists appear as candidates for anti-inflammatory drugs.

6. References

ADAPT Research Group (2008). Cognitive function over time in the Alzheimer's Disease Anti-inflammatory Prevention Trial (ADAPT): Results of a randomized, controlled trial of naproxen and celecoxib. *Arch Neurol*, Vol.65, pp.896–905.

Akama, T.; Baker, S.J.; Zhang, Y.K.; Hernandez, V.; Zhou, H.; Sanders, V.; Freund, Y.; et al. (2009). Bioorganic & Medicinal Chemistry Letters Discovery and structure - activity study of a novel benzoxaborole anti-inflammatory agent (AN2728) for the potential topical treatment of psoriasis and atopic dermatitis. *Bioorganic & Medicinal Chemistry Letters*, Vol.19, No.8, pp. 2129-2132.

Anglicheau, D.; Flamant, M.; Martinez, F. & Schlageter, M.H.; Cassinat, B.; Beaune, P. et al. (2003). Pharmacokinetic interaction between corticosteroids and tacrolimus after renal transplantation. *Nephrology Dialysis Transplantation*, Vol.18, pp. 2409-2414.

Anti, S.M.A.; Giorgi, R.D.N. & Chahade, W.H. (2008). Steroidal antiinflammatory drugs: glucocorticoids. Einstein, Vol.6, No.(Supl 1), pp. 159-165.

Antman, E.M.; DeMets, D. & Loscalzo, J. (2005). Cyclooxygenase inhibition and cardiovascular risk. *Circulation*, Vol. 112, pp. 759-770.

Antman, E.M.; Bennet, J.S.; Daugherty, A.; Furberg, C.; Roberts, H. & Taubert, K.A. (2007) Use of nonsteroidal anti-inflamatory drugs: an update for clinicians: a scientific statement from the American Heart Association. *Circulation*, Vol. 115, No.12, pp. 1634-1642.

Arber, N., Eagle, C.J., Spicak, J., et al. (2006). Celecoxib for the prevention of colorectal adenomatous polyps. *N. Engl. J. Med.*, Vol.355, pp. 885–95

Baldwin, A.S. (1996). The NF-kappa B and I kappa B proteins: new discoveries and insights. *Annual review of immunology*, Vol.14, pp. 649-683.

Barnes, P.J. & Adcock, I.M. (2009). Glucocorticoid resistance in inflammatory diseases. *Review Literature And Arts Of The Americas*, Vol.373, pp.1905-1917.

Berenbaum F. (2004). COX-3: fact or fancy? *Joint Bone Spine*, Vol.71, No.6, pp.451–453.

Bertagnolli, M.M., Eagle, C.J., Zauber, A.G., et al. (2006). Celecoxib for the prevention of sporadic colorectal adenomas. *N Engl J Med*, Vol.355, pp. 873–84

Bresalier, R.S.; Sandler, R.S.; Quan, H.; Bolognese, J.A.; Oxegius, B.; Horgan, K. et al. (2006) Cardiovascular events associated with rofecoxib in a colorectal adenoma chemoprevention trial *N Engl J Med, Vol.*352, pp.1092–1102.

Buttgereit, F.; da Silva, J.A.P.; Boers, M.; Burmester, G.R.; Cutolo, M.; Jacobs, J.; Kirwan, J. et al. (2002). Standardised nomenclature for glucocorticoid dosages and glucocorticoid treatment regimens: current questions and tentative answers in rheumatology. *Annals of the rheumatic diseases*, Vol.61 No.8, pp. 718-722.

Cardozo, A.L.P.; Bolzani, F.C.B.; Stefani, M. & Charlín, R. (2007). Terapéutica Uso sistêmico de corticosteróides: revisão da literatura. *Med Cutan Iber Lat Amer*, Vol.35 No.1, pp. 35-50.

Cevc, G. & Blume, G. (2004). Hydrocortisone and dexamethasone in very deformable drug carriers have increased biological potency , prolonged effect , and reduced therapeutic dosage. *Biochimica et Biophysica Acta*, Vol.1663, pp. 61-73.

Cha, I.Y.; DuBois, R.N. (2007). NSAIDs and Cancer Prevention: Targets Downstream of COX-2. *Annu Rev Med* Vol.58, pp. 239-252.

Chaney, MA. (2002). Corticosteroids and Cardiopulmonary Bypass : A Review of Clinical Investigations. *Chest*, Vol.121, No.3, pp. 921-931.

Charlier, C. & Michaux, C. (2003). Dual inhibition of cyclooxygenase-2 (COX-2) and 5-lipoxygenase (5-LOX) as a new strategy to provide safer non-steroidal anti-inflammatory drugs. *European Journal of Medicinal Chemistry*, Vol.38,No.7-8,pp.645-659.

Chen, CC.; Rosenbloom, CL.; Anderson, DC. & Manning, AM. (1995). Selective inhibition of E-selectin, vascular cell adhesion molecule-1, and intercellular adhesion molecule-1 expression by inhibitors of I kappa B-alpha phosphorylation. *Journal of immunology (Baltimore, Md. : 1950)*, Vol.155, No.7, pp. 3538-3545.

Chung, JH.; Seo, AY.; Chung, SW.; Kim, MK.; Leeuwenburgh, C.; Yu, BP. & Chung, HY. (2008). Molecular mechanism of PPAR in the regulation of age-related inflammation. *Ageing research reviews*, Vol.7, No.2, pp. 126-136.

Collins, T.; Read, MA.; Neish, AS.; Wiiitley, MZ.; Whitley, MZ.; Thanos, D. & Maniatis, T. (1995). Transcriptional regulation of endothelial cell adhesion molecules: NF-kappa B and cytokine-inducible enhancers. *The FASEB journal : official publication of the Federation of American Societies for Experimental Biology*, Vol.9, No.10, pp. 899-909.

Cuzzocrea, S.; Bruscoli, S.; Mazzon, E.; Crisafulli, C.; Donato, V. et al. (2008). Peroxisome Proliferator-Activated Receptor-a Contributes to the Anti-Inflammatory Activity of Glucocorticoids. *Clinical and Experimental Medicine*, Vol.73, No.2, pp. 323-337.

Damiani, D.; Kuperman, H.; Dichtchekenian, V. & Setian, N. (2001). Repercussions of corticotherapy: the cost–benefit ratio. *Pediatria*, No.1, pp. 71-82.

Davenport, MS.; Cohan, RH.; Caoili, EM. & Ellis, JH. (2010). Hyperglycemic consequences of corticosteroid premedication in an outpatient population. *AJR. American journal of roentgenology*, Vol.194, No.6, pp. W483-488.

De Nijs, RN. (2008). Glucocorticoid-induced osteoporosis: a review on pathophysiology and treatment options. *Minerva Med*, Vol.99 No.1, pp. 23-43.

De Paiva, CS. & Pflugfelder, SC. (2008). Rationale for anti-inflammatory therapy in dry eye syndrome. *Inflammation*, Vol.71, pp. 89-95.

Derendorf, H. & Meltzer, E. O. (2008). Review article Molecular and clinical pharmacology of intranasal corticosteroids: clinical and therapeutic implications. *Allergy*, Vol.63, pp. 1292-1300.

Deshmukh, CT. (2007) Minimizing side effects of systemic corticosteroids in children. *Indian J Dermatol Venereol Leprol, Vol.*73, pp. 218-221.

Farrell, RJ. & Kelleher, D. (2003). Mechanism of Steroid Action and Resistance in Inflammation - Glucocorticoid resistance in inflammatory bowel disease. *Journal of Endocrinology*, Vol.178, pp. 339-346.

Feghali, CA.; Wright, TM. (1997). Cytokines in acute and chronic inflammation. *Frontiers in bioscience : a journal and virtual library*, Vol.2, pp. 12-26.

Fernandes, AM.; Cardoso, F.; Valera, P. & Anselmo-Lima, WT. (2008). Mechanism of action of glucocorticoids in nasal polyposis. *Rev Bras Otorrinolaringol*, 74(2), 279-283.

Fingar, VH.; Taber, SW.; Buschemeyer, WC.; Ten Tije, A.; Cerrito, PB.; Tseng, M. et al. (1997). Constitutive and stimulated expression of ICAM-1 protein on pulmonary endothelial cells in vivo. *Microvascular research*, Vol.54, No.2, pp 135-44.

Fitzgerald, DA. (2004) Coxibs and cardiovascular disease. *N Engl J Med*. Vol.351, pp.1709 - 1711.

Flammer, J. R. & Rogatsky, I. (2011). Minireview: Glucocorticoids in autoimmunity: unexpected targets and mechanisms. *Mol Endocrinol*, Vol.25, No.7, pp. 1075-1086.

Frank, PG. & Lisanti, MP. (2008). ICAM-1: role in inflammation and in the regulation of vascular permeability. *American journal of physiology. Heart and circulatory physiology*, Vol.295, No.3, pp. H926-H927.

Gilmore, TD. (2006). Introduction to NF-kappaB: players, pathways, perspectives. *Oncogene,* Vol.25, No.51, p. 6680-4.

Gladding, PA.; Webster, MWI.; Farrell, HB.; Zeng, ISL.; Park, R. & Ruijne, N. (2008). The antiplatelet effect of six non-steroidal antiinflammatorydrugs and their pharmacodynamic interaction with aspirin in healthy volunteers. *Am J Cardiol* Vol.101, pp. 1060–1063.

Goodman, L. S.; Brunton, L. L. & Chabner, B. (2010). *Goodman & Gilman's The pharmacological basis of therapeutics* (p. 1808). McGraw-Hill Medical.

Graham, D.; Campen, D.; Hui, R.; Spence, M.; Cheethan, C.; Levy, G. et al. (2005) Risk of acute myocardial infarction and sudden cardiac death in patients treated with cyclo-oxygenase 2 selective and non-selective non-steroidal anti-inflammatory drugs: nested case-control study. *The lancet on-line,* Vol.365, pp. 475-481.

Grbović, L. & Radenković, M. (2005). Therapeutic use of glucocorticoids and immunosuppressive agents. *Srpski arhiv za celokupno lekarstvo,* Vol.133, pp. 67-73.

Grosser, T.; Fries, S. & FitzGerald, G.A. (2006). Biological basis for the cardiovascular consequences of COX-2 inhibition: therapeutic challenges and opportunities. *The Journal of clinical investigation,* Vol.116, No.1, pp. 4-15.

Guay-Woodford L.M. (1998). Bartter syndrome: Unraveling the pathophysiologic enigma. *Am J Med,* Vol. 105, pp.151-161.

Hagan, J.B.; Taylor, R.L. & Singh, R.J. (2011). Assessment of synthetic glucocorticoids in asthmatic sputum. *Allergy Rhinol,* Vol.2 No.1, pp. 33-35.

Hofstadler G.; Tulzer G.; Altmann R.; Schmitt K.; Danford D.; Huhta JC. Spontaneous closure of the human fetal ductus arteriosus: a cause of fetal congestive heart failure.(1996) *Am J Obstet Gynecol.* Vol.174, No.3, pp. 879-883.

Holdgate A, Pollock T. (2004) Systematic review of the relative efficacy of non-steroidal anti-inflammatory drugs and opioids in the treatment of acute renal colic. *BMJ,* Vol.328, No.7453, pp. 1401.

Hollis Eden Pharmaceutical Annual Report, 2007

Inotai, A.; Hankó, B.; Mészáros, Á. (2010). Trends in the non-steroidal anti-inflammatory drug market in six Central - Eastern European countries based on retail information y. *Parmamacoepidemiology and Drug Safety,* Vol.19, No.2, pp.183-190.

Jakubowski, J.A.; Vaillancourt R. & Deykin D. (1988). Interaction of ethanol, prostacyclin, and aspirin in determining human platelet reactivity in vitro. *Arteriosclerosis,* Vol.8, pp. 436–441.

Jiang, C.; Ting, A. T. & Seed, B. (1998). PPAR-gamma agonists inhibit production of monocyte inflammatory cytokines. *Nature,* Vol.391, No.6662, pp. 82-86.

Jungnickel P.W., Maloley P.A., Vander Tuin E.L., et al. (1997). Effect of two aspirin pretreatment regimens on niacin-induced cutaneous reactions. *J Gen Intern Med,* Vol.12, pp.591–596.

Keenan, R.T.; O'brien, W.R.; Lee, K.H.; Crittenden, D.B.; Fisher, M.C.; Goldfarm, D.S. et al. Prevalence of Contraindications and Prescription of Pharmacologic Therapies for Gout. (2011) *The American journal of medicine,* Vol.124, No.2, pp. 155-162.

Kopf, M.; Bachmann, M.F.; Marsland, B.J. (2010). Averting inflammation by targeting the cytokine environment. *Nature reviews. Drug discovery,* Vol.9, No.9, pp. 703-718.

Kujubu, D.A.; Herschman, H.R. (1992). Dexamethasone inhibits mitogen induction of the TIS10 prostaglandin synthase/cyclooxygenase gene. *J Biol Chem*, No.267, No.12, pp. 7991-7994.

Kulkarni, R.G.; Achaiah, G.; Sastry, G.N. (2006). Novel targets for antiinflammatory and antiarthritic agents. *Current pharmaceutical design*, Vol.12, No.19, pp. 2437-54.

Kurth T.; Glynn R.J.; Walker A.M.; Chan K.A.; Buring J.E.; Hennekens C.H. & Gaziano J.M. (2003). Inhibition of clinical benefits of aspirin on first myocardial infarction by nonsteroidal antiinflammatory drugs. *Circulation;* Vol.108, pp. 1191–1195.

Laine, L.; Curtis, SP.; Cryer, B.; Kaur, A.; Cannon, C. P. (2010). Risk factors for NSAID-associated upper GI clinical events in a long-term prospective study of 34 701 arthritis patients. *Alimentary pharmacology & therapeutics*, Vol.32, No.10, pp. 1240-1248.

Lewis, J. D.; Lichtenstein, G. R.; Deren, J. J.; Sands, B. E.; Hanauer, S. B.; Katz, J. A.; Lashner, B.; et al. (2008). Rosiglitazone for active ulcerative colitis: a randomized placebo-controlled trial. *Gastroenterology*, Vol.134, No.3, pp. 688-695.

Liang, HL.; Ouyang, Q. (2008). A clinical trial of combined use of rosiglitazone and 5-aminosalicylate for ulcerative colitis. *World journal of gastroenterology : WJG*, Vol.14, No.1, pp. 114-119.

Löwenberg, M.; Stahn, C.; Hommes, DW. & Buttgereit, F. (2007). Novel insights into mechanisms of glucocorticoid action and the development of new glucocorticoid receptor ligands. *Arthritis & Rheumatism*, Vol.73, pp. 1025-1029.

Maneechotesuwan, K.; Ekjiratrakul, W.; Kasetsinsombat, K.; Wongkajornsilp, A. & Barnes, PJ. (2010). Statins enhance the anti-inflammatory effects of inhaled corticosteroids in asthmatic patients through increased induction of indoleamine 2 , 3-dioxygenase. *Journal of Allergy and Clinical Immunology*, Vol.126, No.4, pp. 754-762.

Martin, H. (2010). Role of PPAR-gamma in inflammation. Prospects for therapeutic intervention by food components. *Mutation Research/Fundamental and Molecular Mechanisms of Mutagenesis*, Vol.690, No.1-2, pp. 57-63.

Maeda, A.; Tsuruoka, S.; Ushijima, K.; Kanai, Y.; Endou, H.; Saito, K.; Miyamoto, E. & Fujimura, A. (2010). Drug interaction between celecoxib and methotrexate in organic anion transporter 3-transfected renal cells and in rats in vivo. *European journal of pharmacology*, Vol.640, No.1-3, pp. 168-171.

McAdam B.F., Catella-Lawson F., Mardini I.A., et al (1999). Systemic biosynthesis of prostacyclin by cyclooxygenase (COX)-2: The human pharmacology of a selective inhibitor of COX-2. *Proc Natl Acad Sci U S A*, Vol.96, pp. 272–277.

Meade, E.A.; Smith, W.L. & DeWitt, D.L. (1993). Differential inhibition of prostaglandin endoperoxide synthase (cyclooxygenase) isozymes by aspirin and other non-steroidal anti-inflammatory drugs. *The Journal of biological chemistry*, Vol.268,Vol.9,pp.6610-6614.

Melnikova, I. (2010). Pain market. *Nature reviews. Drug discovery*, Vol.9, No.8, pp. 589-590.

Menezes, G.B.; Cara, D.C. & Rezende, RM. (2009). Anti-inflammatory drugs: Basic knowledge to a safe prescription. *Odontol. clín.-cient*, Vol.8, No.1, pp. 7-12.

Moraes, L.A.; Piqueras, L. & Bishop-Bailey, D. (2006). Peroxisome proliferator-activated receptors and inflammation. *Pharmacology & therapeutics*, Vol.110, No.3, pp. 371-385.

Neeck, G.; Renkawitz, R. & Eggert, M. (2002). *Cytokines, Cellular & Molecular Therapy*, Vol.7, No.2, pp. 61-69.

Niedner, R. (2001). Therapie mit systemischen Glukokortikoiden. *Hautarzt*, Vol.52, pp. 1062-1072.

Olaison, G.; Sjödahl, R. & Tagesson, C. (1990). Glucocorticoid treatment in ileal Crohn's disease: relief of symptoms but not of endoscopically viewed inflammation. *Gut*, Vol.31 No.3, pp. 325-328.

O'Neill, L.A.J. (2008). The interleukin-1 receptor/Toll-like receptor superfamily: 10 years of progress. *Immunological reviews*, Vol.226, pp. 10-18.

Paul-Clark, M.J.; Mancini, L.; Del Soldato, P.; Flower, R.J. & Perretti, M. (2002). Potent antiarthritic properties of a glucocorticoid derivative, NCX-1015, in an experimental model of arthritis. *Proceedings of the National Academy of Sciences of the United States of America*, Vol.99, No.3, pp. 1677-1682.

Pountos, I.; Georgouli, T.; Howard, B. & Giannoudis, P.V. (2011) Nonsteroidal anti-inflammatory drugs: prostaglandins, indications, and side effects. International *Journal of Interferon, Cytokine and Mediator Research*, Vol.3, pp. 19–27.

Prasit, P. (1999). The discovery of rofecoxib, [MK 966, VIOXX®, 4-(4'-methylsulfonylphenyl)-3-phenyl-2(5H)-furanone], an orally active cyclooxygenase-2 inhibitor. *Bioorganic & Medicinal Chemistry Letters*, Vol.9, No.13, pp. 1773-1778.

Rao, P.N.P. & Knaus, E.E. (2008). Evolution of Nonsteroidal Anti-Inflammatory Cyclooxygenase (COX) Inhibition and Beyond Drugs (NSAIDs): *J Pharm Pharmaceut Sci*, Vol.11, No.2, pp. 81-110.

Ricote, M.; Li, A.C.; Willson, T.M.; Kelly, C.J. & Glass, C.K. (1998). The peroxisome proliferator-activated receptor-gamma is a negative regulator of macrophage activation. *Nature*, Vol.391, *No*.6662, pp. 79-82.

Rizzo, G. & Fiorucci, S. (2006). PPARs and other nuclear receptors in inflammation. *Current opinion in pharmacology*, Vol.6, No.4, pp. 421-427.

Robbins, S.L.; Kumar, V.; Abbas, A.K.; Cotran, R.S. & Fausto, N. (2010). *Robbins and Cotran pathologic basis of disease* (p. 1450).

Rottier, B.L. & Duiverman, E.J. (2009). Anti-inflammatory drug therapy in asthma. *Clinical Immunology*, Vol.10, pp. 214-219.

Kremers, H.M.; Reinalda, M.S.; Crowson, C.S.; Davis, J.M.; Hunder, G.G. & Gabriel, S.E. (2007). Glucocorticoids and Cardiovascular and Cerebrovascular Events in Polymyalgia Rheumatica. *Arthritis & Rheumatism*, Vol.57 No.2, pp. 279-286.

Salvarani, C.; Cantini, F.; Boiardi, L. & Hunder, G.G. (2002). Polymyalgia Rheumatica and Giant-Cell Arteritis. *N Engl J Med*, Vol.347, PP. 261-271.

Secoli, S.R. (2010) Polifarmácia: interações e reações adversas no uso de medicamentos por idosos. *Revista Brasileira de Enfermagem*, Vol.63, No.1, pp. 136-140.

Seeling, C.B.; Maloley, P.A.; Campbell, J.R. (1990). Nephrotoxicity Associated with concomitant ACE inhibitor and NSAID therapy. *Southern Medical Journal*. Vol.83, No.10, pp. 1144-1148.

Shiri, R.; Koskimäki, J.; Häkkinen, T.L.J.; Tammaela, A.; Auvinen, A.; Hakama, M. (2006) Effect of Nonsteroidal Anti-inflamatory Drug Use on the Incidence of Erectile Dysfunction. *The Journal of Urology*, Vol.175, pp. 1812-1816.

Siew, C.N.G.; Francis, K.L.C. (2010) NSAID-induced Gastrointestinal and Cardiovascular Injury. *Curr Opin Gastroenterol*, Vol.26, No.6, pp.611-617.

Swartz, S.L.; Dluhy, R.G. (1978) Corticosteroids: clinical pharmacology and therapeutic use. *Drugs*, Vol.16, pp. 238-255

Tanaka, K.I.; Suemasu, S.; Ishihara, T.; Tasaka, Y.; Arai, Y.; Misushima, T. (2009) Inhibition of both COX-1 and COX-2 and resulting decrease in the level of prostaglandins E2 is responsible for non-steroidal anti-inflammatory drug (NSAID)-dependent exacerbation of colitis. *European Journal of Pharmacology*, Vol.603, pp. 120–132.

Thomsen, O.O.; Cortot, A.; Jewell, D.; Wright, J.P.; Winter, T. et al. (1998). A comparison of budesonide and mesalamine for active Crohn's disease. International Budesonide-Mesalamine Study Group.*The New England journal of medicine*,Vol.339,No.6,pp.370-374.

Timóteo, R.P. & Dos Santos, D. S. F. de A. V. (2009). Physical activity against reduction of mass bone induced for glucocorticoids. *ConScientiae Saúde*, Vol.8, No.1, pp. 139-144.

Topol, E.J. (2004) Failing the public health: rofecoxib, Merck, and the FDA. *N Engl J Med*. Vol.351, pp.1707–1709.

United States Food and Drug Administration [FDA], Center for Drug Evaluation and Research, U.S. Department of Health and Human Services. (2011) Approved Drug Products with Therapeutic Equivalence Evaluations, 31th ed. U.S. Department of Health and Human Services, Washington, D.C.

Vane, J.R. (2000). The fight against rheumatism: from willow bark to COX-1 sparing drugs. *Journal of physiology and pharmacology : an official journal of the Polish Physiological Society*, Vol.51, pp. 573-586.

Vane, JR. (1971). Inhibition of Prostaglandin Synthesis as a Mechanism of Action for Aspirin-like Drugs. *Nature*, Vol.231, No.25, pp. 232-235.

Waddell, W.R., Ganser, G.F., Cerise, E.J., Loughry, R.W. (1989). Sulindac for polyposis of the colon. *Am J Surg* Vol. 157, pp. 175–79

Waddell, W.R., Loughry, R.W. (1983). Sulindac for polyposis of the colon. *J Surg Oncol* Vol.24, pp.83–87

Winkelmayer, W.C.; Waikar, S.S., Mogun, H. & Solomon D.H. (2008) Nonselective and cyclooxygenase-2-selective NSAIDs and acute kidney injury. *Am J Med*. Vol.121, No.12, p.1092–1098.

Worobec A.S. (2000); Treatment of systemic mast cell disorders. Hematol Oncol Clin *North Am*, Vol.14, pp.659–687.

Yeh, R.K.; Chen, J.; Jennie, L.; Williams, J.L.; Baluch, M.; Hundleym T.R.; Hundley, R.E.; Rosenbaum, R.E.; Srinivas, K.; Tragano, F.; Benardini, F.; Soldato, P.D.; Kashfi, K.; Rigas, B. (2004) NO-donating nonsteroidal antiinflammatory drugs (NSAIDs) inhibit colon cancer cell growth more Potently than traditional NSAIDs: a general pharmacological property? *Biochemical Pharmacology* Vol.67, pp. 2197–2205

Zele, T.V.; Gevaert, P.; Holtappels, G.; Beule, A.; Wormald, P.J.; Mayr, S. et al. (2010). Oral steroids and doxycycline: Two different approaches to treat nasal polyps. *Journal of Allergy and Clinical Immunology*, Vol.125, No.5, pp. 1069-1076.

Zoorob, R.J. & Cender, D. (1998). A different look at corticosteroids. *American family physician*, Vol.58, No.2, pp. 443-50.

7

House Dust Mite Immunotherapy in Iraqi Patients with Allergic Rhinitis and Asthma

Abdulghani Mohamad Alsamarai, Amina Hamed Ahmad Alobaidi, Sami Mezher Alrefaiei and Amar Mohamed Alwan
Departments of Medicine, Biochemistry and Otolaryngology, College of Medicine, Tikrit University, Tikrit Iraq

1. Introduction

Respiratory allergy (allergic rhino conjunctivitis and allergic asthma), is community encountered medical condition that cause substantial morbidity and mortality worldwide [1]. Asthma is still remains a concerning and coasty epidemic that is largely unexplained [2]. In Iraq, both allergic rhinitis and asthma cause poor performance at work and school and diminished quality of life [3]. Suspected allergen(s) avoidance is the first-line treatment for these conditions. However, in many cases, exposure to a particular allergen cannot be completely avoided [4]. Pharmacotherapy, whether that reversing inflammation or controlling the effect of released mediators are not always fully effective or well tolerated [4]. Allergen immunotherapy is widely accepted as an efficacious treatment in allergic rhinitis and asthma [5-9]. Well characterized dust mite extracts have shown significant benefit by reducing symptoms, medication requirements and sensitivity to dust mite allergens [10]. Recent studies of specific immunotherapy using standardized extracts also showed improvement in symptoms, medication and bronchial hyperresponsiveness [10-13]. However, Adkinson et al [14] were unable to show any significant improvement in symptoms, medication use, peak flow rate, BHR or rate of asthma remission following multiple allergens SIT in asthmatic children.

More recent studies in children and adults show additional positive outcomes of SIT which are decreased tendency for additional environmental sensitization [15], as well as a decreased incidence of asthma in treated allergic rhinitis patients [16]. Although the documented effectiveness of SIT in the treatment of allergic rhinitis and allergic asthma, the real life efficacy and use of this treatment option is severely limited by perceived low patient compliance [17, 18], adverse local and systemic side effects [19, 20] and significant delay in effect after the initiation of therapy, all of which may lead to relatively low adherence rate [8].

Although there is much and convincing evidence for SIT effectiveness and efficacy from international studies only single study has prospectively investigated the real-life efficacy in Iraqi patients [21]. This prospective study of patients undergoing SIT in an office setting to produce practical data of efficacy of house dust mite extracts for allergic patients in Iraq.

Objectives: To

1. Determine the therapeutic efficacy of house dust mite immunotherapy in Iraqi patients with allergic rhinitis and asthma.
2. Clarify whether specific immunotherapy of therapeutic benefits in patient with asthma and allergic rhinitis.

2. Patients and methods

2.1 Patients

From January 2000 to December 2008, we selected 822 patients with allergic rhinitis and asthma to receive subcutaneous specific immunotherapy according to European Academy of Allergy and Clinical Immunology (EAACI) guidelines [22] in a double blind placebo controlled clinical trial. Subjects were recruited from asthma clinic in the city of Tikrit, Iraq, only subjects who fulfilled the GINA guidelines for mild to moderate asthma and/or allergic rhinitis [23] and had positive skin prick-test to *Dermatophagoides pteronyssinus* and/or *D. farines* were included.

Subjects excluded if their PEER of <80% of predicted value recorded on 3 occasions during the 2 week prior to randomization, with positive SPT to animals and pets at home; asthma exacerbation during the last month prior to first visit, forced expiratory volume at 1 second (FEV1) of <60% predicted during the screening visits, had any serious chronic underlying illness. Patients were evaluated by medical history, clinical examination and skin prick test with common allergen. All data were collected prospectively, including information on exposure, social factors, additional diagnosis and medication usage, family history of allergic diseases, exposure to house pets, active or passive smoking, measures of treatment efficacy, and patients' satisfaction as well as local and systemic reactions to the SIT shots. The protocol was approved by Tikrit University College of Medicine Ethical Committee and informed written consent taken from each patient. After patient selection, they were randomized to SIT and/or placebo and pharmacotherapy. The two groups were comparable at baseline (Table-1).

Variable	Immunotherapy	Placebo	P value
Patients no.	411	411	NS
Female/Male	198/213	194/217	NS
Defaulted	73(18%)	94(23%)	NS
Patients for analysis	338(82%)	317(77%)	NS
Age range	6-65	6-65	NS
Age mean	32±15	31±18	NS
Clinical history			
AR	52(15%)	54(17%)	NS
Asthma	115(34%)	107(34%)	NS
AR+ Asthma	171(51%)	156(49%)	NS
Use of medication			
Antihistamine	270(80%)	269(85%)	NS
Glucocorticoids	135(39%)	127(40%)	NS
B2-mimetics	166(49%)	149(47%)	NS
Mast cell stabilizer	101(30%)	111(35%)	NS

Table 1. Patient characteristics.

2.2 Asthma and allergic rhinitis diagnosis

The diagnosis of asthma and classification was performed by specialist physicians based on the National Heart Blood and Lung Institute / World Health Organization (NHLBI/WHO) workshop on the Global Strategy for Asthma [24]. Allergic rhinitis diagnosis was performed according to previously reported guidelines [25].

2.3 Lung function test

Computerized Spirometer (Autosphiror, Discom-14, Chest Corporation, and Japan) was used for measurement of FEV1 predicted percent of the patients at their enrollment in the study and when indicated according to studies design.

2.4 Skin prick test

The skin prick tests were performed for all patients and control and evaluated in accordance with European Academy of Allergy and Clinical Immunology subcommittee on allergy standardization and skin tests using standards allergen panel (Stallergen, France). The panel for skin test include: dust mite (Dermatophagoides farina, Dermatophagoides peteronyssinus), Aleternaria, Cadosprium, Penicillum mixture, Aspergillus mixture, Grasses mixture, Feather mixture, Dog hair, Horse hair, Cat fur, Fagacae, Oleaceae, Betulaceae, Plantain, Bermuda grass, Chenopodium and Mugworth. All tests were performed in the outpatient Asthma and Allergy Centre, Mosul by a physician using a commercial allergen extracts (Stallergen, France) and a lancet skin prick test device. A wheal diameter of 3 mm or more in excess of the negative control was considered as positive test result.

2.5 Allergen extracts for SCIT

Therapeutic vaccines containing allergen extracts were purchased from Stallergen, France. Both aqueous and glycenerated extracts were used to achieve a concentrate of 1:100 w/v of the mixed extract. In standardized extracts the stock formulation was prepared by tenfold dilution. Separate vial was used for allergen extract to reduce proteolysis degradation. All extracts were stored at 8 ^{0}C . Therapeutic vaccine varied with each individual patient based on specific allergen identified during testing. Moist patients received a variety of aeroallergen combination.

2.6 SCIT protocol

The treatment protocol is of two stage, the attack and maintenance stages. The attack treatment with gradual increase in dose and concentration of vaccine content were carried weekly for a period of 20 weeks. The vaccine is injected by deep subcutaneous route in the posterior aspect of upper arm. The maintenance treatment dose given in a constant dose every 15 days and then every 4 or 6 weeks interval. The interval between two maintenance injections must not exceed 6 weeks. Local reaction size was measured 20 minutes after each injection. Observed large local reactions (more than 20 mm wheal size) mandated a repeat of the same dose on the next visit, while systemic allergic reactions (skin, respiratory, cardiovascular, and / or gastrointestinal) required a two fold reduction in vaccine concentration. Maintenance dose was set in most cases at 0.5 of the stock standardized extracts.

2.7 Immunotherapy schedule

Immunotherapy was given in term of conventional schedule. Conventional Immunotherapy build- up was typically given as injection per week until the maintenance dose was reached and it was given once monthly. Allergen vaccines were administered subcutaneously according to EAACI guidelines [26] after the patients had given their informed consent.

3. Evaluation of treatment efficacy

3.1 Symptom score

A 10 cm visual analogue scales from 0=absent to 10=sever symptoms, for each symptom: rhinorrhoea, nasal congestion, nasal itching, ocular itching, sneezing, asthma symptoms (chest tightness, shortness of breath, cough) and wheezing as recommended by the ARIA review [27]. A change of 2 or more points on this scale is considered a clinically significant change with consequent significant change in the patient quality of life.

3.2 Medication score

Medication usage was recorded by patients on a VAS from 0=no medication to 10=repeated daily use of nasal corticosteroids, antihistamine oral medication, eye drops, inhaler corticosteroids, systemic corticosteroids, and beta agonists.

Patients graded their symptoms retrospectively at each visit. The use of rescue medication was recorded on the diary card in addition to regular medications.

3.3 Determination of serum eosinophil cationic protein

Serum ECP was determined by ELISA kit (MBL MESCACUP ECP TEST) from Medical and Biological Laboratories Co. LTD, Japan. Serum ECP determined by ELISA kit (MBL MESCACUP ECP TEST) from Medical and Biological Laboratories Co, LTD, Japan. This ELISA detects s human ECP with a minimum detection limit of 0.125 ng/ml. The test performed according to the instruction of manufacturer. Briefly, In the wells coated with antihuman ECP monoclonal antibody, 100 ul of diluted serum samples (1:5 sample diluents) or standards were added and incubated for 60 minutes at room temperature (20 - 25 0C). After washing for 4 times, a 100ul of peroxidase conjugated antihuman ECP polyclonal antibody is added into the wells and incubated for 60 minutes at room temperature. After another 4 times washing, a 100 ul of peroxidase substrate reagent is added to each well and the plate incubated for 10 minutes at room temperature. The add 100 ul of stop solution (0.5 mol/l H2SO4) and read the absorbance at 450 nm using a microplate reader. The concentration of ECP is calibrated from a standard curve based on reference standards.

3.4 Statistical analysis and data collection

The results of the study are reported as ratios and/or percentage of the entire cohort. Paired sample t-test was used for the comparison of symptoms and medication scores. Chi square test was used for comparison of the SPF and pulmonary function test in both groups, using SPSS computer package. P values of < 0.05 were considered significant.

4. Results

A total of 822 patients were randomized into two treatment groups (411 for each). Of them 167 subject defaulted during the trial (73 subjects, 18% in the SIT group; 94 subjects, 23% in placebo group). In most cases this was due to logistical barriers, work schedule, travel distance to the clinic and patients and some doctors wrong opinion regarding SIT. Thus 655 subjects were eligible for analysis (338 subjects, 82% in the SIT group; 317 subjects, 77% in the placebo group), with age range of 6-65 years (Mean 32±15 for SIT group and 31±18 for the placebo group), completed at least 3 years of treatment. There was no significant difference in the frequency of AR, Asthma and AR with asthma between immunotherapy and placebo groups.

4.1 Asthma group

A negative PFT was demonstrated in 87% of asthmatic patients receiving SIT and in 91% of patients in placebo group (P=0.0001). In addition PFT improvement was demonstrated in 67% in SIT group and in 19% of placebo group (P=0.0001). Symptom score reduced from 7.56±1.84 to 3.30±1.74 in SIT group (P=0.0001), while it was reduced from 7.63±1.66 to 7.11±2.65 in placebo group (P=0.08). Medication score significantly declined from 5.38±1.12 to 2.20±0.90 in SIT group. While in placebo it was reduced from 5.30±1.41 to 4.94±1.31 in the placebo group (P=0.05). Combined symptom and medication score significantly (P=0.0000) declined from 6.64±1.48 to 2.73±0.97 in SIT group. In placebo group the reduction was not significant (P=0.99). Serum ECP reduced significantly (P=0.000) in both SIT (29.3±7.21 to 15.3±4.11) and placebo (27.1±6.14 to 17.2±3.27). Table -2.

Variables	Immunotherapy	Placebo	P value
No of patients	115	107	
SPT negative	87%	9.1%	0.0001
PFT improvement	67%	19%	0.0001
Symptom score			
Pre- treatment	7.56(0.84)	7.63(0.66)	0.49
Post-treatment	3.30(0.74)	5.56(0.65)	0.0001
P value	0.0001	0.0004	
Medication score			
Pre-treatment	5.38(1.12)	5.30(1.01)	0.94
Post-treatment	2.20(0.90)	3.84(1.11)	0.001
P value	0.0003	0.002	
Combined symptom and medication score			
Pre-treatment	6.64(1.48)	6.47(1.47)	0.39
Post -treatment	2.73(0.97)	4.70(1.25)	0.0001
P value	0.0001	0.0001	
ECP			
Pre -treatment	29.3(7.21)	27.1(6.14)	0.01
Post -treatment	15.3(4.11)	17.2(3.27)	0.0002
P value	0.0001	0.0001	

Table 2. Response to SCIT in patients with asthma.

4.2 Allergic rhinitis group

After 3 years of intervention, negative SPT demonstrated in 81% of patients receiving SIT and in 19% of placebo group (P=0.000). Symptom score reduced significantly (P=0.0001) from 6.61±1.62 to 2.71±0.74 in SIT group. The reduction of symptom score in placebo group was not significant (6.67±1.37 to 6.00±1.16, P=0.99). Furthermore, medication score declined significantly (P=0.0001) from 5.35±1.85 to 2.21±1.87 in SIT group, while the reduction was not significant (P=0.98) in placebo group.

In addition, combined medication and symptom score was significantly reduced (P=0.0001) from 6.12±1.7 to 2.52±1.78 in SIT group, while the reduction in placebo group was not significant. Serum ECP reduced significantly in both SIT (19.3±7.01 to 14.2±5.10, P=0.0001) and placebo group (20.1±5.30 to 17.3±6.31, P=0.014) Table -3.

Variables	Immunotherapy	Placebo	P value
No of patients	52	54	
SPT negative	81%	19%	0.0001
Symptom score			
Pre-treatment	6.61(1.62)	6.67(1.37)	0.76
Post -treatment	2.71(0.74)	5.64(1.16)	0.0001
P value	0.0001	0.0001	
Medication score			
Pre -treatment	5.35(1.85)	5.3(2.27)	0.85
Post -treatment	2.21(0.87)	4.10(2.44)	0.0001
P value	0.0001	0.009	
Combined symptom and medication score			
Pre-treatment	6.12(1.7)	6.16(1.75)	0.86
Post -treatment	2.52(0.78)	5.10(1.80)	0.0001
P value	0.0001	0.002	
ECP			
Pre-treatment	19.3(7.01)	20.1(5.30)	0.37
Post -treatment	14.2(5.10)	17.3(6.31)	0.0001
P value	0.0001	0.014	

Table 3. Response to SCIT in patients with allergic rhinitis.

4.3 Patients with both allergic rhinitis and asthma

PFT improvement was demonstrated in 65% of SIT group while it was 25% in placebo group (P=0.0001). In addition, negative SPT was demonstrated in 78% of patients receiving SIT, while the corresponding value was 23% in placebo group (P=0.0001).

Symptom score declined significantly (P=0.0001) from 7.56±1.87 to 3.42±1.55 in SIT group, while the reduction in placebo group was not significant (P=0.052).

Medication score reduced significantly (P=0.0001) from 5.22±2.72 to 2.72±1.53 in SIT, but the reduction in placebo group was not significant (5.30±1.99 to 4.99±1.86, P=0.10).

Combined symptom and medication score reduced significantly (P=0.0001) from 6.72±1.51 to 3.18±1.63 in SIT, while the reduction in placebo group was not significant (6.32±2.72 to 6.32±1.99, P=0.31).

Serum ECP reduced significantly (P=0.0001) in both SIT (34.2±13.2 to 16.3±6.72) and placebo group (31.1±11.7 to 19.2±5.4) Table -4.

Variables	Immunotherapy	Placebo	P value
No of patients	171	156	
SPT negative	78%	23%	0.0001
PFT improvement	65%	25%	0.0001
Symptom score			
Pre -treatment	7.56(0.87)	7.35(0.84)	0.06
Post - treatment	3.43(0.55)	5.69(0.87)	0.0001
P value	0.0001	0.0001	
Medication score			
Pre -treatment	5.22(0.89)	5.30(0.79)	0.48
Post -treatment	2.72(0.53)	4.26(0.86)	0.0001
P value	0.0001	0.0001	
Combined symptom and medication score			
Pre-treatment	6.72(1.51)	6.62(1.29)	0.59
Post -treatment	3.18(0.63)	5.19(1.10)	0.0001
P value	0.0001	0.0001	
ECP			
Pre -treatment	34.2(13.20)	31.1(11.7)	0.34
Post -treatment	16.3(6.72)	19.2(5.4)	0.0005
P value	0.0001	0.0001	

Table 4. Response to SCIT in patients with asthma and allergic rhinitis.

4.4 All patients

We combined the data of the three groups together. There was a significant decline (P<0.0001) in symptom score from baseline value to that of after 3 years intervention in the SIT (P=0.0001, 7.29±1.2 to 3.18±1.54), but not in the placebo treated subjects (7.23±2.89 to 6.93±1.85, P=0.12). Medication score significantly (P=0.0001) declined in SIT (5.38±1.05 to 2.42±1.66), and placebo (5.31±2.38 to 4.82±2.14, P=0.03).

The SIT resulted in significant (P=0.0001) decline in combined symptom and medication score (6.61±1.46 to 2.91±1.68). In addition, placebo group demonstrated a significant reduction (P=0.03) in combined medication and symptom score (6.27±2.37 to 5.88±2.2).Serum ECP reduced significantly (P=0.0001) in both SIT (30.2±7.9 to 15.6±2.32) and placebo (27.9±6.37 to 18.2±5.8) groups. Table -5.

Variables	Immunotherapy	Placebo	P value
No of patients	338	317	
SPT negative	82%(5)	17%(7)	0.0001
PFT improvement	66(2)	22(4)	0.0001
Symptom score			
Pre -treatment	7.29(1.20)	7.23(0.99)	0.48
Post -treatment	3.18(0.54)	5.63(0.85)	0.0001
P value	0.0001	0.0001	

Variables	Immunotherapy	Placebo	P value
Medication score			
Pre -treatment	5.38(1.05)	5.31(1.08)	0.62
Post treatment	2.42(0.66)	4.10(1.15)	0.0001
P value	0.0001	0.0001	
Combined symptom and medication score			
Pre -treatment	6.61(1.46)	6.54(1.37)	0.71
Post -treatment	2.91(0.68)	5.10(1.20)	0.0001
P value	0.0001	0.0001	
ECP			
Pre -treatment	30.2(7.9)	27.9(6.37)	0.01
Post -treatment	15.6(2.32)	18.2(5.8)	0.0001
P value	0.0001	0.0001	

Table 5. Response to SCIT in all patients.

4.5 Percentage and amount of score changes

The SIT resulted in significantly (P=0.0001) greater subjective rating of improvement than placebo treatment in all four parameters (symptom score, medication score, combined symptom and medication score, and serum ECP). Whether the analysis performed for each disease condition alone (allergic rhinitis, asthma, both allergic rhinitis and asthma) or combined in one group (all patients).

The results are summarized in Table -6.

Variables	Immunotherapy	Placebo	P value
No of patients	338	317	
SPT negative	277	54	0.0001
PFT improvement	223	70	0.0001
Asthma group			
Symptom score	4.17(55.2%)	2.07(27%)	0.0001
Medication score	3.18(59.1%)	1.46(27.5%)	0.0001
Both scores	3.73(56.2%)	1.77(27.4%)	0.0001
ECP	15.3(52.2%)	9.9(36.5%)	0.0001
Allergic rhinitis group			
Symptom score	3.91(59.2%)	1.03(15.4%)	0.0001
Medication score	3.14(59%)	1.20(22.6%)	0.0001
Both scores	3.60(59%)	1.06(17.2%)	0.0001
ECP	5.10(26.4%)	2.80(14%)	0.0001
Allergic rhinitis and Asthma group			
Symptom score	4.13(55%)	1.66(22.5%)	0.0001
Medication score	2.50(48%)	1.04(20%)	0.0001
Both scores	3.54(53%)	1.43(22%)	0.0001
ECP	17.90(52.3%)	11.90(38.3%)	0.0001
All patients			
Symptom score	4.11(56.4%)	1.60(22.1%)	0.0001

Variables	Immunotherapy	Placebo	P value
Medication score	2.96(55%)	1.21(23%)	0.0001
Both scores	3.7(56%)	1.44(22%)	0.0001
ECP	14.60(48.3%)	9.70(35%)	0.0001

Table 6. Reduction in clinical scores following SIT in patients with asthma and allergic rhinitis.

5. Discussion

Despite numerous studies, the role of IT in the management of asthma remains controversial [28, 29], and interpretation of published reports varies considerably, presumably because of personal bias [30]. The variability in response to SIT in allergic diseases as reported in the literature may be due to uncontrolled factors that differ for people receiving the same therapy [30]. These factors are environmental control measures, degree of allergen exposure, type of allergen exposure, presence of allergenic sensitivities not incorporated into the treatment; non-allergenic triggers of asthma such as infection or exposure chemical sensitizer, genetic influence and source of vaccine used in IT. Furthermore, the outcome of the treatment trial influenced by allergen specificity used in the treatment as well as the dose and treatment schedule employed in the course.

This is the first clinical trial that evaluated the effectiveness of SIT in Iraq, and includes a large treatment group, in which the outcome measured using objective criteria.

The current study shows conclusively that house dust mite SIT results in significant improvement in allergic rhinitis and asthma, symptoms and reduction in rescue medication requirement. The results of this study differ from that of less successful studies [14, 31] with a population more heterogeneous in their allergen sensitivities. In our study we used a single allergen for treatment, as the house dust mite, Dermatophagoides, was by far the most important allergen in our study population. However, this study finding was in agreement to that reported by others [10, 32-36].

Immunotherapy has been established as efficacious treatment for allergic rhinitis by seasonal pollens, dust mite, and animal allergens, some studies show controversial findings [30]. A recent review [37] concluded that immunotherapy is highly effective in the treatment of allergic rhinitis. Several reported studies have shown that immunotherapy is effective for the treatment of AR, both in adults and children [14, 38, 39].

This study indicated that HDM immunotherapy significantly reduced symptom score, medication score and serum ECP level. Furthermore, in patients with both AR and asthma, HDM IT significantly reduced the symptom score, medication score and serum ECP mean level. However, the response was superior in group of patients with AR alone as compared to group of patients with AR and asthma. This finding is consistent with that reported by others [33].

Avoidance and medication provide suboptimal control of AR in up to 40% of some patient populations [40]. However, this study demonstrated that HDM IT induced a 59% reduction in combined symptom & medication score in patients with allergic rhinitis, while the corresponding value was 53% for patients group with asthma and AR. The reported studies indicated efficacy of SIT in AR in adults and children [9, 41-45]. There are clinical and immunological evidence that supports the long term efficacy of SIT [46].

In our study we don't use BHR to a direct stimulus such as methacholine or histamine since it has poor correlations with indices of airway inflammation such as sputum eosinophils [47-49]. Thus we used serum ECP because it is a better marker of airway inflammation in asthma as in correlates with sputum eosinophils [49] and PFT following IT and medication [50]. Serum ECP level decreased after 2 years of immunotherapy in perennial allergic rhinitis [51] and asthma [50]. However, the rise in serum ECP after allergen challenge was significantly attenuated after just 1 year of immunotherapy in asthmatic patients [52]. Our study indicated a significant decrease in serum ECP in both SIT and placebo treated subject. However, the reduction was significantly higher in SIT group as compared to placebo group for patients with AR, Asthma, and AR with Asthma and when the data of patients pooled together. In placebo treated group decline in serum ECP may be due to treatment with inhaled corticosteroids.

When the data of three disease groups pooled together, the symptom score, medication score, combined score and serum ECP significantly reduced in SIT as compared to placebo treatment group. Furthermore, SPT negative results and PFT improvement were significantly higher in SIT compared to placebo group.

In this study SIT induces a significant reduction in all parameters used in the study whether the patients were with AR, asthma or both combined together. SIT shows overall percent reduction of 54%, while it was 17.5% in placebo group.

Based on the finding of this and other studies, single allergen SIT is likely to be beneficial to patients with AR, asthmatic and with both, sensitized to a dominant allergen. However, there are other drugs such as inhaled long acting B_2-agonist and anileukotriens agents that might be better at symptom control and lung function improvement, SIT has some unique benefits [10].

Haugaard et al [53], reported that SIT reduce airway sensitivity to allergens, which may lead subsequently to reduction in frequency of exacerbation and severity of asthma triggered by allergen exposure. In addition, the effect of SIT may persist for at least 5-6 years after the end of treatment [53]. Furthermore, SIT reduces the conversion of AR to asthma [51] and prevents the development of new sensitization [44].

Different studies show controversial outcome for SIT. Failure to respond to SIT may be due to: inadequate dose of allergen, missing allergens not identified during the allergy evaluation, inadequate environmental control, and exposure to non allergenic triggers.

Systemic adverse reactions were developed in 62 (15.1%) individuals from the 411 subjects included in the study. None of the developed systemic reactions had life threatening reactions. House dust mite was with a predictive value for development of systemic adverse reactions (OR=2.3, p=0.0001) [54]. However, this study indicated that HDM specific immunotherapy was with good tolerance

6. Conclusion

HDM immunotherapy for 3 years significantly reduced symptom and medication use in AR, asthma and patients with both conditions, and prevent the consequent development of asthma in patients with AR. This was associated with a greater subjective improvement in asthma control.

7. References

[1] Bousquet J, Michel FB, Vignola AM. Allergen immunotherapy : therapeutic vaccine for asthma. Clin Allergy Immunol 2004;18:511-528.

[2] Eder W, Ege MJ, von Mutius E. The asthma epidemic. N Eng J Med 2006;355:2226-2235.

[3] Alsamarai AGM, Alwan AM, Ahmad AH, et al. The relationship between asthma and allergic rhinitis in the Iraqi population. Allergology International 2009; 58: 4: 549-555.

[4] Rank MA, James TCL. Allergen immunotherapy. Mayo Clin Proc 2007; 82:1119-1123.

[5] Bousquet J, LockeyR, MallingHJ. World Health Organization Position Paper. Allergen Immunotherapy: therapeutical vaccines for allergic diseases. Allergy 1998; 53: 112-121.

[6] Calderon MA, Alves B, Jacobson M, et al. Allergen injection immunotherapy for seasonal allergic rhinitis. Cochrane Database Syst Rev 2007; CD 001936.

[7] Abramson M, Puy R, Weiner J. Allergen immunotherapy for asthma. Cochrane Database System Rev 2003; (4):CD001186.

[8] Zeldin Y, Weiler Z, Magen E, Tiosano L, Kidon MI. Safety and efficacy of allergen immunotherapy in the treatment of allergic rhinitis and asthma in real life. IMAJ 2008; 10:869-872.

[9] Ross RN, Nelson HS, Finegold I. Effectiveness of specific immunotherapy in the treatment of allergic rhinitis: an analysis of randomized, prospective, single- or double blind, placebo controlled studies. Clin Ther 2000; 22:342-350.

[10] Wang H, Lin X, Hao C, et al. A double blind, placebo-controlled study of house dust mite immunotherapy in Chinese asthmatic patients. Allergy 2006; 61:191-197.

[11] Pifferi M, Baldini G, Marrazzini G, et al. Benefits of immunotherapy with a standardized Dermatophagoides peteronyssinus extract in asthmatic children: a three year prospective study. Allergy 2002; 57:785-790.

[12] Pichler CE, Helbling A, Pichler WJ. Three years of specific immunotherapy with house dust mite extracts in patients with rhinitis and asthma: significant improvement of allergen specific parameters and nonspecific bronchial hyperreactivity. Allergy 2001; 56:301-306.

[13] Maesterelli P, Zanolla L, Marcella P, Fabbri L. Effect of specific immunotherapy added to pharmacologic treatment and allergen avoidance in asthmatic patients allergic to house dust mite. J Allergy Clin Immunol 2004; 113:643-649.

[14] Adkinson NF, Eggleston PA, Eney D, et al. A controlled trial of immunotherapy for asthma in allergic children. N Eng J Med 1997; 336:324-331.

[15] Passalacqua G, Durham SR. Allergic rhinitis and its impact on asthma update: allergen immunotherapy. J Allergy Clin Immunol 2007; 119:881-891.

[16] Jacobsen L, Niggemann B, Dreborg S, et al. Specific immunotherapy has long term preventive effect of seasonal and perennial asthma: 10 year follow up on the PAT study. Allergy 2007; 62:943-948.

[17] Cohn JR, Pizzi A. Determinants of patient's compliance with allergen immunotherapy. J Allergy Clin Immunol 1993; 91:734-737.

[18] Tinkelman DG, Cole WQ, Tunno J. Immunotherapy: a one year prospective study to evaluate risk factors of systemic reactions. J Allergy Clin Immunol 1995; 95:8-14.
[19] Taubi E, Kessel A, Blant A, Golan TD. Follow-up after systemic adverse reactions of immunotherapy. Allergy 1999; 54:617-620.
[20] Tamir R, Levy I, Duer S, et al. Immediate adverse reactions to immunotherapy in allergy. Allergy 1992; 47: 260-263.
[21] Alzakar E, Alsamarai A. Efficacy of immunotherapy for treatment of asthma in children. Asthma Allergy Proceeding 2010. Accepted for publication.
[22] Malling HG, Weeke B. Immunotherapy. Position Paper of the EAACI. Allergy 1993; 48[suppl 14]:9-35.
[23] National Institute of Health. Global initiative for asthma. AHLBI Publ. No.95-3659. Bethesda, MD USA: NHLBI, 1995:6.
[24] Global Initiative for Asthma. Global Strategy for Asthma Management and Prevention. NHLBI/WHO WorkshopReport.NIH Publication 02-3659. Bethesda. MD: NHLBI, 2002.
[25] Dykeewicz M, Fineman S, Skoner D, et.al. Diagnosis and management of rhinitis. Complete guidelines of the joint task fore on practice parameters in allergy, asthma, and immunology. Ann Allergy, Asthma, Immunol 1998; 81:478.
[26] Joint Task Force on Practice Parameters; American Academy of Allergy, Asthma and Immunology; American College of Allergy, Asthma and Immunology; Joint Council of Allergy, Asthma and Immunology. Allergen immunotherapy: a practice parameter second update. J Allergy Clin Immunol 2007; 120:S25-85.
[27] Bousquet I, Khaltaev N, Cruz AA, et al. Allergic rhinitis and its impact on asthma (ARIA) 2008 update. Allergy 2008; 63 (suppl 86):8-160.
[28] Norman PS. Immunotherapy: past and present. J Allergy Clin Immunol 1998; 102: 1-10.
[29] Barnes PJ. Is there a role for immunotherapy in the treatment of asthma? N Am J Respir Crit Care Med 1996; 154:1227-1228.
[30] Canadian Asthma Guidelines. CMAJ 1999; 161 :(11 Suppl):S21-23.
[31] Hommers L, Ellert U, Scheidt-Nave C, Langen U. Factors contributing to conductance and outcome of specific immunotherapy: Data from the German National Health Interview and Examination Survey 1998. Euro J Public Health 2006; 17:278-284.
[32] Polzehl D, Keck T, Richelmann H. Analysis of the efficacy of specific immunotherapy with house dust mite extracts in adults with allergic rhinitis and / or asthma. Laringorhinotologie 2003; 82:272-280.
[33] Farid R, Ghasemi R, Rahimi M, et al. evaluation of six years allergen immunotherapy in allergic rhinitis and allergic asthma. I J Allergy Asthma Immunol 2006; 5:29-31.
[34] Peroni DG, Piacentini GL, Martinati LC, et al. Double blind trial of house dust mite immunotherapy in asthmatic children resident at high altitude. Allergy 1995; 50:925-930.
[35] Costa JC, Placedo JL, Silva JP, et al. Effects of immunotherapy on symptoms PEFR, spirometry and airway responsiveness in patients with allergic asthma to house dust mite (D. peteronyssinus) on inhaled steroid therapy. Allergy 1996; 51:238-244.
[36] Cantani A, Arccse G, Luccnti P, et al. A three year prospective study of specific immunotherapy to inhalant allergens: evidence of safety and efficacy in 300 children with allergic asthma. J Investig Allergol Clin Immunol 1997; 7:90-97.
[37] Huggins JL, Looney RJ. Allergen immunotherapy. Am Fam Physician 2004; 70:689-696.

[38] Verhagen J, Taylor A, Akdis CA, Akdis M. Targets in allergen directed immunotherapy. Expert Opinion Ther Target 2005; 9:217-224.

[39] Verhagen J, Taylor A, Akdis CA, Akdis M. Advances of allergen specific immunotherapy Targets in allergen directed immunotherapy. Expert Opinion Biol Ther 2005; 5:537-544.

[40] White P, Smith H, Webley F, Frew A. A survey of the quality of information leaflets on hay fever available from general practices and community pharmacies. Clin Exper Allergy 2004; 34:1438-1443.

[41] Frew AJ, Powell RJ, Corrigan cJ, Durham SR. Efficacy and safety of specific immunotherapy with SQ allergen extract in treatment of resistant seasonal allergic rhinoconjuctivitis. J Allergy Clin Immunol 2006; 117:319-325.

[42] Durham SR, Walker SM, Varga EM, et al. Long-term clinical efficacy of grass pollen immunotherapy. N Eng J Med. 1999;341:468-475

[43] Pajno G, Barberio G, Deluca F, et al. Prevention of new sensitization in asthmatic children monosensitized to house dust mite by specific immunotherapy. Asix-year follow-up study. Clin Exp Allergy 2001; 31:1392-1397.

[44] Des RA, Paradis L, Menardo JL, et al. Immunotherapy with a standardized Dermatophagoides peteronyssinus extract. VI. Specific immunotherapy prevents the onset of new sensitizations in children. J Allergy Clin Immunol 1997; 99:450-453.

[45] Purello-D'Ambrosio F, Gangemi S, Merendino R, et al. Prevention of new sensitizations in monosensitized subjects submitted to specific immunotherapy or not: a retrospective study. Clin Exper Allergy 2001;31:1295- 1302.

[46] Frank E. Retrospektine Untersuchung uber die hyposensibilisierungsbehandlung von Milbenallergikern mit Novo-Helisen Depot. Allergologie 1994;17:154-159.

[47] Polosa R, Ciamarra I, Mangano G, Prosperini G, Pistorio MP, Vancheri C et al. Bronchial hyperresponsiveness and airway inflammation markers in nonasthmatics with allergic rhinitis. Eur Respir J 2000; 15:30–35.

[48] Van Den Berge M, Meijer RJ, Kerstjens HA, de Reus DM, Koeter GH, Kauffman HF et al. PC20 Adenosine 5¢-monophosphate is more closely associated with airway inflammation in asthma than PC20 methacholine. Am J Respir Crit Care Med 2001; 163:1546– 1550.

[49] Alvarez MJ, Olaguibel JM, Garcia BE, Rodriquez A, Tabar AI, Urbiola E. Airway inflammation in asthma and perennial allergic rhinitis: relationship with nonspecific bronchial responsiveness and maximal airway narrowing. Allergy 2000; 55:355–362.

[50] Alsamarai AGM, Alobaidi AH, Alsamarai AKY. Association between serum ECP and FEV1 in asthma. P Med Health Sci 2008; 2:49-54.

[51] Ohashi Y, Nakai Y, Kakinoki Y, Ohno Y, Sakamoto H, Kato A et al. Effect of immunotherapy on serum levels of eosinophil cationic protein in perennial allergic rhinitis. Ann Otol Rhinol Laryngol 1997; 106:848–853.

[52] Arvidsson MB, Lowhagen O, Rak S. Allergen specific immunotherapy attenuates early and late phase reactions in lower airways of birch pollen asthmatic patients: a double blind placebo controlled study. Allergy 2004; 59:74–80.

[53] Haugaard L, Dahl R, Jacobsen L. A controlled dose-response study of immunotherapy with standardized, partially purified extract of house dust mite: clinical efficacy and side effects. J Allergy Clin Immunol 1993; 91:709–722.

[54] Alsamarai AM, Alobaidi AHA, Alwan AM, Abdulaziz ZH, Dawood ZM (2011) Systemic Adverse Reaction to Specific Immunotherapy. J Allergy Ther 2:111. doi:10.4172/2155-6121.1000111

Section 5

Up-to-Date in Antihypertensive Therapy

8

Efficacy of Aliskiren/Hydrochlorothiazide Combination for the Treatment of Hypertension: A Meta-Analytical Revision

Manuel Morgado[1,2], Sandra Rolo[2] and Miguel Castelo-Branco[1,2]
[1]*CICS-UBI - Health Sciences Research Centre, University of Beira Interior, Av. Infante D. Henrique, Covilhã*
[2]*Hospital Centre of Cova da Beira, E.P.E., Quinta do Alvito, Covilhã*
Portugal

1. Introduction

Hypertension is a major risk factor in the development of cardiovascular disease, with myocardial infarction, stroke and renal failure being one of the most important health problems worldwide due to its high prevalence and deleterious impact on the population in terms of excessive morbidity and mortality. Currently, hypertension is estimated to affect approximately 30% of the US and European population and 1 thousand million people worldwide and, as the population ages, this number is expected to increase even further (Wolf-Maier et al., 2003; Kearney et al., 2005; Yoon et al., 2010). Moreover, despite advances in treatment of the condition, hypertension control rates continue to be suboptimal in both the US and Europe as only about one third have their blood pressure (BP) reduced to the recommended levels by the 7th Joint National Committee (JNC-7) to under 140/90 mm Hg for uncomplicated hypertension, and less than 130/80 mmHg for those with diabetes mellitus or renal disease (Chobanian et al., 2003).

Hypertension is a controllable disease and effective pharmacological therapies have been available for nearly 50 years. Socio-economic conditions, medication non-adherence, inadequate prevention strategies and resistant hypertension have all been implicated as barriers to adequate BP control. The major pharmacological strategies currently used for hypertension management include volume control with diuretics, suppression of central and peripheral sympathetic nervous system activity with beta-blockers and alfa-blockers, vasodilation with ion channel manipulation and blockade of renin-angiotensin-aldosterone system (RAAS). Since monotherapy controls the BP of less than 50% of treated hypertensive patients (Materson et al., 1993; Cushman et al., 2002), combination therapy with two or more antihypertensive medications with complementary mechanisms is often required to achieve BP control to recommended levels (Chobanian et al., 2003; Mancia et al., 2007). At present, the most widely used antihypertensive combinations involve hydrochlorothiazide (HCTZ) and drugs that block the RAAS, such as angiotensin-converting enzyme (ACE) inhibitors and angiotensin II type-1 receptor blockers (ARBs).

Recently a new blocker of the RAAS, aliskiren, has been developed and approved by the US Food and Drug Administration (FDA, on 5th March 2007) and by the European Medicines Agency (EMEA, on 22nd August 2007) for the treatment of essential hypertension. Aliskiren is an oral direct renin inhibitor, the rate-limiting enzyme in the production of the end product of the RAAS cascade, angiotensin II (Ang II), a potent vasoactive peptide. Aliskiren is a long-acting antihypertensive (half-life ≈ 40 hours) and has been shown in several clinical trials to be effective in lowering BP, safe and well tolerated in daily doses of 150 and 300 mg (approved once-daily doses) (Musini et al., 2009). In a recent systematic review and meta-analysis of six double-blind randomized clinical trials to quantify the systolic and diastolic BP (SBP and DBP) lowering efficacy of aliskiren in the treatment of adults with essential hypertension, the obtained weighted mean differences with 95% CI (confidence interval) were: aliskiren 150 mg, -5.5 (-6.5, -4.4)/-3.0 (-3.7, -2.3) mm Hg; aliskiren 300 mg, -8.7 (-9.7, -7.6)/-5.0 (-5.6, -4.3) mm Hg (Musini et al., 2009).

Several clinical trials revealed that aliskiren/HCTZ combination therapy reduced SBP and DBP from baseline to a significantly greater extent than placebo, aliskiren monotherapy and HCTZ monotherapy (Chrysant 2008; Baldwin and Plosker 2009). Aliskiren/HCTZ also produced significant additional SBP and DBP reductions in patients inadequately responsive to 4 weeks' prior treatment with aliskiren or HCTZ alone (Baldwin and Plosker 2009). Single-pill combinations (SPCs) of aliskiren/HCTZ (150/12.5 mg, 150/25 mg, 300/12.5 mg, 300/25 mg) have recently been approved by the US FDA (18th January 2008) and by EMEA (16th January 2009) for the treatment of adults with essential hypertension whose BP is not adequately controlled with aliskiren or HCTZ alone, and as a substitution treatment in patients with hypertension adequately treated by the two individual drugs concomitantly at the equivalent fixed dosage. In this chapter, we briefly reviewed the pharmacodynamic and pharmacokinetic profile of aliskiren and assessed the antihypertensive efficacy and tolerability of the aliskiren/HCTZ combination therapy in reducing SBP and DBP in patients with mild to moderate hypertension by using a systematic review of the literature and a meta-analytical approach to combine data from different clinical trials.

2. Aliskiren: Pharmacodynamic and pharmacokinetic properties

A schematic of the RAAS is depicted in Figure 1. Renin is an aspartic protease produced by the juxtaglomerular cells in the kidney. This enzyme catalyses the cleavage of angiotensinogen, the only know substrate of renin, to the decapeptide angiotensin I (Ang I). This is the rate-limiting step of RAAS activation. In the presence of ACE, Ang I is converted into the octapeptide hormone Ang II, a potent vasoconstrictor that mediates its activity through the type-1 angiotensin II (AT1) receptor. Binding of Ang II to AT1 receptor increases BP, and promotes aldosterone secretion from adrenal cortex, sodium reabsorption in renal proximal tubules, and catecholamine release from pre-synaptic nerve endings and adrenal medulla (Kim and Iwao 2000). Pathological activation of RAAS can result in high BP with consequent end-organ damage.

Several drugs can inhibit the RAAS cascade but redundant biochemical pathways limit the potential beneficial effects of these drugs.

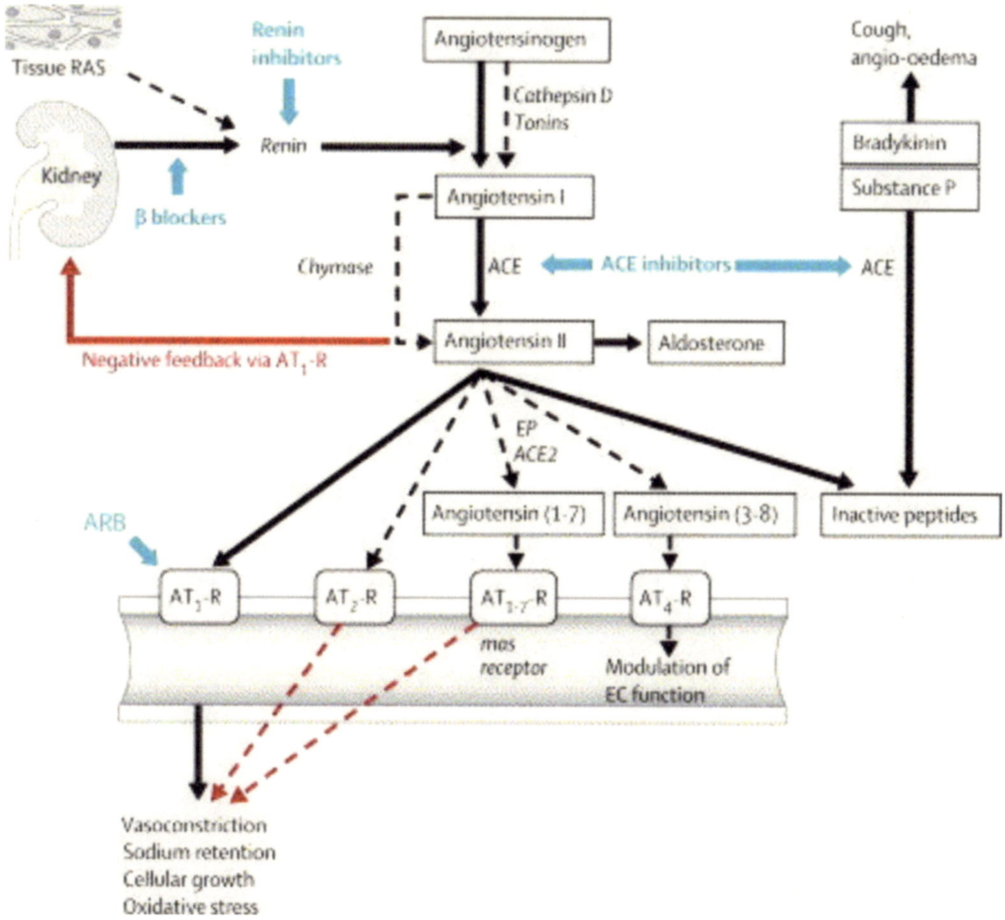

Fig. 1. The renin-angiotensin-aldosterone system (Staessen et al., 2006). Black arrows show stimulation and red arrows show inhibition. Dotted lines show alternative pathways mainly documented in experimental studies. Beta-blockers, renin inhibitors, inhibitors of angiotensin-converting enzyme (ACE) and angiotensin II type-1 receptor blockers (ARB) reduce the activity of the renin-angiotensin system (RAS). Abbreviations: AT-R, angiotensin receptor; EP, endopeptidases; EC, endothelial cells. From reference Staessen et al., with permission from Elsevier.

ACE inhibitors block the conversion of Ang I to Ang II but non-ACE pathways of Ang II generation such as a chymase and presumably other enzymes pathways present in end organs including heart, kidney and blood vessels get activated under conditions of ACE inhibition (Urata et al., 1996; Hollenberg et al., 1998). The existence of alternative pathways for Ang II generation that are unaffected by ACE inhibitors raises questions about whether ACE is the optimal target for RAAS suppression. Furthermore, ACE inhibitors are not specific for RAAS and can prevent ACE-induced inactivation of bradykinin and substance P that are thought to be responsible for ACE-inhibitor related side effects as cough and angioedema. ARBs exert their effect by blocking AT1 receptors activation by Ang II. This may lead to unbalanced activation of other types of receptors such as type-2 and type-4 Ang

II receptors (AT2 and AT4 receptors). Physiological role of these receptors are not clear but may be important for endothelial function (Wantanabe et al 2005). Over stimulation of AT2 receptors can generate deleterious agents such as oxygen free radicals, pro-inflammatory cytokines and pro-fibrotic mediators and may promote left ventricular hypertrophy (Williams 2001; Azizi et al 2006). On the other hand, beneficial effects such as inhibition of renin synthesis and Ang II formation are also reported following AT2 receptor activation (Siragy et al 2005). Both ACE inhibitors and ARBs stimulate renal renin production by interrupting the normal feedback suppression of renin secretion from the kidneys. The reactive rise in circulating active renin leads to greater generation of Ang II via pathways dependent or independent of ACE.

2.1 Pharmacodynamic properties of aliskiren

Recently, a new blocker of RAAS, aliskiren, has been developed and approved for the treatment of hypertension. Aliskiren is a direct inhibitor of renin, the enzyme that catalyses the conversion of angiotensinogen to Ang I. This is the rate limiting step in the production of the end product of RAAS cascade, which makes renin inhibition an attractive option for effective RAAS blockade. Renin is measured as plasma renin concentration (PRC) and plasma renin activity (PRA). PRC measures the actual amount of renin in plasma regardless of its enzymatic activity and is expressed as either µU/mL or pg/mL. PRA denotes the enzymatic activity of renin and is measured as the rate of Ang I production after adding serum to angiotensinogen and is expressed as ng/ml/hour. Like ACE inhibitors and ARBs, aliskiren can reactively lead to an increase in PRC. However, unlike these other inhibitors of the RAAS, the effects of renin are suppressed with aliskiren, resulting in a reduction in PRA.

Aliskiren is a small molecular weight, orally active, non-peptide direct renin inhibitor with very high affinity and specificity for human and primate renin (Wood et al., 2003). It is significantly less active against renin from dogs, rats, rabbits, pigs and cats, which made the process of conducting preclinical experimental studies a challenging one (Wood et al., 2003). As a result, these preclinical studies have been performed in marmosets (primates) and double-transgenic rats that express the human renin and human angiotensinogen genes (Pilz et al., 2005; Wood et al., 2005).

Aliskiren is a potent inhibitor of renin with an IC_{50} (concentration inhibiting 50% of activity) of 0.6 nmol/L. Aliskiren oral doses of 3 and 10 mg/kg completely suppressed PRA for 24 hours in mildly sodium depleted marmosets (Wood et al., 2005; Vaidyanathan et al., 2006; O'Brien et al., 2007; Vaidyanathan et al., 2007a; Vaidyanathan et al., 2007b). It decreased PRA, Ang I and Ang II levels in normotensive volunteers in a dose dependent manner but caused a 10-fold increase in PRC (Nussberger et al., 2002). A decrease in plasma and urine aldosterone levels were also noted with daily aliskiren doses of 80 mg and above (Nussberger et al., 2002).

Effects of various medications on RAAS pathway are shown in Table 1. With the exception of beta-blockers, all other agents blocking RAAS and diuretics including HCTZ increase PRC. Aliskiren and ACE inhibitors achieve this by decreasing Ang II levels and ARBs by blocking inhibitory effects of Ang II on AT1 receptors on juxtaglomerular cells. Diuretics increase PRC by inducing volume depletion. The extent of PRC elevation is more marked when aliskiren is combined with HCTZ. PRA is increased by ACE inhibitors, ARBs and

HCTZ while aliskiren use alone and in combination with HCTZ is associated with a decrease in PRA. Other agents that can decrease PRA include beta-blockers and central alfa-2 receptor agonists.

Antihypertensive medications	Enzymes		Substrates	End-products			
	PRC	PRA	Angiotensinogen	Ang I	Ang II	Ang_{1-7}	Aldosterone
Beta-blockers	↓	↓	–	↓	↓	↓	↓
ACE inhibitors	↑	↑	↓	↑	↓	↑	↓
ARBs	↑	↑	↓	↑	↑	↑	↓
Aliskiren	↑↑	↓↓	-	↓	↓	↓	↓
HCTZ	↑	↑	↓	↑	↑	↑	↑
Aliskiren/HCTZ combination	↑↑↑	↓	–	–	–	–	–

Abbreviations: ACE, angiotensin-converting enzyme; Ang I, angiotensin I; Ang II, angiotensin II; Ang 1–7, angiotensin 1–7; ARBs, angiotensin II type-1 receptor blockers; HCTZ, hydrochlorothiazide; PRA, plasma renin activity; PRC, plasma renin concentration; ↑, increased; ↓, decreased; –, unchanged or unknown. Adapted from (Sureshkumar 2008).

Table 1. Antihypertensive medication effects on RAAS pathway

2.2 Pharmacokinetic properties of aliskiren

The pharmacokinetic properties of aliskiren have been studied in animals, healthy human subjects, patients with compromised liver and kidney function, and subjects with mild hypertension (Waldmeier et al., 2007). Aliskiren has a poor bioavailability (2-6%), but this is compensated by its high solubility and the already mentioned high inhibitory effect (IC_{50} = 0.6 nM) from *in vitro* inhibition of human renin (Wood et al., 2005; Azizi et al., 2006).

After oral administration, peak plasma concentrations (Cmax) of aliskiren are reached within 1–3 hours (Vaidyanathan et al., 2006; Zhao et al., 2006). When taken with a high-fat meal, the mean area under the plasma concentration–time curve (AUC) and Cmax of aliskiren are decreased by 71% and 85%, respectively (Novartis_Europharm_Limited 2007. Available at http://www.ema.europa.eu/docs/pt_PT/document_library/EPAR_-_Product_Information/human/000780/WC500047010.pdf. Accessed on 27th August 2011). Steady state is achieved after approximately 7 days with once daily dosing (Nussberger et al., 2002). Aliskiren is not extensively bound (49.5%) to plasma proteins (Novartis Europharm Limited, 2007). The volume of distribution at steady state is 135 L (Novartis Europharm Limited, 2007).

Aliskiren undergoes minimal hepatic metabolism. *In vitro* studies indicate that aliskiren is a substrate of the cytochrome P450 (CYP) 3A4 isoenzyme; however, it is neither an inhibitor nor an inducer of CYP isoenzymes (Vaidyanathan et al., 2006). Aliskiren is primarily eliminated by the hepatobiliary route as unmetabolized drug. Less than 1% of an orally administered dose is excreted in the urine as unchanged drug (Waldmeier et al., 2007). After oral administration of a single 300-mg dose of aliskiren to healthy volunteers, the mean ± SD clearance corrected for bioavailability [i.e., clearance/drug bioavailability (Cl/F)] was 234 ± 137 L/hour (Zhao et al., 2006). The terminal half-life of aliskiren ranges from 24–40 hours (Nussberger et al., 2002; Azizi et al., 2004; Zhao et al., 2006). This half-life, which is longer than the 24-hour dosing interval, is consistent with the observation that plasma concentrations of aliskiren have been shown to accumulate by about 2-fold at steady state compared with administration of a single dose (Vaidyanathan et al., 2006).

3. Aim of the review

The aim of this review was to assess the antihypertensive efficacy and tolerability of the aliskiren/HCTZ combination therapy (as a combination of the individual components or as SPCs) in reducing SBP and DBP in patients with mild to moderate hypertension by using systematic analysis of the literature and meta-analytical approach to combine data from different randomized, double-blind, clinical trials.

4. Methodology for selection of clinical trials and data analysis

A literature search to identify clinical trials using aliskiren in combination with HCTZ for the treatment of hypertension was conducted on July 2011 to obtain all published study reports that met our inclusion criteria.

4.1 Inclusion and exclusion criteria

We included all articles in the literature written in any of the major languages. To be included in our review studies were required to be randomized, double-blind, clinical trials using aliskiren in combination with HCTZ (as a combination of the individual components or as SPCs) for the treatment of hypertension. Additionally, studies were included if they evaluated the antihypertensive efficacy [outcome measure) of aliskiren/HCTZ in patients with mild or moderate essential hypertension (SBP 140-179 mm Hg and/or DBP 90-109 mm Hg, as defined in current international guidelines (Mancia et al., 2007)] and patient age ≥ 18 years. Articles were automatically excluded if their results were not reported or had been presented in forms such as abstracts, letters, or commentaries.

4.2 Literature search strategy

We searched the following electronic databases: International Pharmaceutical Abstracts, MEDLINE, The Cochrane Library and ISI Web of Knowledge. Each database was independently searched by 2 reviewers for articles published from 2000 to and including June 30, 2011, using the search terms *aliskiren, aliskiren/hydrochlorothiazide, aliskiren-hydrochlorothiazide, aliskiren in combination with hydrochlorothiazide, renin inhibitor*. The reviewers selected articles based on the predefined inclusion/exclusion criteria and results were matched. A consensus method was applied to judge any article selection divergences. The rationale for decisions was discussed until reviewers agreed on the final decision. A third author was called to resolve any remaining discrepancies concerning article eligibility.

Selected articles' references and reviews of the subject were hand searched for additional studies that were not obtained through our initial electronic search.

4.3 Data extraction

The following information was gathered for each clinical trial: author names, year of publication, study design and duration, setting, characteristics of the patients enrolled, sizes of the treatment groups, daily treatment regimens and primary endpoint. Outcomes extracted from articles included mean and variation of SBP and DBP at baseline and final assessments for each group, responder rate (DBP < 90 mm Hg or ≥10 mm Hg reduction from baseline) and BP control rate (SBP < 140 mm Hg and DBP < 90 mm Hg). Changes from baseline in PRA and PRC with aliskiren/HCTZ and with either component alone were also extracted whenever reported, as well as adverse events recorded during the trials. During the data extraction phase, we wrote to corresponding authors of studies to request missing data and clarify study details.

4.4 Quality assessment

The quality of selected articles was assessed by the same principles used in article selection and data extraction (i.e., 2 independent reviewers), and was based on the Jadad et al. method to measure the risk of bias (Jadad et al., 1996). Their 3-item quality assessment checklist evaluates the following methodological parameters: controlled trial, random allocation of treatments, double-blind follow-up, dropout rate, intention-to-treat (ITT) analysis and absence of other biases. Quality scores were presented as proportions of the total possible score (i.e., 5) of the quality assessment scale (where 100% represents the maximum quality). The scores were categorized according to the following criteria: weak (<60%), fair (60%), good (80%), or very good (100%).

4.5 Analysis method

For trials meeting the criteria for inclusion in the analysis, the efficacy of treatment was evaluated via measurements of SBP and DBP at the start of the trial (baseline) and after 8 weeks of therapy. The meta-analytical approach therefore compared the efficacy of each aliskiren/HCTZ dose combination in reducing SBP and DBP over this period of time. The analysis method used was based on calculation of the mean BP reduction for a set of aliskiren/HCTZ dose combinations evaluated, by weighting the combined data for the trial size using the following formula: (BP reduction [trial 1] • number of patients [trial 1] +…+ BP reduction [trial n] • number of patients [trial n])/total number of patients (trial 1 +…+ trial n).

5. Results

A completed QUOROM flow chart (Moher et al., 1999) of the literature search strategy applied and results found is depicted in Figure 2. Initially, 52 potentially relevant RCTs were identified that appeared to meet the inclusion criteria and were screened for retrieval based on their titles and abstracts. Thirty-six of those articles were excluded for not evaluating aliskiren in combination with hydrochlorothiazide. The remaining 16 articles were retrieved for full-text review. Eleven of those articles were excluded for the following reasons: two had data that were not extractable (Andersen et al., 2008; Andersen et al., 2009), three presented excluded study designs (O'Brien et al., 2007; Chrysant et al., 2008; Littlejohn et al., 2009), one enrolled patients with severe hypertension (Strasser et al., 2007), four appeared only in the abstract form (Sica et al., 2006; Gradman et al., 2007; Prescott et al., 2007; Calhoun et al., 2008) and one was indexed in MEDLINE in duplicate (Nickenig et al., 2008). Therefore, after exclusion criteria were applied, a total of 5 studies involving a total of 5508 patients were included in this analysis [20-24].

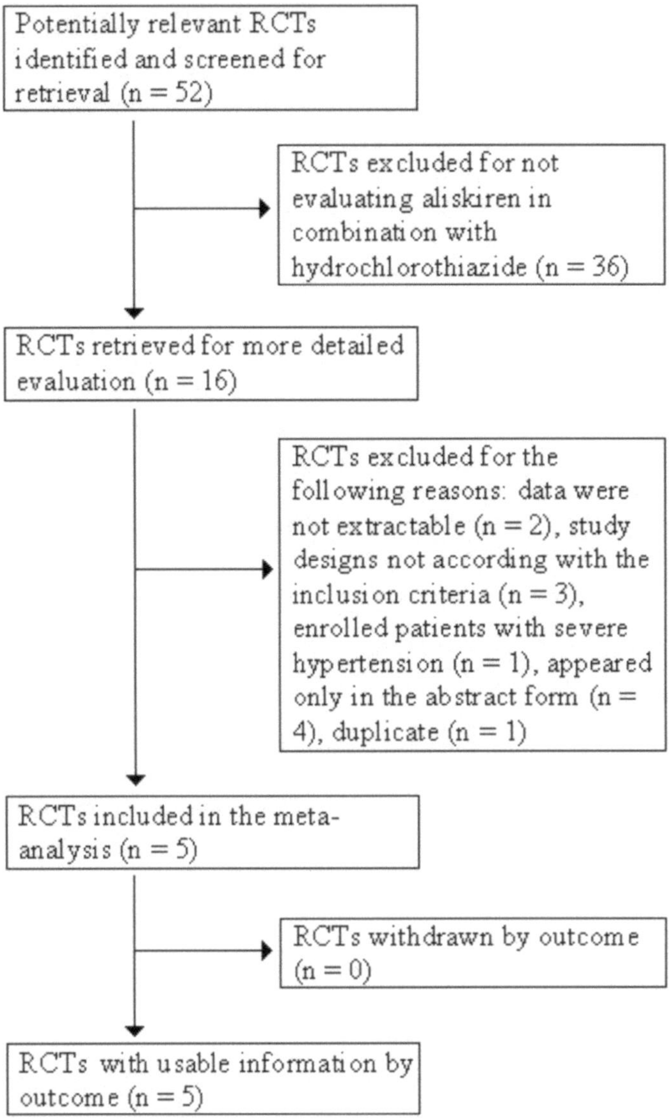

Fig. 2. Quorom flow chart of literature search strategy applied and results. Five double-blind randomized controlled trials met the inclusion criteria, using aliskiren in combination with HCTZ for the treatment of hypertension.

Table 2 presents the overall characteristics of the evaluated studies. The average sample size was 1102 ± 947 (mean ± SD), with a median of 722 and range from 489–2776 patients. All included studies were randomized, double-blind, multicenter clinical trials, proceeded by a single-blind, placebo (Villamil et al., 2007) / active comparator (Jordan et al., 2007; Nickenig et al., 2008; Blumenstein et al., 2009; Geiger et al., 2009), run-in period of 2-4 weeks. Moreover, all five studies specified the change from baseline (start of double-blind treatment) in mean sitting DBP (msDBP) at 8 weeks as the primary endpoint.

Reference (Year)	Study Design, Duration, Setting, BP measurement, No of patients	Demographics and Baseline Characteristics[a]	Daily Treatment Regimens	Primary End Point	Quality Score[b]
Villamil (2007)	Randomized, double-blind, placebo-controlled, multicenter; 8 wks; clinic; trough BP; n=2776	Age ≥ 18 yrs. Eligibility for single-blind phase: msDBP ≥95 and <110 mmHg (baseline). Eligibility for double-blind phase: msDBP ≥95 and <110 mmHg after 2 or 4 wks on placebo. Mean age 55 yrs; 55% men; 86% Caucasian.	Single-blind, placebo run-in period (2 wks or 4 wks): Placebo. Double-blind treatment (8 wks): Placebo; Aliskiren 75, 150, 300mg; HCTZ 6.25, 12.5, 25mg; Aliskiren/HCTZ 75/6.25, 75/12.5, 75/25, 150/6.25, 150/12.5, 150/25, 300/12.5, 300/25mg.	Change in msDBP from baseline (start of double-blind treatment) to wk 8 endpoint (aliskiren monotherapy vs placebo; combination therapy vs respective monotherapies)	60%[c]
Jordan (2007)	Randomized, double-blind, multicenter; 12 wks; clinic; trough BP; n=489	Age ≥ 18 yrs. Eligibility for single-blind phase: msDBP ≥95 and <110 mmHg (baseline). Eligibility for double-blind phase: msDBP ≥90 and <110 mmHg. BMI ≥ 30 kg/m²; Mean age 54 yrs; 44% men; 99.6% Caucasian.	Single-blind treatment (4 wks): HCTZ 25mg. Double-blind treatment (first 4 wks - next 8 wks): Placebo–HCTZ 25 - 25mg; Aliskiren/HCTZ 150/25 - 300/25mg; Irbesartan/HCTZ 150/25 – 300/25 mg; Amlodipine/HCTZ 5/25 – 10/25mg.	Change in msDBP from baseline (start of double-blind treatment) to wk 8 endpoint (aliskiren/HCTZ 300/25 mg vs placebo–HCTZ 25 mg)	100%
Nickenig (2008)	Randomized, double-blind, multicenter; 8 wks; clinic; trough BP; n=880	Age ≥ 18 yrs. Eligibility for single-blind phase: msDBP ≥95 and <110 mmHg or msDBP ≥85 and <110 mmHg if treated for HT within the 4 wks prior to screening (baseline). Eligibility for double-blind phase: msDBP ≥90 and <110 mmHg after 4 wks of aliskiren 300 mg monotherapy. Mean age 55 yrs;55% men;83% Caucasian.	Single-blind treatment (4 wks): Aliskiren 300mg. Double-blind treatment (8 wks): Aliskiren 300mg; Aliskiren/HCTZ 300/12.5, 300/25mg.	Change in msDBP from baseline (start of double-blind treatment) to wk 8 endpoint (aliskiren monotherapy vs combination therapy)	100%
Blumenstein (2009)	Randomized, double-blind, multicenter; 8 wks; clinic; trough BP; n=722	Age ≥ 18 yrs. Eligibility for single-blind phase: patients with HT, who were newly diagnosed, untreated or treated at the time of screening. Newly diagnosed pts or pts who had not been treated for HT in the 4 wks prior to screening had to have msDBP ≥95 and <110 mmHg at the time of the screening. Eligibility for double-blind phase: msDBP ≥90 and <110 mmHg after 4 wks of HCTZ 25 mg monotherapy. Mean age 54 yrs; 59% men;91% Caucasian.	Single-blind treatment (4 wks): HCTZ 25mg. Double-blind treatment (8 wks): HCTZ 25mg; Aliskiren/HCTZ 150/25, 300/25mg.	Change in msDBP from baseline (start of double-blind treatment) to wk 8 endpoint (HCTZ monotherapy vs combination therapy)	100%

Reference (Year)	Study Design, Duration, Setting, BP measurement, No of patients	Demographics and Baseline Characteristics[a]	Daily Treatment Regimens	Primary End Point	Quality Score[b]
Geiger (2009)	Randomized, double-blind, multicenter; 8 wks; clinic; trough BP; n=641	Age ≥ 18 yrs. Eligibility for single-blind phase: pts with mild to moderate HT taking antihypertensive agents. Eligibility for double-blind phase: msDBP ≥95 and <110 mmHg after 4 wks of HCTZ monotherapy. Mean age 53 yrs; 57% men; 86% Caucasian.	Single-blind treatment (4 wks): HCTZ 12.5mg for 1 wk followed by HCTZ 25mg for 3 wks. Double-blind treatment (8 wks): HCTZ 25mg; Aliskiren/HCTZ 150/25mg for 4 wks followed by 300/25mg for another 4 wks; Valsartan/HCTZ 160/25mg for 4 wks followed by 320/25mg for another 4 wks; Aliskiren/Valsartan/HCTZ 150/160/25mg for 4 wks followed by 300/320/25mg for another 4 wks.	Change in msDBP from baseline (start of double-blind treatment) to wk 8 endpoint (aliskiren/HCTZ and valsartan/HCTZ vs aliskiren/valsartan/HCTZ)	60%[d]

[a]In each published clinical trial, patient baseline and demographic characteristics were comparable for all treatment groups.
[b]The percentage of the total possible score (i.e., 5) of the quality assessment scale applied (100% represents the maximum quality).
[c]Method to generate the sequence of randomization and method of double blind were not described; additionally, some information on outcome variability was not provided.
[d]Method to generate the sequence of randomization and method of double blind were not described.
Abbreviations: BP, blood pressure; HCTZ, hydrochlorothiazide; HT, hypertension; msDBP, mean sitting diastolic blood pressure; pts, patients; wk, week.

Table 2. Published clinical trials of aliskiren/HCTZ for treatment of mild to moderate hypertension

Secondary efficacy measures included the change in mean sitting SBP (msSBP) (Jordan et al., 2007; Villamil et al., 2007; Nickenig et al., 2008; Blumenstein et al., 2009; Geiger et al., 2009), the proportion of patients with successful response to treatment (defined as msDBP < 90 mmHg and/or a ≥ 10 mmHg reduction from baseline) (Jordan et al., 2007; Villamil et al., 2007) and the proportion of patients attaining BP control (defined as msDBP < 90 mmHg and msSBP < 140 mm Hg) (Jordan et al., 2007; Villamil et al., 2007; Nickenig et al., 2008; Blumenstein et al., 2009; Geiger et al., 2009). Two trials used the SPC (Jordan et al., 2007; Villamil et al., 2007), and three combined the individual components (Nickenig et al., 2008; Blumenstein et al., 2009; Geiger et al., 2009), with aliskiren and HCTZ administered orally as single daily doses in all studies. One trial enrolled obese hypertensive patients only (obesity defined as body mass index of ≥ 30 kg/m^2) (Jordan et al., 2007), although in the remaining four trials subgroups of patients with obesity were also present. In the five included clinical trials patient demographics and baseline characteristics were similar across treatment groups. Brief details of the characteristics of each individual trial and treatment group, including mean patient ages, sex ratios, body mass index / obesity and baseline SBP and DBP are provided in Table 3.

Reference	Pts., n	Treatment and daily dose (mg)	Patient age (years)	Sex ratio (M/F)	BMI (kg/m²)	Obese (BMI ≥ 30 kg/ m²) (%)	SBP baseline (mm Hg)	DBP baseline (mm Hg)
Villamil (2007)	195	Placebo	54.4	109/86	NR	40.5	152.7	99.3
	184	Aliskiren 75	55.0	103/81	NR	41.8	153.2	99.4
	185	Aliskiren 150	53.5	112/73	NR	32.4	153.4	98.8
	183	Aliskiren 300	54.2	99/84	NR	38.8	154.4	99.3
	194	HCTZ 6.25	55.2	109/85	NR	41.2	153.4	99.3
	188	HCTZ 12.5	55.4	103/85	NR	38.8	153.4	99.1
	176	HCTZ 25	55.1	92/84	NR	32.4	154.5	99.1
	188	Aliskiren/HCTZ 75/6.25	55.1	108/80	NR	37.8	154.5	98.9
	193	Aliskiren/HCTZ 75/12.5	54.4	101/92	NR	39.9	154.0	100.0
	186	Aliskiren/HCTZ 75/25	54.7	101/85	NR	38.7	152.9	99.0
	176	Aliskiren/HCTZ 150/6.25	53.9	96/80	NR	37.5	153.3	99.0
	186	Aliskiren/HCTZ 150/12.5	54.7	98/88	NR	35.5	154.1	99.1
	188	Aliskiren/HCTZ 150/25	53.7	104/84	NR	37.8	153.2	98.4
	181	Aliskiren/HCTZ 300/12.5	55.5	89/92	NR	42.0	153.2	99.5
	173	Aliskiren/HCTZ 300/25	54.8	98/75	NR	41.0	154.6	99.3
Jordan (2007)	122	HCTZ 25	55.2±12.3	52/70	34.0±4.1	NR	149.5±11.3	97.2±4.6
	122	Aliskiren/HCTZ 300/25	53.1±11.9	60/62	34.8±5.2	NR	149.4±11.6	96.8±4.9
	119	Irbesartan/HCTZ 300/25	53.0±11.0	48/71	34.3±4.7	NR	149.1±13.4	96.6±4.4
	126	Amlodipine/HCTZ 10/25	55.2±11.9	53/73	34.5±4.1	NR	149.8±11.5	96.7±5.0
Nickenig (2008)	298	Aliskiren 300	55.5±10.6	159/139	29.2±4.5	NR	149.8±12.6	95.5±4.4
	293	Aliskiren/HCTZ 300/12.5	54.9±10.5	155/138	29.2±4.9	NR	150.3±12.5	95.5±4.3
	289	Aliskiren/HCTZ 300/25	54.4±10.3	172/117	28.9±4.6	NR	150.8±12.8	95.8±4.7
Blumenstein (2009)	246	HCTZ 25 mg	52.9±11.5	143/103	29.7±5.0	NR	151.8±11.9	96.3±4.9
	244	Aliskiren/HCTZ 150/25	53.6±11.1	144/100	28.9±4.7	NR	151.2±12.7	96.1±4.9
	232	Aliskiren/HCTZ 300/25	54.1±9.5	140/92	29.9±5.0	NR	151.1±12.3	96.1±4.6
Geiger (2009)	152	HCTZ 25	52.6±9.93	94/58	31.8±6.13	NR	154.1±12.61	99.9±4.33
	166	Aliskiren/HCTZ 300/25	52.3±10.90	92/74	31.3±6.28	NR	153.3±12.68	99.3±4.10
	155	Valsartan/HCTZ 320/25	55.0±11.40	88/67	31.3±5.85	NR	156.7±12.49	99.9±3.97
	168	Aliskiren/Valsartan/HCTZ 300/320/25	52.9±10.83	91/77	31.9±6.21	NR	152.7±11.64	99.2±3.70

Values are mean ±SD unless otherwise stated.
Abbreviations: BMI, body mass index; DBP, diastolic blood pressure; F, female; HCTZ, hydrochlorothiazide; M, male; NR, not reported; Pts, patients; SBP, systolic blood pressure.

Table 3. Main patient baseline and demographic characteristics by treatment group of the included clinical trials (randomized population)

The average quality score of study reporting was 84% ± 22% (range 60–100%), which could be categorized as very good. One study failed to report all information on data variability (Villamil et al., 2007), which prevented the use of an approximation for standard error of the mean (SEM) or confidence interval (CI) estimation, when calculating some weighted average reductions in SBP and DBP. We contacted the corresponding author of this study by email to request missing data on SEM as well as on BP control rate at endpoint for each aliskiren/HCTZ, aliskiren and HCTZ daily doses tested, but no response was provided.

Table 4 details results from clinical trials on the efficacy of aliskiren/HCTZ in reducing BP. In the only placebo-controlled study (and also the largest of the RCTs), aliskiren/HCTZ combination reduced SBP and DBP from baseline to a significantly ($p \leq 0.0001$) greater extent than placebo in patients with mild to moderate hypertension (Villamil et al., 2007).

Reference	Patients, n (ITT)	Treatment and daily dose (mg)	Change in SBP from baseline at endpoint (mm Hg)	Change in DBP from baseline at endpoint (mm Hg)	Responder rate (%)	BP control rate at endpoint (%)
Villamil (2007)	192	Placebo	-7.5	-6.9	45.8	28.1
	183	Aliskiren 75	-9.4	-8.7±0.59[a]	51.9	(29.0
	183	Aliskiren 150	-12.2[b]	-8.9±0.59[a]	51.9	to
	180	Aliskiren 300	-15.7[c]	-10.3±0.60[c]	63.9[b]	[c] 46.7)
	194	HCTZ 6.25	-11.0[a]	-9.1±0.58[a]	53.6	(32.5
	188	HCTZ 12.5	-13.9[c]	-10.1±0.59[c]	60.6[a]	to
	173	HCTZ 25	-14.3[c]	-9.4±0.61[a]	59.0[a]	37.8)
	187	Aliskiren/HCTZ 75/6.25	-14.3 ±0.93[c,d]	-10.8[c,d]	61.5[a]	
	189	Aliskiren/HCTZ 75/12.5	-15.6[c]	-11.1[c]	63.5[b]	[a]
	186	Aliskiren/HCTZ 75/25	-17.3[c,d]	-11.5[c,d]	70.4[c,d]	[a,d]
	173	Aliskiren/HCTZ 150/6.25	-15.3[c]	-10.4±0.59[c]	58.4[a]	[a] (37.4
	184	Aliskiren/HCTZ 150/12.5	-17.6[c,d]	-11.9[c,d]	69.6[c]	[a,d] to
	187	Aliskiren/HCTZ 150/25	-19.5[c,d]	-12.7[c,d]	71.1[c,d]	[a,d] 59.5)
	180	Aliskiren/HCTZ 300/12.5	-19.8[c,d]	-13.9[c,d]	80.6[c,d]	[a,d]
	173	Aliskiren/HCTZ 300/25	-21.2±0.97[c,d]	-14.3±0.61[c,d]	76.9[c,d]	[a,d]
Jordan (2007)	117	HCTZ 25	-8.6±1.00	-7.9±0.73	59.0	34.2
	113	Aliskiren/HCTZ 300/25	-15.8±1.01[e]	-11.9±0.74[e]	73.5[f]	56.6[g]
	117	Irbesartan/HCTZ 300/25	-15.4±1.00[h]	-11.3±0.72[h]	70.9[h]	54.7[h]
	122	Amlodipine/HCTZ 10/25	-13.6±0.98[h]	-10.3±0.71[h]	68.0[h]	45.1[i]
Nickenig (2008)	296	Aliskiren 300	-8.0±0.9	-7.4±0.5	62.2	40.9
	292	Aliskiren/HCTZ 300/12.5	-13.5±0.9[j]	-10.5±0.5[j]	73.3[k]	57.9[j]
	284	Aliskiren/HCTZ 300/25	-15.9±0.9[j]	-11.0±0.6[j]	77.1[j]	60.2[j]
Blumenstein (2009)	244	HCTZ 25 mg	-7.1±0.7	-4.8±0.4	47.1	25.8
	242	Aliskiren/HCTZ 150/25	-12.9±0.7[l]	-8.5±0.4[l]	67.4[l]	48.8[l]
	232	Aliskiren/HCTZ 300/25	-16.7±0.7[l,m]	-10.7±0.4[l,n]	78.5[l]	58.2[l,o]
Geiger (2009)	151	HCTZ 25	-6±1.12	-6±0.70	NR	20.53
	164	Aliskiren/HCTZ 300/25	-15 ±1.08[l]	-11±0.67[l]	NR	40.85[l]
	154	Valsartan/HCTZ 320/25	-18 ±1.12[l]	-14±0.70[l]	NR	48.70[l]
	168	Aliskiren/Valsartan/HCTZ 300/320/25	-22±1.07[l,p,q]	-16±0.67[l,p,q]	NR	66.67[l,p,r]

Changes in blood pressure are presented as the least-squares mean changes (with ± SEM, whenever provided by the authors).
[a]P < 0.05, [b]P < 0.001, [c]P ≤ 0.0001 vs placebo; [d]P < 0.05 vs each component monotherapy; [e]P < 0.0001 vs HCTZ 25 mg; [f]P < 0.05 vs HCTZ 25 mg; [g]P = 0.0005 vs HCTZ 25 mg; [h]P > 0.05 vs aliskiren/HCTZ 300/25 mg; [i]P = 0.052 vs aliskiren/HCTZ 300/25 mg; [j]P < 0.001 vs aliskiren 300 mg; [k]P = 0.002 vs aliskiren 300 mg; [l]P < 0.001 vs HCTZ 25 mg; [m]P = 0.009 vs aliskiren/HCTZ 150/25 mg; [n]P < 0.001 vs aliskiren/HCTZ 150/25 mg; [o]P = 0.033 vs aliskiren/HCTZ 150/25 mg; [p]P < 0.001 vs aliskiren/HCTZ 300/25 mg; [q]P < 0.01 vs valsartan/HCTZ 320/25 mg; [r]P < 0.001 vs valsartan/HCTZ 320/25 mg.
Abbreviations: BP, blood pressure; DBP, diastolic blood pressure; HCTZ, hydrochlorothiazide; ITT, intention-to-treat analysis; NR, not reported; SBP, systolic blood pressure.

Table 4. Clinical trial data on the efficacy of aliskiren/HCTZ in reducing blood pressure

Furthermore, aliskiren/HCTZ combination (at all but the 75/12.5 mg and 150/6.25 mg dosages, both of which are not commercially available) decreased SBP and DBP from baseline to a significantly ($p < 0.05$) greater extent than the component monotherapies (Villamil et al., 2007). In the other selected RCTs, all of which with an active comparator and a non-responder study design (Jordan et al., 2007; Nickenig et al., 2008; Blumenstein et al., 2009; Geiger et al., 2009), aliskiren/HCTZ combination was an effective treatment option, producing significantly additional reductions in SBP and DBP in patients with mild to moderate hypertension inadequately responsive to 4 weeks' prior treatment with aliskiren

(Nickenig et al., 2008) or HCTZ (Jordan et al., 2007; Blumenstein et al., 2009; Geiger et al., 2009) alone. In the five included RCTs, BP control rates were also significantly higher with all aliskiren/HCTZ combinations commercially available than with placebo, aliskiren alone and HCTZ alone. One of the included studies did not report the BP response rate (Geiger et al., 2009), in the remaining four studies, BP response rates were also significantly higher with all aliskiren/HCTZ combinations commercially available than with placebo; however, only the three higher dosages of aliskiren/HCTZ combinations yielded significantly higher BP response rates than the component monotherapies (Jordan et al., 2007; Villamil et al., 2007; Nickenig et al., 2008; Blumenstein et al., 2009).

Two studies also compared the efficacy of aliskiren/HCTZ 300/25 mg combination in reducing and controlling BP with other treatment combinations (amlodipine/HCTZ 10/25 mg, irbesartan/HCTZ 300/25 mg, valsartan/HCTZ 320/25 mg and aliskiren/valsartan/HCTZ 300/320/25 mg) (Jordan et al., 2007; Geiger et al., 2009). Only the last combination yielded significantly greater decreases in SBP and DBP and higher BP control rates than the aliskiren/HCTZ 300/25 mg combination (Geiger et al., 2009).

Aliskiren/HCTZ combination evaluated	Number of clinical trials	Total number of patients	Change in SBP from baseline at endpoint (mm Hg)	Change in DBP from baseline at endpoint (mm Hg)	BP control rate (%)[a]
Aliskiren/HCTZ 150/12.5 mg	1	184	-17.6	-11.9	[37.4, 59.5][a]
Aliskiren/HCTZ 150/25 mg	2	429	-15.8	-10.3	[43.8, 53.5][a]
Aliskiren/HCTZ 300/12.5 mg	2	472	-15.9	-11.8	[50.1, 58.5][a]
Aliskiren/HCTZ 300/25 mg	5	966	-16.9±0.4	-11.6±0.3	[51.9, 55.9][a]

Changes in blood pressure are presented as the weighted least-squares mean changes ± SEM (not all variability information was provided in the trial of Villamil (2007), preventing the use of an approximation for SEM or confidence intervals estimation for the first three aliskiren/HCTZ dose combinations).
[a]The range presented is due to the trial of Villamil (2007), which presented the range of BP control rate for aliskiren/HCTZ combination, without specify the values for each dose combination.
Abbreviations: BP, blood pressure; DBP, diastolic blood pressure; HCTZ, hydrochlorothiazide; SBP, systolic blood pressure.

Table 5. Weighted average reductions from baseline of SBP and DBP and BP control rate for each aliskiren/HCTZ combination commercially available

The Q statistic for heterogeneity of effects was not significant, both for SBP ($\chi^2 = 1.14$, $p = 0.89$) and for DBP ($\chi^2 = 0.62$, $p = 0.96$); therefore we considered the study results to be combinable and a fixed-effects model was used in the analysis. Table 5 presents the weighted mean reductions from baseline of SBP and DBP and BP control rate for each aliskiren/HCTZ combination commercially available. It should be noted that four RCTs were not placebo-controlled and, furthermore, the active comparator (aliskiren or HCTZ) differed in these studies (Jordan et al., 2007; Nickenig et al., 2008; Blumenstein et al., 2009; Geiger et al., 2009). In these circumstances, appraisal of the change from baseline in SBP and DBP achieved by each aliskiren/HCTZ combination allows some appreciation of their antihypertensive efficacy since all data are derived from studies of similar design. Nevertheless, the higher BP reductions reported in the Villamil (2007) trial (Villamil et al., 2007) with aliskiren/HCTZ (a fact also observed with aliskiren and HCTZ monotherapies) must be observed with some caution, as they clearly diverged upward from the results obtained by other authors and yielded an unexpected higher effect of the lowest dose of aliskiren/HCTZ commercially available (150/12.5 mg).

Reference	Pts., n (ITT)	Treatment and daily dose (mg)	Δ in PRA from pretreatment[a] or baseline[b, c] (%)	Δ in PRC from pretreatment[a] or baseline[b,c] (%)	Adverse Events
Villamil (2007)	192	Placebo	+0.7[d]	+30	The overall incidence of treatment-related adverse events (AEs) was slightly higher in the HCTZ (9.3-11.0%) and combination groups (8.7-16.6%) compared with placebo (8.8%) and aliskiren (6.5-9.8%) groups. However, this could not be attributed to any particular AE or class of AE. Hypokalaemia (serum potassium <3.5 mmol/L) occurred with the highest frequency in HCTZ 12.5 and 25mg groups (3.9 and 5.2%, respectively). When these doses of HCTZ were administered in combination with aliskiren, the frequency of hypokalaemia decreased to 0.7-2.0% for the combination groups with HCTZ 12.5mg and to 2.2-3.4% for the combination groups with HCTZ 25mg.
	183	Aliskiren 75	-54.2	+164	
	183	Aliskiren 150	-65.1	+192	
	180	Aliskiren 300	-57.6	+348	
	194	HCTZ 6.25	+3.5	+10[e]	
	188	HCTZ 12.5	+44.7	+26[e]	
	173	HCTZ 25	+71.9	+108	
	187	Aliskiren/HCTZ 75/6.25	-54.5	PRC increased in all combination groups and was related to dosages of both drugs.	
	189	Aliskiren/HCTZ 75/12.5	NR		
	186	Aliskiren/HCTZ 75/25	NR		
	173	Aliskiren/HCTZ 150/6.25	NR		
	184	Aliskiren/HCTZ 150/12.5	-49.6		
	187	Aliskiren/HCTZ 150/25	NR		
	180	Aliskiren/HCTZ 300/12.5	NR		
	173	Aliskiren/HCTZ 300/25	-62.3	+1211	
Jordan (2007)	117	HCTZ 25	+46.3[f]	NR	Amlodipine/HCTZ group had the highest rate of AEs (45.2%) because of a higher incidence of peripheral edema. Incidence of AEs in the other treatment groups was: 39.3% - aliskiren/HCTZ; 38.5% - HCTZ; 36.1% - Irbesartan/HCTZ. The proportion of patients experiencing nasopharyngitis, dizziness and hyperkalaemia were slightly higher in aliskiren/HCTZ group (8.2%, 3.3% and 5.7%, respectively).
	113	Aliskiren/HCTZ 300/25	-45.0[f]	NR	
	117	Irbesartan/HCTZ 300/25	+536.6[f]	NR	
	122	Amlodipine/HCTZ 10/25	+195.6[f]	NR	
Nickenig (2008)	296	Aliskiren 300	NR	NR	Aliskiren/HCTZ SPC treatment showed similar tolerability to aliskiren monotherapy. Headache, hypercholesterolemia and nasopharyngitis occurred in ≥2% of patients in any treatment group. The proportion of patients with hypokalaemia was lower in the aliskiren/HCTZ 300/12.5 mg group (0.4%) and aliskiren 300 mg monotherapy group (0.4%) than in the aliskiren/HCTZ 300/25 mg group (2.5%).
	292	Aliskiren/HCTZ 300/12.5	NR	NR	
	284	Aliskiren/HCTZ 300/25	NR	NR	

Reference	Pts., n (ITT)	Treatment and daily dose (mg)	Δ in PRA from pretreatment[a] or baseline[b, c] (%)	Δ in PRC from pretreatment[a] or baseline[b,c] (%)	Adverse Events
Blumenstein (2009)	244 242 232	HCTZ 25 Aliskiren/HCTZ 150/25 Aliskiren/HCTZ 300/25	NR NR NR	NR NR NR	Aliskiren/HCTZ SPC treatment showed similar tolerability to HCTZ alone and a numerically lower incidence of hypokalaemia (aliskiren/HCTZ, 1.3-2.2%; HCTZ alone, 3.4%). AEs reported in ≥2% of patients in any treatment group were nasopharyngitis, dizziness, back pain and vertigo.
Geiger (2009)	151 164 154 168	HCTZ 25 Aliskiren/HCTZ 300/25 Valsartan/HCTZ 320/25 Aliskiren/Valsartan/HCTZ 300/320/25	-13.2[g] -40.5[h] +509.5[h] +38.9[g]	-29.1[i] +489.8[j] +561.4[j] +1760.1[j]	Aliskiren/HCTZ SPC treatment showed similar tolerability to HCT alone and a numerically lower incidence of hypokalaemia (aliskiren/HCTZ, 5.0%; HCTZ alone, 9.3%), nasopharyngitis (aliskiren/HCTZ, 3.0%; HCTZ alone, 6.6%) and headache (aliskiren/HCTZ, 2.4%; HCTZ alone, 5.3%).

[a]Jordan (2007); [b]Villamil (2007); [c]Geiger (2009); [d]$P > 0.05$ vs baseline; [e]$P > 0.05$ vs placebo; [f]$P < 0.05$ vs pretreatment; [g]$P > 0.75$ vs baseline; [h]$P < 0.001$ vs baseline; [i]$P \geq 0.05$ vs baseline; [j]$P < 0.05$ vs baseline.
Abbreviations: AE, adverse event; HCTZ, hydrochlorothiazide; ITT, intention-to-treat analysis; NR, not reported; PRA, plasma renin activity; PRC, plasma renin concentration; Pts, patients; SPC, single-pill combination.

Table 6. Changes from baseline in PRA and PRC with aliskiren and HCTZ monotherapy and combination therapy

Some authors also studied changes from pre-treatment (Jordan et al., 2007) (start of single-blind treatment) or baseline (Villamil et al., 2007; Geiger et al., 2009) (start of double-blind treatment) in PRA and PRC with aliskiren and HCTZ monotherapy and combination therapy (Table 6). Aliskiren 75, 150 and 300 mg/day decreased (the geometric) PRA from baseline by 54.2%, 65.1% and 57.6%, respectively (Villamil et al., 2007). Conversely, HCTZ monotherapy significantly increased PRA at 12.5 and 25 mg/day dosages (Jordan et al., 2007; Villamil et al., 2007). When combined, aliskiren/HCTZ significantly reduced PRA from pretreatment (by 45%) (Jordan et al., 2007) and baseline (by 40.5-62.3%) (Villamil et al., 2007; Geiger et al., 2009), whereas combined treatment with amlodipine/HCTZ, irbesartan/HCTZ and valsartan/HCTZ significantly increased PRA (Jordan et al., 2007; Geiger et al., 2009). Aliskiren elevated PRC from baseline in a dose-dependent manner, with increases of 164%, 192% and 348% at dosages of 75, 150 and 300 mg/day, respectively (Villamil et al., 2007). HCTZ 25 mg/day increased PRC by 108%, whereas lower dosages did not cause alterations in PCR that significantly differed from placebo. All aliskiren/HCTZ combinations significantly increased PCR (Villamil et al., 2007; Geiger et al., 2009), the magnitude of increases was related to the dosages of both components, with the most marked increase (1211% from baseline) occurring in the aliskiren/HCTZ 300/25 mg group (Villamil et al., 2007). Furthermore, increases in PRC in several combination groups were considerably greater than the sum of the increases seen with each component (Villamil et al., 2007). It should be noted that Geiger *et al* measured the baseline PRA and PCR at the end of the 4-week single-blind HCTZ period (Geiger et al., 2009). Therefore, the effect of HCTZ on PRA and PRC might have been stabilized with this initial therapy and no further changes after the 8-week additional HCTZ treatment was observed (Geiger et al., 2009).

Table 6 also describes the most common adverse events reported in the clinical trials. Aliskiren/HCTZ, as a SPC or as a combination of the individual components concurrently administered, was generally well tolerated in the five clinical trials reviewed. The majority of adverse events were mild and transient in nature, with the most commonly reported events including nasopharyngitis (Jordan et al., 2007; Villamil et al., 2007; Nickenig et al., 2008; Blumenstein et al., 2009; Geiger et al., 2009), headache (Jordan et al., 2007; Villamil et al., 2007; Nickenig et al., 2008; Blumenstein et al., 2009; Geiger et al., 2009), dizziness (Jordan et al., 2007; Blumenstein et al., 2009), back pain (Blumenstein et al., 2009), vertigo (Blumenstein et al., 2009) and hypercholesterolemia (Nickenig et al., 2008).

The proportion of patients experiencing hypokalaemia (defined as serum potassium levels <3.5 mmol/L) were numerically lower with aliskiren/HCTZ than with HCTZ alone (Villamil et al., 2007; Blumenstein et al., 2009; Geiger et al., 2009). The proportion of patients with hypokalaemia was also lower in the aliskiren/HCTZ 300/12.5 mg group (0.4%) and aliskiren 300 mg monotherapy group (0.4%) than in the aliskiren/HCTZ 300/25 mg group (2.5%) (Nickenig et al., 2008). In obese hypertensive patients, hypokalaemia occurred in 4.9% patients of the aliskiren/HCTZ group versus 2.5%, 10.3% and 4.1% of patients treated with irbesartan/HCTZ, amlodipine/HCTZ or HCTZ alone, respectively (Jordan et al., 2007).

6. Discussion

SPCs of aliskiren/HCTZ has recently been introduced in European Union for the second-line treatment of adults with essential hypertension whose BP is not adequately controlled with either drug alone, or as a substitution treatment in patients with hypertension adequately treated by the two individual drugs concomitantly at the equivalent fixed dosage. To our knowledge, this study represents the first published meta-analytical approach to the efficacy of aliskiren/HCTZ in reducing BP in patients with mild to moderate hypertension. Although other reviews dealing with the same topic are available in the literature, no study has provided a synthesis of data from clinical trials.

The five studies included in this systematic review are short-term (8-12 weeks) randomized, double-blind, clinical trials with a similar design and comparable primary endpoints and secondary efficacy measures. All studies compared the change in SBP and DBP from baseline (start of double-blind treatment) to week 8 endpoint in each aliskiren/HCTZ combination group with that in placebo and/or aliskiren monotherapy and/or HCTZ monotherapy group. Patient demographics and baseline characteristics were also similar across treatment groups in all included studies, except that one study included obese patients only (Jordan et al., 2007). The average quality of the articles was considered to be very good.

In this study we chose to present the results by way of weighted average sums of BP reductions over 8 weeks, a period consistent with current clinical recommendations for assessing the clinical efficacy and tolerability of antihypertensive drugs following their initiation (Chobanian et al., 2003; Mancia et al., 2007). The weighted means method, which has been used in other meta-analyses (Conlin et al., 2000; Baguet et al., 2005; Baguet et al.,

2007), takes into account the different sizes of trials and provides results that are easy to interpret clinically.

In all clinical trials selected for analysis, commercially available aliskiren/HCTZ combinations (150/12.5 mg, 150/25 mg, 300/12.5 mg and 300/25 mg) provided clinically significant additional SBP and DBP reductions and improved BP control rates over aliskiren or HCTZ monotherapy, which demonstrates that aliskiren/HCTZ SPCs are a effective treatment option for patients with mild to moderate hypertension who do not achieve BP control with aliskiren 300 mg or HCTZ 25 mg alone. A meta-analysis of 354 randomized clinical trials involving more than 40,000 treated patients with hypertension revealed that the additional reduction in BP achieved with antihypertensive combination therapy versus monotherapy provide a reduced risk of stroke and ischemic heart events (Law et al., 2003). In another meta-analysis, examining individual data from one million adults in 61 prospective studies, it was found that, at ages 40-69 years, each increase of 20 mm Hg usual SBP (or, approximately equivalently, 10 mm Hg usual DBP) is associated with more than a twofold difference in the stroke death rate, and with twofold differences in the death rates from ischaemic heart disease and from other vascular causes (Lewington et al., 2002). Thus, the additional mean BP reductions of up to 8.0/4.8 mmHg (versus HCTZ 25 mg) or 6.0/3.1 mmHg (versus aliskiren 300 mg) provided by aliskiren/HCTZ 300/25 mg in the present analysis might be expected to reduce the risk of cardiovascular mortality. However, long-term and large-scale studies analysing the effects of aliskiren/HCTZ combination therapy on clinical outcomes are required to confirm this hypothesis.

The capacity of aliskiren to enhance the antihypertensive efficacy of HCTZ reflects its complementary mode of action, targeting the RAAS at its point of activation and thus suppressing PRA. HCTZ monotherapy increased PRA, as a result of stimulated renin release in response to reduced intravascular volume. The addition of aliskiren counteracted this effect, resulting in a significant ($p < 0.05$) overall decrease in PRA compared with HCTZ monotherapy (Jordan et al., 2007; Villamil et al., 2007; Geiger et al., 2009). Furthermore, aliskiren effectively inhibited the renin enzyme, despite marked elevation in PRC, to produce an overall reduction in PRA from baseline. This contrasts to agents that block the RAAS at other points, such as ACE inhibitors and ARBs, which induce increases in PRA in parallel with PRC (Nussberger et al., 2002; Jordan et al., 2007; Geiger et al., 2009).

Aliskiren/HCTZ was generally well tolerated in the clinical trials reviewed and not associated with a notably higher incidence of adverse events than treatment with either component alone. These results are consistent with a long-term open-label study in 1955 hypertensive patients showing that aliskiren/HCTZ free combinations were well tolerated over up to 12 months of treatment (Sica et al., 2006; Gradman et al.,) 2007). In three included trials, when aliskiren and HCTZ was administered in combination, aliskiren opposed the adverse hypokalaemic effects of HCTZ (Villamil et al., 2007; Blumenstein et al., 2009; Geiger et al., 2009). The safety profile of an aliskiren/valsartan/HCTZ combination was also investigated in one clinical trial and was similar to the 2-drug combinations (aliskiren/HCTZ or valsartan/HCTZ), with a greater BP-lowering effect in patients not adequately responding to HCTZ monotherapy (Geiger et al., 2009).

Most patients with hypertension will require combination treatment with two or more antihypertensive medications in order to achieve BP control to recommended levels

(Chobanian et al., 2003; Mancia et al., 2007). A meta-analysis of adherence studies showed that the use of SPC regimens reduced the rate of non-compliance by 24–26% compared with respective free combinations (Bangalore et al., 2007). Aliskiren/HCTZ SPCs therefore offers the convenience of a single-tablet once daily treatment regimen, which may improve treatment compliance and subsequent BP control.

The limitations of this study should be noted. Firstly, the intervention effect size as reported above (Tables 2 and 3) could be an overestimate due to publication bias since the manufacturer (Novartis Pharmaceuticals Corporation) sponsored four (Jordan et al., 2007; Nickenig et al., 2008; Blumenstein et al., 2009; Geiger et al., 2009) of the included published studies and one author of the remaining study (Villamil et al., 2007) is employee of Novartis Pharmaceuticals Corporation. It is possible that less optimistic studies have not been published and therefore not included in our analysis. Secondly, because the BP lowering efficacy estimate is limited to 8 weeks, we cannot extrapolate our results to the longer term benefits of the treatments on cardiovascular morbidity and mortality. However, in this regard, the 2007 European Society of Hypertension (ESH)/European Society of Cardiology (ESC) guidelines are pertinent, which state that the size of BP reduction is more important than the class used for cardiovascular event reduction (Mancia et al., 2007). Thirdly, an overall of 87% patients included in the RCTs analysed were Caucasian, which greatly limits the extraction of conclusions for hypertensive patients of other races/ethnicities. Actually, blacks are known to have a less responsive renin-angiotensin-aldosterone system (He et al., 2001) and ACE inhibitors and angiotensin receptor antagonists are less effective in this subpopulation (Cushman et al., 2000; Brewster et al., 2004). One other limitation is based on the fact that there is only one clinical trial investigating the antihypertensive efficacy of the lowest dose of aliskiren/HCTZ commercially available (150/12.5 mg), which, additionally, lacks information on outcome variability (SEM or CI) (Villamil et al., 2007). This fact was responsible for an unexpected higher efficacy of aliskiren/HCTZ 150/12.5 mg in reducing SBP and DBP, when compared with higher combination dosages (Table 5). Further studies are required to accurately evaluate the dose-related antihypertensive efficacy of the commercially available aliskiren/HCTZ combinations.

7. Conclusion

In conclusion, aliskiren/HCTZ combinations commercially available were effective and generally well tolerated in clinical trials evaluating its antihypertensive effects in adults with mild to moderate hypertension and in hypertensive patients with obesity, providing clinically significant additional BP reductions and improved BP control rates in patients who are inadequately controlled with aliskiren or HCTZ monotherapy. The aliskiren/HCTZ SPCs present the convenience of a once-daily single-tablet treatment regimen, which may improve treatment adherence and subsequent BP control. Further studies are required to evaluate the relative benefits of the aliskiren/HCTZ SPCs with generically available alternatives. Also, long-term trials evaluating the efficacy and tolerability of this combination therapy would be of interest to establish the ultimate effects of treatment on the cardiovascular morbidity and mortality of hypertension.

8. Acknowledgements

We thank Novartis Farma SA for supporting the article processing charge.

9. References

Andersen, K., M. H. Weinberger, C. M. Constance, M. A. Ali, J. Jin, M. F. Prescott, et al. (2009). Comparative effects of aliskiren-based and ramipril-based therapy on the renin system during long-term (6 months) treatment and withdrawal in patients with hypertension, J Renin Angiotensin Aldosterone Syst 10(3): 157-67.

Andersen, K., M. H. Weinberger, B. Egan, C. M. Constance, M. A. Ali, J. Jin, et al. (2008). Comparative efficacy and safety of aliskiren, an oral direct renin inhibitor, and ramipril in hypertension: a 6-month, randomized, double-blind trial, J Hypertens 26(3): 589-99.

Azizi, M., J. Menard, A. Bissery, T. T. Guyenne, A. Bura-Riviere, S. Vaidyanathan, et al. (2004). Pharmacologic demonstration of the synergistic effects of a combination of the renin inhibitor aliskiren and the AT1 receptor antagonist valsartan on the angiotensin II-renin feedback interruption, J Am Soc Nephrol 15(12): 3126-33.

Azizi, M., R. Webb, J. Nussberger and N. K. Hollenberg (2006). Renin inhibition with aliskiren: where are we now, and where are we going?, J Hypertens 24(2): 243-56.

Baguet, J. P., B. Legallicier, P. Auquier and S. Robitail (2007). Updated meta-analytical approach to the efficacy of antihypertensive drugs in reducing blood pressure, Clin Drug Investig 27(11): 735-53.

Baguet, J. P., S. Robitail, L. Boyer, D. Debensason and P. Auquier (2005). A meta-analytical approach to the efficacy of antihypertensive drugs in reducing blood pressure, Am J Cardiovasc Drugs 5(2): 131-40.

Baldwin, C. M. and G. L. Plosker (2009). Aliskiren/hydrochlorothiazide combination: in mild to moderate hypertension, Drugs 69(7): 833-41.

Bangalore, S., G. Kamalakkannan, S. Parkar and F. H. Messerli (2007). Fixed-dose combinations improve medication compliance: a meta-analysis, Am J Med 120(8): 713-9.

Blumenstein, M., J. Romaszko, A. Calderon, K. Andersen, G. Ibram, Z. Liu, et al. (2009). Antihypertensive efficacy and tolerability of aliskiren/hydrochlorothiazide (HCT) single-pill combinations in patients who are non-responsive to HCT 25 mg alone, Curr Med Res Opin 25(4): 903-10.

Brewster, L. M., G. A. van Montfrans and J. Kleijnen (2004). Systematic review: antihypertensive drug therapy in black patients, Ann Intern Med 141(8): 614-27.

Calhoun, D. A., A. S. Villamil, S. G. Chrysant, S. G. Chrysant, S. G. Chrysant, S. G. Chrysant, et al. (2008). Antihypertensive efficacy of aliskiren/hydrochlorothiazide (HCT) combinations in patients with stage 2 hypertension: subgroup analysis of a randomized, double-blind, factorial trial [abstract no. P-209], Hypertension 52(4): e97.

Chobanian, A. V., G. L. Bakris, H. R. Black, W. C. Cushman, L. A. Green, J. L. Izzo, Jr., et al. (2003). Seventh report of the Joint National Committee on Prevention, Detection, Evaluation, and Treatment of High Blood Pressure, Hypertension 42(6): 1206-52.

Chrysant, S. G. (2008). Aliskiren-hydrochlorothiazide combination for the treatment of hypertension, Expert Rev Cardiovasc Ther 6(3): 305-14.

Chrysant, S. G., A. V. Murray, U. C. Hoppe, D. Dattani, S. Patel, H. Hsu, et al. (2008). Long-term safety, tolerability and efficacy of aliskiren in combination with valsartan in patients with hypertension: a 6-month interim analysis, Curr Med Res Opin 24(4): 1039-47.

Conlin, P. R., J. D. Spence, B. Williams, A. B. Ribeiro, I. Saito, C. Benedict, et al. (2000). Angiotensin II antagonists for hypertension: are there differences in efficacy?, Am J Hypertens 13(4 Pt 1): 418-26.

Cushman, W. C., C. E. Ford, J. A. Cutler, K. L. Margolis, B. R. Davis, R. H. Grimm, et al. (2002). Success and predictors of blood pressure control in diverse North American settings: the antihypertensive and lipid-lowering treatment to prevent heart attack trial (ALLHAT), J Clin Hypertens (Greenwich) 4(6): 393-404.

Cushman, W. C., D. J. Reda, H. M. Perry, D. Williams, M. Abdellatif and B. J. Materson (2000). Regional and racial differences in response to antihypertensive medication use in a randomized controlled trial of men with hypertension in the United States. Department of Veterans Affairs Cooperative Study Group on Antihypertensive Agents, Arch Intern Med 160(6): 825-31.

Geiger, H., E. Barranco, M. Gorostidi, A. Taylor, X. Zhang, Z. Xiang, et al. (2009). Combination therapy with various combinations of aliskiren, valsartan, and hydrochlorothiazide in hypertensive patients not adequately responsive to hydrochlorothiazide alone, J Clin Hypertens (Greenwich) 11(6): 324-32.

Gradman, A. H., R. E. Kolloch, M. Meyers, M. Meyers, M. Meyers, M. Meyers, et al. (2007). Aliskiren in combination with hydrochlorothiazide is effective and well tolerated during long-term treatment of hypertension [abstract no. P-384], J Clin Hypertens (Greenwich 9(5 Suppl. A): 160.

Gradman, A. H., R. E. Kolloch, M. Meyers, M. Meyers, M. Meyers, M. Meyers, et al. () 2007). Aliskiren in combination with hydrochlorothiazide is effective and well tolerated during long-term treatment of hypertension [abstract no. P-384], J Clin Hypertens (Greenwich 9(5 Suppl. A): 160.

He, F. J., N. D. Markandu and G. A. MacGregor (2001). Importance of the renin system for determining blood pressure fall with acute salt restriction in hypertensive and normotensive whites, Hypertension 38(3): 321-5.

Hollenberg, N. K., N. D. Fisher and D. A. Price (1998). Pathways for angiotensin II generation in intact human tissue: evidence from comparative pharmacological interruption of the renin system, Hypertension 32(3): 387-92.

Jadad, A. R., R. A. Moore, D. Carroll, C. Jenkinson, D. J. Reynolds, D. J. Gavaghan, et al. (1996). Assessing the quality of reports of randomized clinical trials: is blinding necessary?, Control Clin Trials 17(1): 1-12.

Jordan, J., S. Engeli, S. W. Boye, S. Le Breton and D. L. Keefe (2007). Direct Renin inhibition with aliskiren in obese patients with arterial hypertension, Hypertension 49(5): 1047-55.

Kearney, P. M., M. Whelton, K. Reynolds, P. Muntner, P. K. Whelton and J. He (2005). Global burden of hypertension: analysis of worldwide data, Lancet 365(9455): 217-23.

Kim, S. and H. Iwao (2000). Molecular and cellular mechanisms of angiotensin II-mediated cardiovascular and renal diseases, Pharmacol Rev 52(1): 11-34.

Law, M. R., N. J. Wald, J. K. Morris and R. E. Jordan (2003). Value of low dose combination treatment with blood pressure lowering drugs: analysis of 354 randomised trials, Bmj 326(7404): 1427.

Lewington, S., R. Clarke, N. Qizilbash, R. Peto and R. Collins (2002). Age-specific relevance of usual blood pressure to vascular mortality: a meta-analysis of individual data for one million adults in 61 prospective studies, Lancet 360(9349): 1903-13.

Littlejohn, T. W., 3rd, P. Trenkwalder, G. Hollanders, Y. Zhao and W. Liao (2009). Long-term safety, tolerability and efficacy of combination therapy with aliskiren and amlodipine in patients with hypertension, Curr Med Res Opin 25(4): 951-9.

Mancia, G., G. De Backer, A. Dominiczak, R. Cifkova, R. Fagard, G. Germano, et al. (2007). 2007 Guidelines for the Management of Arterial Hypertension: The Task Force for the Management of Arterial Hypertension of the European Society of Hypertension (ESH) and of the European Society of Cardiology (ESC), J Hypertens 25(6): 1105-87.

Materson, B. J., D. J. Reda, W. C. Cushman, B. M. Massie, E. D. Freis, M. S. Kochar, et al. (1993). Single-drug therapy for hypertension in men. A comparison of six antihypertensive agents with placebo. The Department of Veterans Affairs Cooperative Study Group on Antihypertensive Agents, N Engl J Med 328(13): 914-21.

Moher, D., D. J. Cook, S. Eastwood, I. Olkin, D. Rennie and D. F. Stroup (1999). Improving the quality of reports of meta-analyses of randomised controlled trials: the QUOROM statement. Quality of Reporting of Meta-analyses, Lancet 354(9193): 1896-900.

Musini, V. M., P. M. Fortin, K. Bassett and J. M. Wright (2009). Blood pressure lowering efficacy of renin inhibitors for primary hypertension: a Cochrane systematic review, J Hum Hypertens 23(8): 495-502.

Nickenig, G., V. Simanenkov, G. Lembo, P. Rodriguez, T. Salko, S. Ritter, et al. (2008). Efficacy of aliskiren/hydrochlorothiazide single-pill combinations in aliskiren non-responders, Blood Press 17 Suppl 2: 31-40.

Novartis_Europharm_Limited (2007. Available at http://www.ema.europa.eu/docs/pt_PT/document_library/EPAR_-_Product _Information/ human/000780/WC500047010.pdf. Accessed on 27th August 2011). Rasilez - Summary of Product Characteristics E. P. A. R. Human Medicines, European Medicines Agency.

Nussberger, J., G. Wuerzner, C. Jensen and H. R. Brunner (2002). Angiotensin II suppression in humans by the orally active renin inhibitor Aliskiren (SPP100): comparison with enalapril, Hypertension 39(1): E1-8.

O'Brien, E., J. Barton, J. Nussberger, D. Mulcahy, C. Jensen, P. Dicker, et al. (2007). Aliskiren reduces blood pressure and suppresses plasma renin activity in combination with a thiazide diuretic, an angiotensin-converting enzyme inhibitor, or an angiotensin receptor blocker, Hypertension 49(2): 276-84.

Pilz, B., E. Shagdarsuren, M. Wellner, A. Fiebeler, R. Dechend, P. Gratze, et al. (2005). Aliskiren, a human renin inhibitor, ameliorates cardiac and renal damage in double-transgenic rats, Hypertension 46(3): 569-76.

Prescott, M. F., S. W. Boye, S. Le Breton, S. Le Breton, S. Le Breton, S. Le Breton, et al. (2007). Antihypertensive efficacy of the direct renin inhibitor when added to hydrochlorothiazide treatment in patients with extreme obesity and hypertension [abstract no. 1014-169], J Am Coll Cardiol 49(9 Suppl. A): 370.

Sica, D., A. Gradman, O. Lederballe, O. Lederballe, O. Lederballe, O. Lederballe, et al. (2006). Aliskiren, a novel renin inhibitor, is well tolerated and has sustained BP-lowering effects alone or in combination with HCTZ during long-term (52 weeks) treatment of hypertension [abstract no. P-797], Eur Heart J 27(Suppl): 121.

Staessen, J. A., Y. Li and T. Richart (2006). Oral renin inhibitors, Lancet 368(9545): 1449-56.

Strasser, R. H., J. G. Puig, C. Farsang, M. Croket, J. Li and H. van Ingen (2007). A comparison of the tolerability of the direct renin inhibitor aliskiren and lisinopril in patients with severe hypertension, J Hum Hypertens 21(10): 780-7.

Sureshkumar, K. K. (2008). Renin inhibition with aliskiren in hypertension: focus on aliskiren/hydrochlorothiazide combination therapy, Vasc Health Risk Manag 4(6): 1205-20.

Urata, H., H. Nishimura and D. Ganten (1996). Chymase-dependent angiotensin II forming systems in humans, Am J Hypertens 9(3): 277-84.

Vaidyanathan, S., H. Bigler, C. Yeh, M. N. Bizot, H. A. Dieterich, D. Howard, et al. (2007a). Pharmacokinetics of the oral direct renin inhibitor aliskiren alone and in combination with irbesartan in renal impairment, Clin Pharmacokinet 46(8): 661-75.

Vaidyanathan, S., J. Jermany, C. Yeh, M. N. Bizot and R. Camisasca (2006). Aliskiren, a novel orally effective renin inhibitor, exhibits similar pharmacokinetics and pharmacodynamics in Japanese and Caucasian subjects, Br J Clin Pharmacol 62(6): 690-8.

Vaidyanathan, S., V. Warren, C. Yeh, M. N. Bizot, H. A. Dieterich and W. P. Dole (2007b). Pharmacokinetics, safety, and tolerability of the oral Renin inhibitor aliskiren in patients with hepatic impairment, J Clin Pharmacol 47(2): 192-200.

Villamil, A., S. G. Chrysant, D. Calhoun, B. Schober, H. Hsu, L. Matrisciano-Dimichino, et al. (2007). Renin inhibition with aliskiren provides additive antihypertensive efficacy when used in combination with hydrochlorothiazide, J Hypertens 25(1): 217-26.

Waldmeier, F., U. Glaenzel, B. Wirz, L. Oberer, D. Schmid, M. Seiberling, et al. (2007). Absorption, distribution, metabolism, and elimination of the direct renin inhibitor aliskiren in healthy volunteers, Drug Metab Dispos 35(8): 1418-28.

Wolf-Maier, K., R. S. Cooper, J. R. Banegas, S. Giampaoli, H. W. Hense, M. Joffres, et al. (2003). Hypertension prevalence and blood pressure levels in 6 European countries, Canada, and the United States, Jama 289(18): 2363-9.

Wood, J. M., J. Maibaum, J. Rahuel, M. G. Grutter, N. C. Cohen, V. Rasetti, et al. (2003). Structure-based design of aliskiren, a novel orally effective renin inhibitor, Biochem Biophys Res Commun 308(4): 698-705.

Wood, J. M., C. R. Schnell, F. Cumin, J. Menard and R. L. Webb (2005). Aliskiren, a novel, orally effective renin inhibitor, lowers blood pressure in marmosets and spontaneously hypertensive rats, J Hypertens 23(2): 417-26.

Yoon, S. S., Y. Ostchega and T. Louis (2010). Recent trends in the prevalence of high blood pressure and its treatment and control, 1999-2008, NCHS Data Brief(48): 1-8.

Zhao, C., S. Vaidyanathan, C. M. Yeh, M. Maboudian and H. Armin Dieterich (2006). Aliskiren exhibits similar pharmacokinetics in healthy volunteers and patients with type 2 diabetes mellitus, Clin Pharmacokinet 45(11): 1125-34.

Section 6

Up-to-Date in Ulcer with Venous Origin Therapy

9

LavTIME – A Brand-New Treatment Method of Lasting Wounds – A Multi-Centre Randomized Double-Blind Study on Effectiveness of Polyhexanide and Betaine in Ulcers' Healing with Venous Origin

Z. Rybak[1], G Krasowski[2,4], R. Wajda[2] and P. Ciesielczyk[3]
[1]Department of Experimental Surgery and Biomaterials Research Wrocław Medical University
[2]County Hospital, Krapkowice
[3]Ars Medica Wrocław
[4]University of Technology, Opole
Poland

1. Introduction

In ulcers' healing the organic contaminations causes a problem that are not scrupulously removed by patients or medical personnel, particularly, where approximately 90 % patients suffering from the disease have been cured in an open system care. Secondly, up to the latest days there was no appropriate medicine effectively supporting wound's cleaning. Necrotic organic substances remaining in the wound do activate a holder's immunological system and promote bacteria, fungi, and virus increments, in which environment reactive oxygen species are created. These very aggressive substances destroy healthy tissues and favour accumulating significantly extensive amount of granulocytes which, in turn, affect micro-obstructions and micro-clots in the wound's edge area. The mentioned circumstances suspend the healing or even preclude this process. Another issue is, that majority of patients do not rinse up the whole wound surface while the edges only or they do not change bandages sufficiently often. A commonly used salt to rinse the wound is a physiological salt or Ringer's liquid. However, these are the liquids which do not contain a conservation mean. Therefore, outstaying usually in an open way for many days, or more often in a room temperature, the solutions can be secondarily contaminated. What is more, patients often use a tap water which is also bacterially contaminated. Having in mind a nature of the wound's protein components, which are strongly associated with a substratum via fibrins, it is not indifferent what the wound is rinse up with (1,2,3,4).

In the study, the Authors present a new tactics against lasting wounds. It relies on supplementing the TIME procedure by the Lav acronym which means lavage (washing, cleaning) in the first instance, before wound treatment. Moreover, an effectiveness of wound cleaning from the organic elements including bacteria using a physiological salt (NaCl) and Prontosan (polyhexanide+betaine) has been reported (5,6).

2. Material and method

In the study have been enrolled 60 patients (19 males and 41 females, 47-83 of age with 58.5 average). Retired persons (52 patients) were predominant in the group, widowers (43), alone (39) and inhabitants of a >100 thou. population city (38). All the patients have been suffering from thrombosis for 2-15 years. In the color duplex Doppler's test in all the patients signs of post thrombotic syndrome with damage of venous valves on different levels of the extremity has been diagnosed. A valve damage in femoral vein was predominant in 49 patients (formerly treated but unsuccessfully).

	Male	Female	Total
Gender	19	41	60
Retired	14	38	52
Widower	9	34	43
Alone	7	32	39
Citizen of > 100 thou. population city	12	26	38
Kind of profession a/ physical worker, farmer b/ office worker c/ student	 11 6 2	 27 14 0	 38 20 2
Age	56 +/- 14	63 +/- 14	
Median	55	62	
Range	(20-87)	(24-88)	
BMI	27,3 +/- 5,3	28,7 +/- 5,1	
Median	25	27	
Range	(16,2-38,2)	(15,7-39,1)	

Table 1. The patient demographics

In the study 30 patients were taken into account with 44 ulcers' histories (158 visit records). From the preliminary set of 60 patients, those were excluded who appeared once or who did not restrict the regimes of the treatment procedure. After decoding the bottles' containments and appropriate patients' assigning to the groups, it was established that 17 patients were treated by Prontosan, whereas 13 by the 0.9% NaCl solution, respectively.

Drop out patients are presented in table 2.

	Prontosan group	0.9% NaCl group	Total
Adverse events	3	2	5
Major protocol violation	2	4	6
Patient wished to leave study	3	5	8
Patient not compliant	4	3	7
Significant concomitant illness	1	3	4
Treatment failure	0	0	0
Total	13	17	30

Table 2.

2.1 Study design

This study was an open, multicenter, prospective, randomized, double blind, parallel group study on efficacy of Prontosan solution in treatment of venous leg ulcers.

The study was performed in 3 centers and was included a total number of 60 patients. After dropped out 30 patients because of different reasons remaining patients were as follow : 17 patients for Prontosan and 13 for 0.9% NaCl subgroup. Treated venous leg ulcers were classified according to ABI /Ankle-Brachial Index/. The venous leg ulcers were recognized when ABI was higher than or equal to 0,9 and no lymphatic disorders revealed.

All study participants had been treated during 12 weeks or until complete healing is achieved (whichever occurs first).

2.2 Study population

The study population consists of individuals above 18 years of age, in which venous leg ulcers have been identified of the size limited by the size of applied wound dressing and ABI ≥ 0.9.

Exclusion criteria were as follows:

a. hypersensitivity to any of Prontosan® components or to any of wound dressing components,
b. active osteomyelitis in the area of the treated ulcer,
c. active rheumatoidal or collagen disease of blood vessels treated with corticosteroids,
d. neoplastic disease
e. serum proteins < 4 g/dl
f. anemia: < 10g haemoglobin per dl
g. exclusion of phlebotropic, vasorelaxing and reological medicines for the study period
h. diabetic foot
i. lack of compliance of the patient
j. intolerance to compression therapy

2.3 Route of administration

External application.

2.4 Dosage regimen

Either Prontosan® or saline solution (depending on the study group) had been applied at every change of the wound dressing. Frequency of dressing change: every day.

3. Application

1. first, Prontosan/saline solution was used for cleansing of the wound bed; this will be done using sterile gauze & sterile gauze compress soaked in the solution an used to cover the wound for 15 min, then removed from the wound bed
2. next, the polyurethane wound dressing was activated with given solution and used to cover the wound
3. finally, medical compression stockings was used to fasten the wound dressing to the patient's leg.

Prontosan or 0.9% NaCl solution were used to soak and gently remove the wound dressing at the time of each dressing change procedure.

For each patient 10 bottles 350 ml of Prontosan or 0.9% NaCl saline solution were available and used as necessary according to applied randomization scheme.

3.1 Efficacy criteria

Primary efficacy criteria:

1. incidence of infection during treatment period
2. rate of healing of the ulcer in cm^2/week

Secondary efficacy criteria:

1. complete healing of the ulcer - ulcer is defined as completely healed if there is stable wound epithelialization
2. improved state of the ulcer - ulcer is defined as improved if there is decrease in its surface of at least 25% in comparison to the initial findings
3. lack of improvement of the ulcer - defined as the ulcer that do not belong to any of the above listed categories

Tertiary efficacy criteria:

1. incidence of pain during dressing change, comfort for the patient - subjective pain scale used during the course of study - before, during and after each dressing change (CIVIQ questionnaire)
2. incidence of side effects
3. change of clinical symptoms of the ulcer (granulation, epithelialization; computer-aided analysis of digital pictures of the wound).

3.2 Methods of evaluation of the efficacy of treatment include:

- planimetry of the ulcer, software-aided surface evaluation,
- assessment of clinical status of the ulcer (computer-aided analysis of pictures of wound surface)
- assessment of changes in microbial load in the ulcer in first, second & last visit of the study
- photographic documentation of the treatment (done in a standardized way to allow for further computer-aided analysis)
- laboratory tests: full blood count, total proteins

3.3 Safety evaluation

Assessment of differences between measured general health parameters (as listed under laboratory tests) as well as incidence of adverse reactions before and after therapeutical process.

Following the study qualification during the initial visit (D-0), for bacteria culture inoculation, swabs from the wounds were taken and bottles with unknown liquid together with the treatment prescription among the patients were distributed. During the control visits before bandaging a digital photographical documentation of healing was conducted.

The treatment procedure consisted with:

Every day applying wet gauze with the liquid from the bottle. The dressing was on the wound during fifteen minutes than polyurethan wound dressing (Allevyn) was put on. Such dressing was covered by two knee stockings. First was a thrombo profilactic and the second one was Sigvaris 503 class compression. Day by day patient change the dressings according to above mentioned method. To make easier for the patients each one get diary with detail prescription how to use getting materials for the treatment.

The visits' D-13 and D-31, D-58 consisted with: check the wound healing process, make a digital photography, take the culture from the wound bed, put the new dressing on, take used bottles off and give new bottles with the medicament.

The last visit was D-85. During this visit physician estimated the healing process, advers events and ask patients about their satisfaction with the treatment.

4. Statistical analysis

In the statistical analysis, hierarchical (multi-level) modelling has been performed that allows variance in outcome variable (wound surface) to be analysed at multiple hierarchical levels (i.e. time of treatment, treatment groups and their interaction) [Raudenbush S., Bryk A. (2001). Hierarchical Linear Models: Applications and Data Analysis Methods (2nd ed.). Sage Publications, Thousand Oaks CA]. A mixed effects' model has been applied in the study.

A statistical difference between means of the speed of ulcers' healing in Prontosan and NaCl patients has been estimated with the use of Welch's *t*-test that is an adaptation of Student's *t*-test intended for use with two samples having possibly unequal variance [Welch B. (1947). The generalization of "student's" problem when several different population variances are involved. Biometrika 34: 28-35] for details.

A so-called *k*-means algorithm which classifies a given data set (speed of ulcers' healing) through a certain number of clusters (two time bands) [MacQueen J. (1967). Some Methods for classification and Analysis of Multivariate Observations. Proceedings of 5-th Berkeley Symposium on Mathematical Statistics and Probability. Berkeley, University of California Press 1:281-297].

A statistical difference in infection numbers between the selected Prontosan and NaCl patients' visits has been estimated through the Mann-Whitney *U*-test [Mann H., Whitney D. (1947). On a test of whether one of two random variables is stochastically larger than the other. Annals of Mathematical Statistics 18: 50-60], which is a non-parametric test and assesses whether two independent samples of observations (infection numbers in treatment groups) come from the same distribution.

The statistical computation has been conducted in R platform [The R Foundation for Statistical Computing (2008). R version 2.8.1 (2008-12-22)].

The planimetrical estimation of ulcers was carried out based on digital pictures of wounds with the use of the MapInfo 6.5 geographical software.

5. Results

In the group of patients underwent study were 11 smokers but only two smokers belongs to the group of assessed patients, one in group of Prontosan and one in 0.9% NaCl group.

The ulcer location was predominantly in ankle region (49), above ankle (11). Status of the wound before and following treatment are presented in table 3.

Status of the wound	Before treatment Prontosan	Before treatment 0.9% NaCl	After treatment Prontosan	After treatment 0.9% NaCl
necrosis	7	6	0	1
Fibrinogen coating	17	13	0	2
Infection	9	6	2	5
Visible tendoms	5	3	2	2
Fistulas	0	0	0	0
Granulation faze			17	9
Epithelialization faze	0	0	17	3

Table 3.

Total healing rate in the estimated groups is presented in table 4

	Prontosan n = 17	0.9% NaCl n = 13
Total healing of ulcer within 90 days	16	6
85% of ulcer healing	1	3
50% of ulcer healing	0	3
30% of ulcer healing	0	1
Lack of improvement of the ulcer	0	0

Table 4.

All blood and urine tests were in of normal range before and following study procedure.

Only in three patients of Prontosan group appeared adverse events listed in table 5.

	Prontosan n = 17	0.9% NaCl n = 13
Serious adverse events	0	0
Not serious adverse events		
Headache	0	1
Excitation/sleepless	0	0
Stabbing pain of the heart	0	0
Nausea	0	0
Itching	2	3
Eruption of the skin	1	3
Oedema foots and legs	0	2

Table 5.

In the study 30 patients (17 Prontosan and 13 0.9% NaCl) were taken into account with 44 ulceration episodes (mean age = 71.9 +/- 10.7). All together in 2008 and 2009, 158 visits were documented in the form below:

Episode	Treatment	Time since 1st visit [days]	Time between visits [days]	Surface [mm^2]
1	Prontosan	0	0	3006,7
1	Prontosan	42	42	2057
1	Prontosan	75	33	1240,9
1	Prontosan	151	76	183,6
1	Prontosan	186	35	33,4
1	Prontosan	224	38	64,2
2	NaCl	0	0	110,6
2	NaCl	14	14	178,6
2	NaCl	17	3	176
2	NaCl	57	40	45,9
2	NaCl	71	14	30,1
3	NaCl	0	0	286,2
3	NaCl	17	17	198,5
3	NaCl	33	16	133,3
4	NaCl	0	0	476,2
4	NaCl	14	14	510
4	NaCl	70	56	467
4	NaCl	91	21	419,8
*****	*******	*****************	*****************	**********

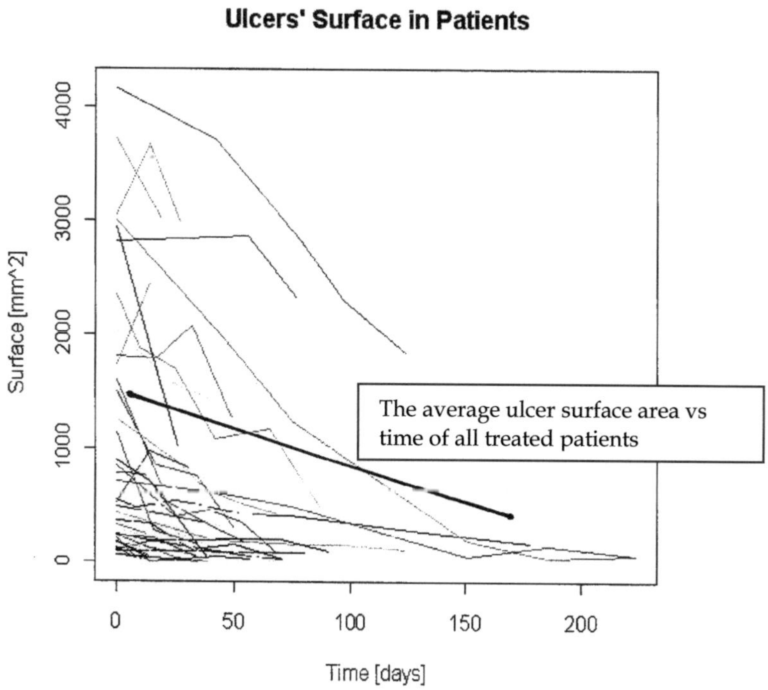

Fig. 1.

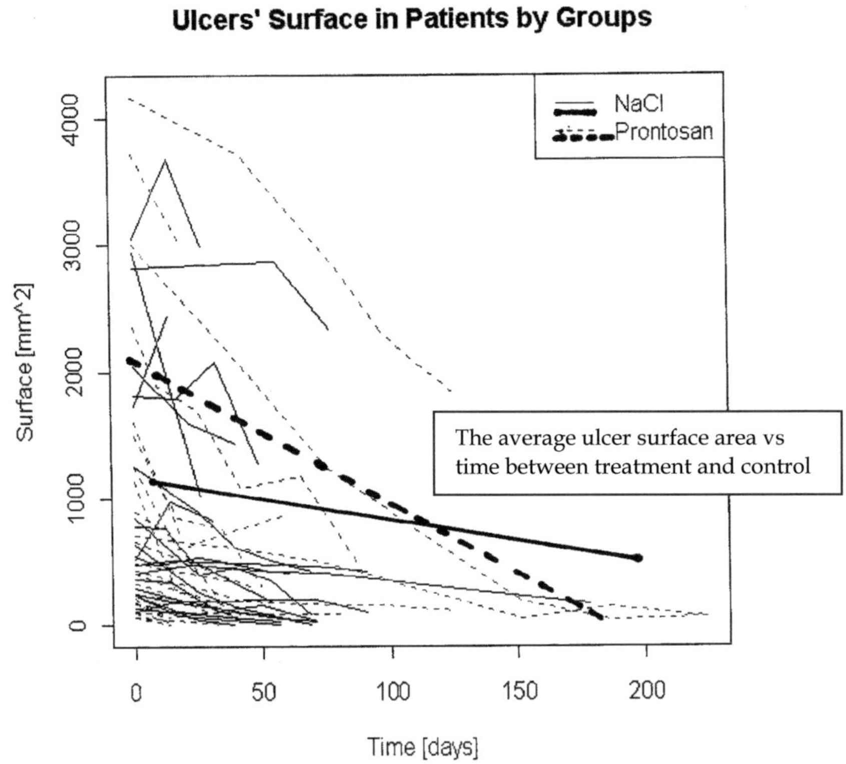

Fig. 2.

The regression estimates of the assumed hierarchical model are reported in Table 6.

Parameter	Value	Std. Error	*p*-value
intercept	1012,796	178,385	<0,0001
time	-4,053	1,168	0,0007
groupProntosan	-86,154	194,633	0,6589
time:groupProntosan	-5,004	1,479	0,0010

Table 6. Hierarchical Modelling Analysis

- A statistically significant reduction of the surface of ulcers in Prontosan and in NaCl patiens was observed approximately 4 mm^2 per day (time);
  Prontosan patients represented a larger reduction of the wound surface during treatment compared to NaCl patients (86 mm^2 in average) , however, the difference was not statistically significant (groupProntosan);
- A statistically significant difference in healing effect in time between the treatment groups was observed and for each therapy increment of one day, the reduction of 5 mm^2 was larger approximately in Prontosan patients compared to NaCl group (time:groupProntosan).

The graphical model of the reduction of ulcers in treatment groups is presented in Figure 3.

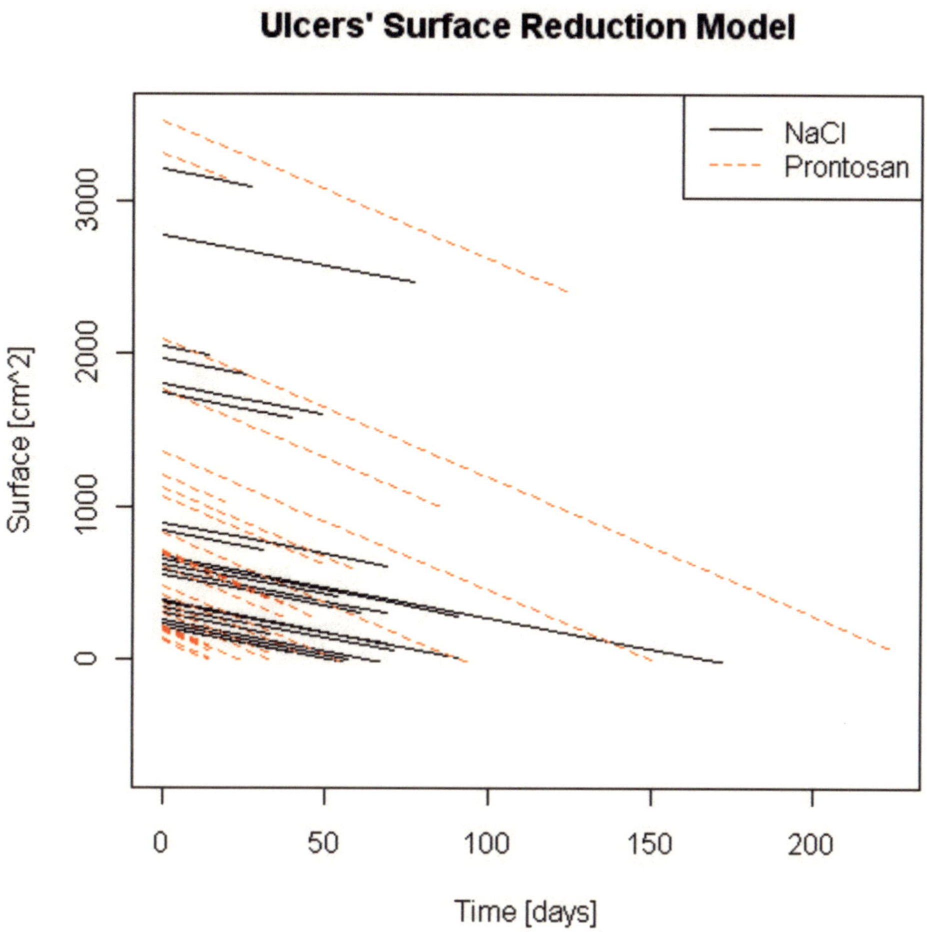

Fig. 3.

The regression model estimates indicate that a particular 1000 mm2 ulcer wound should be approximately healed after 110.4 days of Prontosan therapy whereas 246.8 days with the NaCl treatment.

The estimates of the statistical difference between means of the speed of ulcers' healing in Prontosan and in NaCl patients are presented below

Treatment	Mean	Std. Dev.	*p*-value
Prontosan	13,320	14,763	0,01465
NaCl	5,641	18,124	

Table 7. Ulcers' Healing Speed *t*-test (mm2)

The *t*-test estimates provide evidence of the over twice as high ulcer reduction in Prontosan treatment patients compared to NaCl group. The average healing in Prontosan patients exceeded 13 mm2 per day whereas in NaCl patients it was much below 6 mm2 daily. The difference in means is statistically significant.

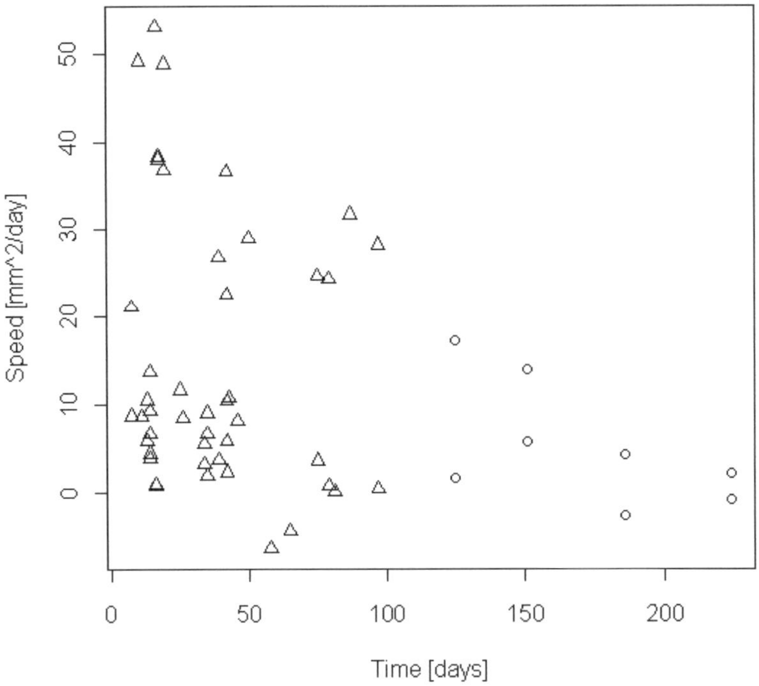

Fig. 4. Time-Speed Clusters of Ulcers' Healing in: Prontosan Patients

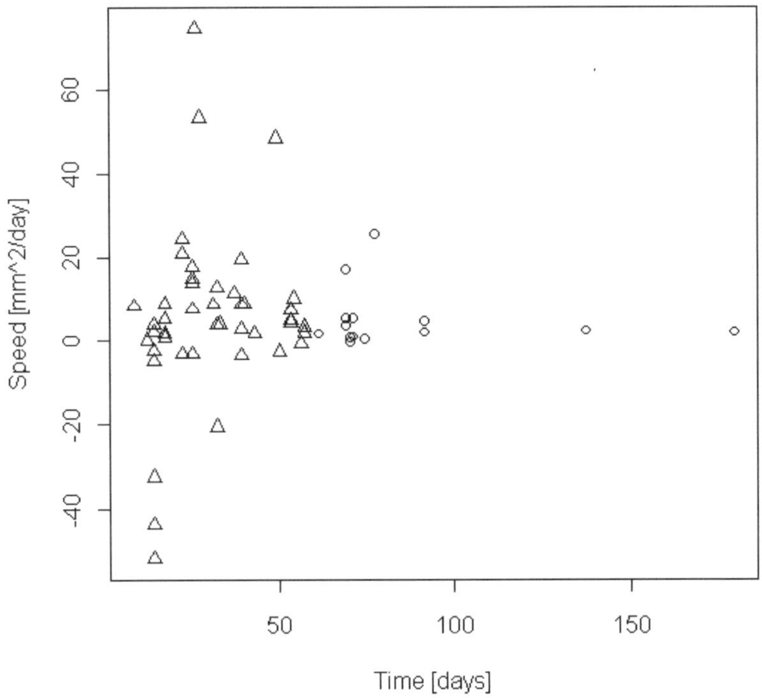

Fig. 5. Time-Speed Clusters of Ulcers' Healing in: NaCl patients

Treatment	Means		
	Cluster 1	Cluster 2	*p*-value
Prontosan	14,770	5,164	0,00931
NaCl	5,730	5,347	0,9152

Table 8. The *t*-test analysis for the time-speed clusters in Prontosan and NaCl patients are given

The outcomes testify that there is a significant difference in means of healing speed in Prontosan patients between the estimated clusters. The obtained time band can be established around the 100 days since the beginning of Prontosan treatment and the average speed of ulcer healing reaches nearly 15 mm^2 per day up to this time border. After this time the speed decreases significantly to 5 mm^2/day. The healing speed in NaCl patients does not vary with time and in both clusters it is slightly above 5 mm^2 per day of treatment.

Treatment	No. of Obs.	Rank Sum	*U* statistic	*Z* statistic	*p*-level
Prontosan	27	509,5	131,5	-3,9054	9,43E-05
NaCl	26	921,5			

Table 9. The *U*-test results for the infection numbers between the selected Prontosan and NaCl patients' visits are reported *U*-Test Infection Numbers Analysis

The results provide evidence of significantly lower infection numbers in Prontosan patients' ulcers in comparison to the NaCl group (nearly twice as low).

6. Discussion

In the study 30 patients were taken into account with 44 ulcers' histories (158 visit records). From the preliminary set of 60 patients, those were excluded who appeared once or who did not restrict the regimes of the treatment procedure. After decoding the bottles' containments and appropriate patients' assigning to the groups, it was established that 17 patients were treated by Prontosan, whereas 13 by the NaCl solution, respectively.

The obtained outcomes provide evidence nearly three times as a higher healing speed in those patients who were treated by Prontosan in comparison to the NaCl group. The cleaning from bacteria tribes was as twice as higher, respectively. In both the analyses the results were statistically significant.

The importance of lavasepsis for the treatment of chronic wounds results from a fundamental, commonly understood and accepted standard, which for wound management field translates as follows: "first wound hygiene, then wound tratment (7)." This principle goes hand in hand with the generally accepted rule of limiting the use of drugs to an essential minimum and giving prophylaxis priority in medicine. What is then the real impact of lavasepsis on the individual elements of the TIME framework?

The effect of lavasepsis on *Tissue management* is many-sided. It softens and separates necroses from healthy tissue, which facilitates their identification and elimination. Furthermore, lavasepsis removes crust, scabs and exudate residues, as well as fibrin coatings from the wound surface (8, 9). Finally, everyday wound lavasepsis secures effective biofilm removal (10). Wound lavasepsis cannot replace surgical interventions or sharp debridement, but it can considerably help in assessment of the wound and in effective employment of the required procedure.

In the area of *Inflammation and infection control*, it is worth emphasising the significance of the aforementioned cleansing properties, namely the removal of wound coatings and biofilm from the wound surface. The use of antiseptics and antibiotics for a wound that is either contaminated or coated with a biofilm is inadequate. It can cause the therapy to be ineffective and increases the likelihood of the development of drug-resistance (12, 14). Wound cleansing or hygiene lowers the microbial load and significantly lowers the risk of complications, including infections. The microcirculation, oxygen and nutrient availability, as well as the effectiveness of patient's immune system are improving. Lavasepsis cannot replace antisepsis, but secures optimal conditions for the use of local and systemic anti-infectives. In this way, it minimizes and streamlines their application.

Maintaining an adequate *Moisture balance* of the wound is an important element of the therapeutic process. Everyday wound lavasepsis helps to remove excessive exudate (also by reinforcing the habit of wound cleansing). It facilitates wound moistening in the case of dry wounds and raises the effectiveness of wound dressings. Lavasepsis is not meant to replace modern wound dressings, which are essential for maintaining a moist wound environment and absorbing excessive exudate. It can, however, prepare the wound bed in a way that ensures optimal therapeutic effect of their application.

Epithelial/edge advancement is an element of the TIME framework, for which lavasepsis is important because of the fact that the removal of wound coatings facilitates the reestablishment of cellular proliferation and angiogenesis. Lavasepsis also removes potential physical barriers to epithelial growth across the wound bed. Finally, optimal wound bed preparation is a prerequisite for effective use of advanced therapies, such as skin transplants and cellular growth factors (11).

Lavasepsis thus has a significant influence on all elements of the TIME framework, being a process of preparing the wound bed *per se*. Thanks to this, it allows one to achieve optimal results from any therapeutic procedures applied at specific stages of wound treatment.

The above outcomes point to the conclusion that a lack of effective wound cleaning from organic elements laying on the wound bed as well as from the remained bacteria (protected by the bacterial biofilm which is difficult to remove using physiological salts) result in significant elongation of the healing time. Prontosan dissolves and removes contaminations from the wound bed, destroys the bacterial biofilm and accelerates the healing of ulcers. Despite of a slightly higher price, the use of Prontosan may importantly reduce sufferance in patients likewise both the costs carried out by their own and the governmental subsidies, taking the time of the medical treatment in mind. Further economical simulation are required to estimate such the profits. Our results were confirmed by other investigators (12).

Lavasepsis is a new term created to describe and delineate a group of products that, according to the authors, brings in a new, desired quality to local treatment of chronic wounds (13). This new quality arises directly from the evolution of the WBP paradigm and TIME framework set earlier by EWMA experts (14). The TIME framework and EWMA recommendations are a good milestone not only for clinical practice, but also for manufacturers who are trying to adopt their product offering to the needs of contemporary medicine. The LAV-TIME concept presented in this paper, extends and supplements the

TIME framework with the new and important element of lavasepsis (15,16,17,18). Although at present there are few products on the market that can be described as "lavaseptics", the rapid development of this group of products is to be expected, and their availability on the medical market will grow. This would certainly be of benefit to the medical world, and most of all to the patients (19,20).

7. Conclusion

1. A statistically significant difference in healing effect in time between the treatment groups was observed and for each therapy increment of one day, the reduction of 5 mm^2 was larger approximately in Prontosan patients compared to NaCl group.
2. The results provide evidence of significantly lower infection numbers in Prontosan patients' ulcers in comparison to the NaCl group.
3. Prontosan appeared as a very good tolerated product for patients without any serious adverse effects. Only three out of seventeen patients have a temporary local problems with Itching (two patients) and eruption of the skin (one patient).
4. 16 patients out of 17 in the Prontosan group were totally healed within 90 days of treatment and only 6 out of 13 were totally healed in NaCl group at the same time.

8. References

[1] Kramer A, „Antiseptika und Händedesinfektionsmittel". W: Korting HC, Sterry W (Hrsg) Therapeutische Verfahren in der Dermatologie. 2001, Blackwell Wissenschaft Berlin, 273-294.

[2] Kramer A, Adrian V, Rudolph P, Wurster S, Lippert H, "Explantationstest mit Haut und Peritoneum der neonatalen Ratte als Voraussagetest zur Verträglichkeit lokaler Antiinfektiva für Wunden und Körperhöhlen". 1988, Chirurg 69, 8:840-845.

[3] Kallenberger A, Kallenberger C, Willenegger H, „Experimentelle Untersuchungen zur Gewebeverträglichkeit von Antiseptika". 1991, Hyg Med 16, 10:383-395.

[4] Sellmer W, „Lokaltherapeutika, speziell Antiseptika, in der Behandlung chronischer Wunden - eine aktuelle Bewertung". 2001, Med Praxis 2: 20-30.

[5] Schmit-Neuerburg KP, Bettag Ch, Schlickewei W, Fabry W, Hanke J, Renzing-Köhler K, Hirche H, Kock H-J, „Wirksamkeit eines neuartigen Antisepticum in der Behandlung kontaminierter Weichteilwunden". 2001, Chirurg 72: 61-71.

[6] Seipp H-M et al., „Wirksamkeit verschiedener Wundspüllösungen gegenüber Biofilmen". 2005, Zeitschrift für Wundheilung, 1, 160-164.

[7] European Wound Management Association (EWMA). Position Document: Wound Bed

[8] Preparation in Practice. London: MEP Ltd. 2004

Ciesielczyk P, Rybak Z, „Prawidłowe przygotowanie łożyska rany i profilaktyka

[9] antybakteryjna - droga do sukcesu w leczeniu ran. Zastosowanie Prontosanu i produktów PVP-jodowych". Streszczenia. II Kongres Naukowo-Szkoleniowy Polskiego Towarzystwa Leczenia Ran. 2007, Leczenie Ran 4(4): 140.

[10] Kramer A et al., "Consensus recommendation on wound antisepsis". 2004, Zeitschrift für Wundheilung 3.

[11] Werner HP, „Die mikrobizide Wirksamkeit ausgewählter Antiseptika". 1992, Hyg Med 17, 2:51-59.

[12] Kramer A, Adrian V, Rudolph P, Wurster S, Lippert H, "Explantationstest mit Haut und Peritoneum der neonatalen Ratte als Voraussagetest zur Verträglichkeit lokaler Antiinfektiva für Wunden und Körperhöhlen". 1988, Chirurg 69, 8:840-845.

[13] Kallenberger A, Kallenberger C, Willenegger H, „Experimentelle Untersuchungen zur Gewebeverträglichkeit von Antiseptika". 1991, Hyg Med 16, 10:383-395.

[14] Sellmer W, „Lokaltherapeutika, speziell Antiseptika, in der Behandlung chronischer Wunden - eine aktuelle Bewertung". 2001, Med Praxis 2: 20-30.

[15] Selvaggi G et al., „The role of iodine in antisepsis and wound management: a reappraisal". 2003, Acta chir. belg 103, 241-247.

[16] Seipp H-M and Stroh A, "Methicillin-resistant S. aureus (MRSA) - Significant reduction of incidence and rate in a maximum-care clinical centre (1994 to 1999)". 1999, Hyg Med 24 (6): 224-237.

[17] Ciesielczyk P., Michalski T., Rybak Z.: LA V-TIME. Ewolucja paradygmatu,2007, Zakażenia;6:104-108.

[18] Rybak Z.: Venous leg ulcers, 2008, Sepsis;1(2):95-98.

[19] Rybak Z., Cisielczyk P.: Lavasepsis as a helpful method in wound treatment, 2008, Dermat. Estet;10(2):104-106.

[20] Kramer A, „Antiseptika und Handedesinfektionsmittel". W: Korting HC, Sterry W (Hrsg) Therapeutische Verfahren in der Dermatologie. 2001, Blackwell Wissenschaft Berlin, 273-294.